AF839488

Applied Physiology to Reduce Ventilator Induced Lung Injury

Gary F. Nieman • Nader M. Habashi

Applied Physiology to Reduce Ventilator Induced Lung Injury

Clinical Applications for the Acutely Injured Lung

Springer

Gary F. Nieman
Department of Surgery
SUNY Upstate Medical University
Syracuse, NY, USA

Department of Clinical Sciences
Cornell University
Ithaca, NY, USA

Nader M. Habashi
School of Medicine
University of Maryland, Baltimore
Baltimore, MD, USA

ISBN 978-3-031-66351-2 ISBN 978-3-031-66352-9 (eBook)
https://doi.org/10.1007/978-3-031-66352-9

© The Editor(s) (if applicable) and The Author(s), under exclusive license to Springer Nature Switzerland AG 2024
This work is subject to copyright. All rights are solely and exclusively licensed by the Publisher, whether the whole or part of the material is concerned, specifically the rights of translation, reprinting, reuse of illustrations, recitation, broadcasting, reproduction on microfilms or in any other physical way, and transmission or information storage and retrieval, electronic adaptation, computer software, or by similar or dissimilar methodology now known or hereafter developed.
The use of general descriptive names, registered names, trademarks, service marks, etc. in this publication does not imply, even in the absence of a specific statement, that such names are exempt from the relevant protective laws and regulations and therefore free for general use.
The publisher, the authors and the editors are safe to assume that the advice and information in this book are believed to be true and accurate at the date of publication. Neither the publisher nor the authors or the editors give a warranty, expressed or implied, with respect to the material contained herein or for any errors or omissions that may have been made. The publisher remains neutral with regard to jurisdictional claims in published maps and institutional affiliations.

This Springer imprint is published by the registered company Springer Nature Switzerland AG
The registered company address is: Gewerbestrasse 11, 6330 Cham, Switzerland

If disposing of this product, please recycle the paper.

This book is dedicated to the giants of science and medicine upon whose shoulders we stand, our colleagues and coworkers, and most importantly our friends and family without whom this book would not have been possible.

Contents

Chapter 1
Unifying Hypothesis of Ventilator-Induced Lung Injury

Introduction

The gradual collapse of lung tissue occurring over hours or days, a characteristic feature of ARDS pathogenesis, has been coined the "VILI Vortex" (Fig. 2.4) [1]. To mitigate ARDS-associated mortality, it is imperative to integrate our understanding of the intricate pathogenesis linked to ARDS, leading to the modification of dynamic alveolar and alveolar duct (acinar) mechanics. Identifying how these alterations predispose the lung to secondary VILI is crucial for formulating a comprehensive hypothesis (Fig. 1.2). This knowledge serves as the foundation for designing a more efficacious Mechanical Breath Profile (MB_P), encompassing airway pressures, volumes, flows, rates, and their application duration during inspiration and expiration. Such a profile is essential for normalizing acinar mechanics and reducing VILI-related mortality.

Protective Mechanical Ventilation for ARDS Patients

The current standard of care for protective lung ventilation aims to reduce VILI in individuals with ARDS by reducing tidal volume (V_T) and plateau pressure (Pplat). The goal is to prevent overdistension of the still-functioning normal lung tissue, often referred to as the "baby lung." Additionally, this approach aims to prevent the progression of lung collapse into the VILI vortex by applying positive end-expiratory pressure (PEEP), with the setting determined based on oxygenation levels. The collapsed atelectatic tissue is allowed to "Rest" by keeping it out of the ventilatory cycle. Despite the clarity of the general approach, specific nominal values for both tidal volume and positive end-expiratory pressure (PEEP) at the initiation of

© The Author(s), under exclusive license to Springer Nature Switzerland AG 2024

G. F. Nieman, N. M. Habashi, *Applied Physiology to Reduce Ventilator Induced Lung Injury*, https://doi.org/10.1007/978-3-031-66352-9_1

lung-protective ventilation, as well as their application throughout the individual course of illness, remain undefined and lack consensus [2].

The ARDS network's low tidal volume (LV_T) method is grounded in the two-compartment model of ARDS pathology. It delineates: (i) a small quantity of normal lung tissue (referred to as the "baby lung") situated in the nondependent compartment and (ii) an affected region characterized by injured, unstable, collapsed, and edematous tissue in the dependent compartment [3]. The decrease in lung volume results in a loss of compliance in the dependent lung compartment, significantly diminishing the total lung volume available for ventilation. Consequently, a primary hypothesis suggests that VILI is predominantly triggered by the overdistension of the compliant normal "baby lung." Conceptually, this overdistension may occur if the remaining healthy lung tissue is ventilated with a standard-size tidal volume (V_T) [3, 4]. Hence, the LV_T method is most accurately described as a "Protect the Baby Lung Approach." The reduction of both the V_T and Pplat aims to "protect" the normal lung tissue from overdistension, allowing the injured tissue to remain collapsed and "rest," while applying positive end-expiratory pressure (PEEP) minimizes progressive lung collapse [2, 5, 6]. The most extreme manifestation of the "Protect the Baby Lung" approach involves employing ultra-low tidal volume (REST Trial) [7] relying on extracorporeal carbon dioxide removal membrane oxygenation (ECCOR) or no V_T relying on extracorporeal membrane oxygenation (ECMO) for blood gas exchange [8]. However, despite its implementation over 20 years ago, most, though not all, randomized controlled trials (RCTs), statistical analyses, and meta-analyses have indicated that this approach, whether with or without ECMO, has not led to a significant reduction in mortality for patients with established acute respiratory distress syndrome (ARDS) [9–22].

A variation of the Protect the Lung Approach, termed the Open Lung Approach (OLA), has been explored. This method incorporates low V_T but also aims to recruit most collapsed lung tissue over a brief duration (e.g., 40 cmH_2O for 40 s—40/40) or minutes using progressive increases in positive end-expiratory pressure (PEEP). The intention is to prevent re-collapse by setting PEEP at a level which results in the best respiratory system compliance (C_{RS}) [21]. Unfortunately, the open lung approach has also not demonstrated a reduction in ARDS-related mortality [21].

The failure of the Protect and Open Lung approaches to reduce ARDS-related mortality may be attributed to the potential inaccuracy of the previously discussed two-compartment ARDS pathology model. This model suggests that the primary mechanism for VILI is the overdistension of the "baby lung." However, recent research reveals a more complex ARDS pathophysiology involving regional alveolar collapse and instability in supposedly normal baby lung tissues. Crucially, these abnormalities are not visible through conventional imaging techniques such as computerized tomography (CT) or X-rays [23–26]. These concealed areas, termed "Hidden Microatelectasis," of alveolar collapse have been identified as a significant factor, making the lung highly susceptible to VILI, as depicted in Fig. 2.8 [27].

Another potential explanation lies in our incomplete understanding of the biophysical mechanisms underlying ventilator-induced lung injury (VILI) at the alveolar level. The lung comprises a highly intricate system of interconnected alveolar architectures, incorporating various cell types, a continuous network of elastin and collagen from the alveolar walls to the visceral pleura, serving as a load-bearing scaffolding, and a dynamic surfactant system [28–33]. These interrelated components play a crucial role in the normal acinar volume change mechanism in response to a spontaneous or mechanical breath in a healthy lung. However, ARDS pathology significantly alters these alveolar mechanics, making the acutely injured lung more susceptible to secondary VILI, as illustrated in Fig. 1.1—**Alveolar Edema**—causing alveolar overdistension (OD)-induced volutrauma and **RACE**-induced atelectrauma.

The latest evidence indicates that the nondependent areas in patients with ARDS may appear as normal lung tissue on X-ray or CT scans. However, it is now understood that this seemingly normal tissue harbors regional hidden microatelectasis. These areas create stress multipliers, concentrating the mechanical power delivered during ventilation specifically to the open alveoli surrounding the collapse, as depicted in Fig. 1.1—**Alveolar Edema** with increased stress shown by the green arrow [27]. Stress multipliers arise from local factors such as pneumonia,

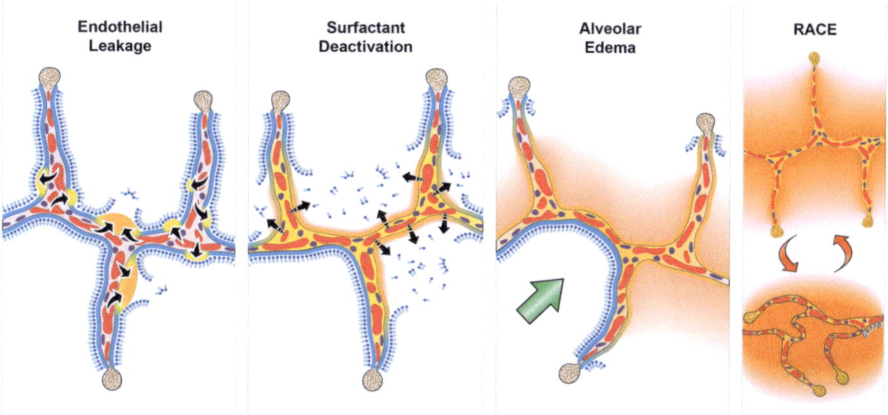

Fig. 1.1 The tetrad of injury at the alveolar level is the hallmark of ARDS pathophysiology. Local (pneumonia) or systemic (sepsis) inflammation results in air-blood barrier disruption leading to **Endothelial Leakage**. Edema fluid [21] moves out of the capillaries (black arrows), disrupting the pulmonary surfactant layer. Extensive edema flooding of the alveolus leads to extensive **Surfactant Deactivation**. **Alveolar Edema** results when the entire alveolus is fluid-filled. This flooding is heterogeneous such that open alveoli adjacent to flooded alveoli generate stress multiplies (green arrow) resulting in mechanical damage (overdistension-induced volutrauma) to the normal air-filled alveoli. Alveoli with a functional surfactant are stable and do not collapse at expiration. Loss of surfactant function severely alters alveolar mechanics, causing repetitive alveolar collapse and expansion (**RACE**) with each breath. RACE is the mechanism of atelectrauma

aspiration, and smoke inhalation or systemic factors like sepsis, trauma, and hemorrhagic shock. These conditions induce inflammation, leading to increased microvascular permeability and regional areas of pulmonary edema or collapse, as illustrated in Fig. 1.1—**Endothelial Leakage**. Edema, in turn, deactivates pulmonary surfactant, triggering alveolar instability, collapse, and flooding, as shown in Fig. 1.1—**Surfactant Deactivation** and **Alveolar Edema**. This cascade ultimately leads to alveolar flooding, altering alveolar mechanics and causing repetitive alveolar collapse and expansion (RACE), resulting in areas of regional alveolar instability, as depicted in Fig. 1.1—**RACE**. This initiates a progressive lung injury termed the Permeability-Originated Obstruction Response (POOR), which worsens as tissue damage extends around the initial pulmonary lesions, as depicted in Fig. 1.2—POOR get POORer [34]. This process leads to a heterogeneity of tissue stiffness between the injured POOR areas and the normal tissue surrounding these primary lesions, as illustrated in Figs. 2.5 and 2.7. Given the interconnected nature of alveolar walls, as shown in Fig. 2.9, this generates intercellular and intracellular stress, resulting in the failure of load-bearing structures during ventilation [35]. As a result, regional stress multipliers, stemming from a high-permeability pulmonary edema, can cause physical injury to the normal surrounding tissue with each mechanical breath. This injury occurs through both RACE-induced atelectrauma and alveolar duct overdistension (OD), commonly known as volutrauma, thereby significantly accelerating the progression of tissue damage (POOR get POORer) initiated by systemic or local inflammation [23–25, 36]. Additionally, the injured, unstable, or flooded acini faces excessive shear or "peeling" stress as microbubbles "peel open" the tissue, leading to atelectrauma, as illustrated in Fig. 1.1—**RACE** [37]. The progression of tissue injury rapidly spreads from the primary lesions in a POOR get POORer sequence (Fig. 4.11) [34]. This cascade triggers the clinical pathogenesis of progressive tissue collapse, driving the lung into the VILI vortex, as illustrated in Fig. 2.4 [1].

As previously discussed, ARDS introduces a heterogeneous lung injury characterized by regional stress multiplication and RACE. When this pathophysiology is coupled with high airway pressure, it creates the "'perfect storm" conducive to damaging lung tissue with each breath. Therefore, applied physiology suggests that preventing VILI requires developing a mechanical breath strategy that eliminates stress multipliers and reduces dynamic strain [38–42], pulling the lung out of the VILI vortex, as depicted in Fig. 2.4. Achieving this objective necessitates a comprehensive analysis of all components in the mechanical breath profile and formulates a ventilator strategy capable of mitigating these primary VILI mechanisms. This suggests that high pressures and volumes will cause minimal lung tissue injury if the tissue does not collapse and reopen with every breath. Thus, it is not so much the static peak-inspiratory and end-expiratory pressures that cause VILI but rather the *dynamic* changes in the microenvironment between these two points [38–43].

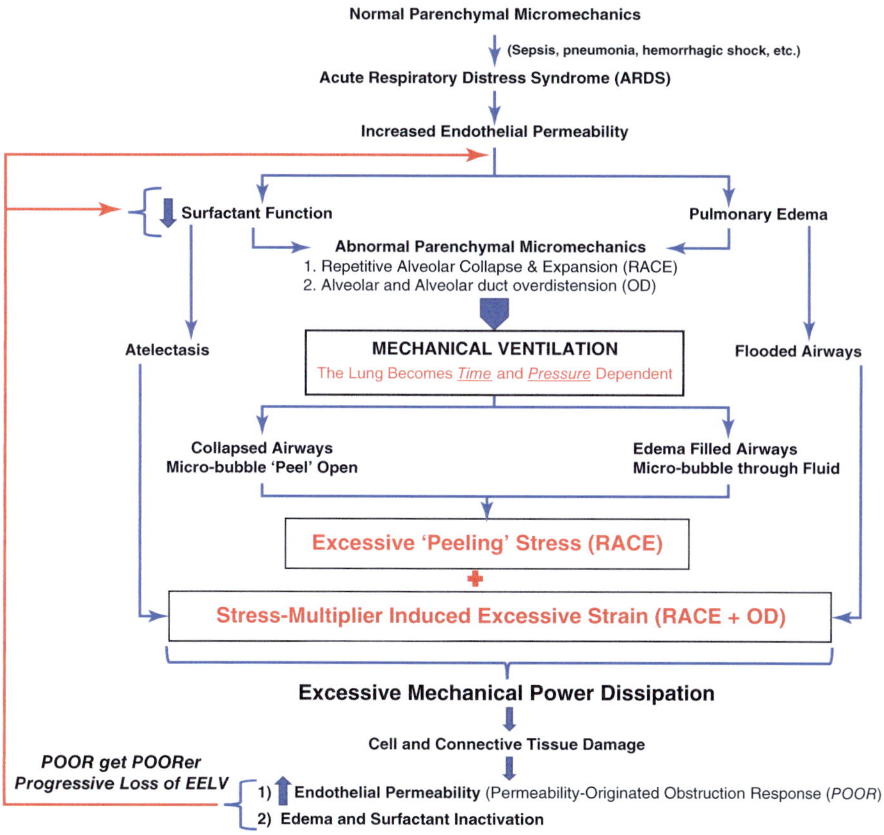

Fig. 1.2 The unifying hypothesis of the mechanisms by which the acute respiratory distress syndrome [2] pathophysiology predisposes the lung to a secondary ventilator-induced lung injury (VILI). A complex cascade of events occurs following injuries such as sepsis, pneumonia, or hemorrhagic shock leading to ARDS. Inflammation from these initiating insults results in *Increased Endothelial Permeability* causing two critical factors, ↓ *Surfactant Function* and *Pulmonary Edema*, resulting in *Abnormal Parenchymal Micromechanics* (alveoli and alveolar ducts). Abnormal parenchymal mechanics result in *Repetitive Alveolar Collapse and Expansion (RACE)* that causes **Atelectrauma** and Alveolar and Alveolar Duct Overdistension (OD) that causes **Volutrauma**. Collapsed and edema-filled alveoli reduce the diffusion surface area of the lung, leading to hypoxia and hypercapnia, necessitating placing the patient on *MECHANICAL VENTILATION*. With the loss of functional surfactant, the lung becomes *Time- and Pressure-Dependent*. This means it will take more time for alveoli to open and less time for them to collapse at any given airway pressure pushing the lung into the VILI vortex (Fig. 2.4). During inspiration, the mechanical ventilator will force an air bubble into collapsed or edema-filled small airways and alveoli, causing an excessive "Peeling" stress as these small airways open or the air bubble is pushed through edema-filled airways (Figs. 4.6 and 4.7). In addition, regional alveolar collapse and instability generate stress multipliers in the adjacent open alveoli, causing both RACE (Fig. 2.6) and OD (Fig. 2.7) of alveoli and alveolar ducts. RACE and OD cause energy dissipation into the tissue with each breath, which is the central mechanism of *Cell and Connective Tissue Damage*. Tissue damage during mechanical ventilation elicits the *Permeability-Originated Obstruction Response (POOR) gets POORer* response causing a rapid spread of injury throughout the lung, resulting in *a Progressive Loss of End-Expiratory Lung Volume (EELV)* (Fig. 4.11), both of which exacerbate ↓ *Surfactant Function* and *Increased Endothelial Permeability* further accelerating VILI-induced tissue injury

Summary

Extensive reviews discuss pulmonary microanatomy, gas exchange, and lung parenchymal mechanics [28–30, 44, 45]. This book will focus on the dynamic physical damage to pulmonary tissue caused by atelectrauma and volutrauma. It will not address the inflammatory injury that has been reviewed in detail elsewhere [6, 46–51]. To generate a sound physiological understanding of the biophysical mechanisms of VILI, multiple systems must be analyzed and integrated, and a unifying hypothesis developed that includes (Fig. 1.2):

- The microanatomy of alveoli and alveolar ducts that form the acinus, which is the functional unit of the lung.
- The dynamic mechanism of acinar volume change in the normal lung.
- The role of pulmonary surfactant in dynamic acinar mechanics.
- The importance of viscoelastic acinar volume change in the normal and acutely injured lung.
- The role of inspiratory and expiratory time on acinar mechanics in the acutely injured lung.
- Altered acinar mechanics as a mechanism of VILI.
- How can all components in the MB_P be optimally set and adjusted to normalize acinar mechanics and minimize VILI-induced lung tissue damage, which is necessary to reduce ARDS-related morbidity and mortality?

Using this unifying hypothesis, we can logically determine what components of the MB_P and which combination will normalize altered acinar mechanics and reduce VILI. By identifying the alterations in dynamic alveolar mechanics caused by ARDS that render the lung so susceptible to VILI, we can begin to design an effective MB_P necessary to reduce VILI intelligently. This book aims to identify how the increase in alveolar-capillary permeability (POOR) by local or systemic inflammation predisposes the lung to a secondary physical injury caused by mechanical ventilation. This pathophysiologic knowledge can then be applied to identify an MB_P that will effectively reduce the tissue damage caused by VILI with the ultimate goal of lowering ARDS-related mortality and improving patient care (Fig. 1.3).

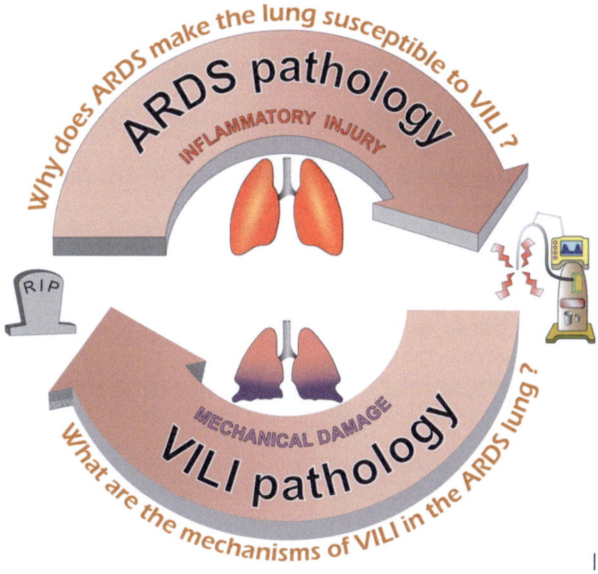

Fig. 1.3 Acute Respiratory Distress Syndrome (ARDS) pathology causes inflammatory injury (red lungs) that leads to altered alveolar and alveolar duct mechanics that render the lung highly susceptible to a secondary ventilator-induced lung injury (VILI). If mechanical ventilation is misapplied, it can cause mechanical damage (partially collapsed lungs) to the inflamed lung that will exacerbate the initial inflammatory lesion, leading to a vicious cycle resulting in high mortality. To block this injury vortex, a mechanical ventilation strategy that normalizes alveolar and alveolar duct mechanics necessary to minimize VILI must be identified

References

1. Marini JJ, Gattinoni L. Time course of evolving ventilator-induced lung injury: the "shrinking baby lung". Crit Care Med. 2020;48(8):1203–9.
2. The Acute Respiratory Distress Syndrome Network. ARDSnet: ventilation with lower tidal volumes as compared with traditional tidal volumes for acute lung injury and the acute respiratory distress syndrome. N Engl J Med. 2000;342(18):1301–8.
3. Gattinoni L, Pesenti A. The concept of "baby lung". Intensive Care Med. 2005;31(6):776–84.
4. Gattinoni L, Pesenti A, Avalli L, Rossi F, Bombino M. Pressure-volume curve of total respiratory system in acute respiratory failure. Computed tomographic scan study. Am Rev Respir Dis. 1987;136(3):730–6.
5. Slutsky AS. Lung injury caused by mechanical ventilation. Chest. 1999;116(1 Suppl):9S–15S.
6. Slutsky AS, Ranieri VM. Ventilator-induced lung injury. N Engl J Med. 2013;369(22):2126–36.
7. https://doi.org/10.1001/jama.2021.13374.
8. Araos J, Alegria L, Garcia P, Cruces P, Soto D, Erranz B, Amthauer M, Salomon T, Medina T, Rodriguez F, et al. Near-apneic ventilation decreases lung injury and fibroproliferation in an acute respiratory distress syndrome model with extracorporeal membrane oxygenation. Am J Respir Crit Care Med. 2019;199(5):603–12.

9. Maca J, Jor O, Holub M, Sklienka P, Bursa F, Burda M, Janout V, Sevcik P. Past and present ARDS mortality rates: a systematic review. Respir Care. 2017;62(1):113–22.
10. Bellani G, Laffey JG, Pham T, Fan E, Brochard L, Esteban A, Gattinoni L, van Haren F, Larsson A, McAuley DF, et al. Epidemiology, patterns of care, and mortality for patients with acute respiratory distress syndrome in intensive care units in 50 countries. JAMA. 2016;315(8):788–800.
11. Phua J, Badia JR, Adhikari NK, Friedrich JO, Fowler RA, Singh JM, Scales DC, Stather DR, Li A, Jones A, et al. Has mortality from acute respiratory distress syndrome decreased over time?: a systematic review. Am J Respir Crit Care Med. 2009;179(3):220–7.
12. Fan E, Brodie D, Slutsky AS. Acute respiratory distress syndrome: advances in diagnosis and treatment. JAMA. 2018;319(7):698–710.
13. Rezoagli E, Fumagalli R, Bellani G. Definition and epidemiology of acute respiratory distress syndrome. Ann Transl Med. 2017;5(14):282.
14. Villar J, Blanco J, Kacmarek RM. Current incidence and outcome of the acute respiratory distress syndrome. Curr Opin Crit Care. 2016;22(1):1–6.
15. McNicholas BA, Rooney GM, Laffey JG. Lessons to learn from epidemiologic studies in ARDS. Curr Opin Crit Care. 2018;24(1):41–8.
16. Raymondos K, Dirks T, Quintel M, Molitoris U, Ahrens J, Dieck T, Johanning K, Henzler D, Rossaint R, Putensen C, et al. Outcome of acute respiratory distress syndrome in university and non-university hospitals in Germany. Crit Care. 2017;21(1):122.
17. Cochi SE, Kempker JA, Annangi S, Kramer MR, Martin GS. Mortality trends of acute respiratory distress syndrome in the United States from 1999 to 2013. Ann Am Thorac Soc. 2016;13(10):1742–51.
18. Pham T, Serpa Neto A, Pelosi P, Laffey JG, De Haro C, Lorente JA, Bellani G, Fan E, Brochard LJ, Pesenti A, et al. Outcomes of patients presenting with mild acute respiratory distress syndrome: insights from the LUNG SAFE study. Anesthesiology. 2018;130:263.
19. Zhang Z, Spieth PM, Chiumello D, Goyal H, Torres A, Laffey JG, Hong Y. Declining mortality in patients with acute respiratory distress syndrome: an analysis of the acute respiratory distress syndrome network trials. Crit Care Med. 2019;47(3):315–23.
20. Combes A, Hajage D, Capellier G, Demoule A, Lavoue S, Guervilly C, Da Silva D, Zafrani L, Tirot P, Veber B, et al. Extracorporeal membrane oxygenation for severe acute respiratory distress syndrome. N Engl J Med. 2018;378(21):1965–75.
21. Cavalcanti AB, Suzumura EA, Laranjeira LN, Paisani DM, Damiani LP, Guimaraes HP, Romano ER, Regenga MM, Taniguchi LNT, Teixeira C, et al. Effect of lung recruitment and titrated positive end-expiratory pressure (PEEP) vs low PEEP on mortality in patients with acute respiratory distress syndrome: a randomized clinical trial. JAMA. 2017;318(14):1335–45.
22. Writing C, Steering Committee for the RCG, Algera AG, Pisani L, Serpa Neto A, den Boer SS, Bosch FFH, Bruin K, Klooster PM, Van der Meer NJM, et al. Effect of a lower vs higher positive end-expiratory pressure strategy on ventilator-free days in ICU patients without ARDS: a randomized clinical trial. JAMA. 2020;
23. Cereda M, Xin Y. Alveolar recruitment and lung injury: an issue of timing and location? Crit Care Med. 2013;41(12):2837–8.
24. Cereda M, Xin Y, Hamedani H, Bellani G, Kadlecek S, Clapp J, Guerra L, Meeder N, Rajaei J, Tustison NJ, et al. Tidal changes on CT and progression of ARDS. Thorax. 2017;72(11):981–9.
25. Cereda M, Xin Y, Hamedani H, Clapp J, Kadlecek S, Meeder N, Zeng J, Profka H, Kavanagh BP, Rizi RR. Mild loss of lung aeration augments stretch in healthy lung regions. J Appl Physiol (1985). 2016;120(4):444–54.
26. Cereda M, Xin Y, Meeder N, Zeng J, Jiang Y, Hamedani H, Profka H, Kadlecek S, Clapp J, Deshpande CG, et al. Visualizing the propagation of acute lung injury. Anesthesiology. 2016;124(1):121–31.
27. Albert K, Krischer JM, Pfaffenroth A, Wilde S, Lopez-Rodriguez E, Braun A, Smith BJ, Knudsen L. Hidden microatelectases increase vulnerability to ventilation-induced lung injury. Front Physiol. 2020;11:530485.

28. Knudsen L, Ochs M. The micromechanics of lung alveoli: structure and function of surfactant and tissue components. Histochem Cell Biol. 2018;150(6):661–76.
29. Weibel ER. Lung morphometry: the link between structure and function. Cell Tissue Res. 2017;367(3):413–26.
30. Hsia CC, Hyde DM, Weibel ER. Lung structure and the intrinsic challenges of gas exchange. Compr Physiol. 2016;6(2):827–95.
31. Toshima M, Ohtani Y, Ohtani O. Three-dimensional architecture of elastin and collagen fiber networks in the human and rat lung. Arch Histol Cytol. 2004;67(1):31–40.
32. Whimster WF. The microanatomy of the alveolar duct system. Thorax. 1970;25(2):141–9.
33. Autilio C, Perez-Gil J. Understanding the principle biophysics concepts of pulmonary surfactant in health and disease. Arch Dis Child Fetal Neonatal Ed. 2019;104(4):F443–51.
34. Gaver DP 3rd, Nieman GF, Gatto LA, Cereda M, Habashi NM, Bates JHT. The POOR get POORer: a hypothesis for the pathogenesis of ventilator-induced lung injury. Am J Respir Crit Care Med. 2020;202(8):1081–7.
35. Suki B, Hubmayr R. Epithelial and endothelial damage induced by mechanical ventilation modes. Curr Opin Crit Care. 2014;20(1):17–24.
36. Cereda M, Xin Y, Emami K, Huang J, Rajaei J, Profka H, Han B, Mongkolwisetwara P, Kadlecek S, Kuzma NN, et al. Positive end-expiratory pressure increments during anesthesia in normal lung result in hysteresis and greater numbers of smaller aerated airspaces. Anesthesiology. 2013;119(6):1402–9.
37. Bilek AM, Dee KC, Gaver DP 3rd. Mechanisms of surface-tension-induced epithelial cell damage in a model of pulmonary airway reopening. J Appl Physiol. 2003;94(2):770–83.
38. Protti A, Andreis DT, Monti M, Santini A, Sparacino CC, Langer T, Votta E, Gatti S, Lombardi L, Leopardi O, et al. Lung stress and strain during mechanical ventilation: any difference between statics and dynamics? Crit Care Med. 2013;41(4):1046–55.
39. Protti A, Andreis DT, Iapichino GE, Monti M, Comini B, Milesi M, Zani L, Gatti S, Lombardi L, Gattinoni L. High positive end-expiratory pressure: only a dam against oedema formation? Crit Care. 2013;17(4):R131.
40. Jain SV, Kollisch-Singule M, Satalin J, Searles Q, Dombert L, Abdel-Razek O, Yepuri N, Leonard A, Gruessner A, Andrews P, et al. The role of high airway pressure and dynamic strain on ventilator-induced lung injury in a heterogeneous acute lung injury model. Intensive Care Med Exp. 2017;5(1):25.
41. Seah AS, Grant KA, Aliyeva M, Allen GB, Bates JH. Quantifying the roles of tidal volume and PEEP in the pathogenesis of ventilator-induced lung injury. Ann Biomed Eng. 2011;39(5):1505–16.
42. Wilson MR, Patel BV, Takata M. Ventilation with "clinically relevant" high tidal volumes does not promote stretch-induced injury in the lungs of healthy mice. Crit Care Med. 2012;40(10):2850–7.
43. Costa ELV, Slutsky A, Brochard LJ, Brower R, Serpa-Neto A, Cavalcanti AB, Mercat A, Meade M, Morais CCA, Goligher E, et al. Ventilatory variables and mechanical power in patients with acute respiratory distress syndrome. Am J Respir Crit Care Med. 2021;204:303.
44. Roan E, Waters CM. What do we know about mechanical strain in lung alveoli? Am J Physiol Lung Cell Mol Physiol. 2011;301(5):L625–35.
45. Suki B, Stamenovic D, Hubmayr R. Lung parenchymal mechanics. Compr Physiol. 2011;1(3):1317–51.
46. Nieman GF, Gatto LA, Habashi NM. Impact of mechanical ventilation on the pathophysiology of progressive acute lung injury. J Appl Physiol. 2015;119(11):1245–61.
47. Cong X, Hubmayr RD, Li C, Zhao X. Plasma membrane wounding and repair in pulmonary diseases. Am J Physiol Lung Cell Mol Physiol. 2017;312(3):L371–91.
48. Uhlig U, Uhlig S. Ventilator-induced lung injury. Compr Physiol. 2011;1:635–61.
49. Reiss LK, Uhlig U, Uhlig S. Models and mechanisms of acute lung injury caused by direct insults. Eur J Cell Biol. 2012;91(6–7):590–601.

50. Curley GF, Laffey JG, Zhang H, Slutsky AS. Biotrauma and ventilator-induced lung injury: clinical implications. Chest. 2016;150(5):1109–17.
51. Wurfel MM. Microarray-based analysis of ventilator-induced lung injury. Proc Am Thorac Soc. 2007;4(1):77–84.

Chapter 2
Current Protective Ventilation Approach

History of Mechanical Ventilation for the ARDS Patient

Application of a mechanical breath to a lung with abnormal alveolar mechanics can result in a secondary ventilator-iduced lung injury (VILI) (Fig. 2.1, Green Box). Large-scale mechanical ventilation can be traced back to 1929, when the first iron lung was widely used for polio patients (Fig. 2.2) [1]. Initially designed to address polio-related mortality, the negative pressure ventilation provided by the iron lung posed logistical challenges. The response to the polio outbreak in the early 1950s saw the introduction of positive-pressure mechanical ventilation.

Initially, it was believed that polio patients were succumbing to kidney failure, as evidenced by symptoms such as excessive sweating, elevated plasma CO_2, and hypertension. However, it was later recognized that these symptoms were indicative of respiratory failure. Despite initial resistance from the clinical establishment against tracheostomy and positive pressure ventilation for polio-induced respiratory paralysis, it eventually became a primary treatment option. This acceptance was marked by a significant drop in mortality from 87% to 40% [2]. However, the demand for positive pressure ventilators far exceeded the available supply, necessitating manually ventilating thousands of polio patients.

It's crucial to note that the lungs of these polio patients were typically normal, and positive pressure ventilation or manual bagging served to compensate for paralyzed respiratory muscles rather than to address an acutely injured lung. Consequently, ventilator-induced lung injury (VILI) was not a prevalent concern. Additionally, hand-bagged polio patients were often centralized within the hospital for logistical efficiency, giving rise to the inception of the first Intensive Care Unit (ICU).

Positive pressure mechanical ventilation has been a subject of investigation for many decades, with studies examining its advantages and drawbacks. As early as 1938,

---

Supplementary Information The online version contains supplementary material available at https://doi.org/10.1007/978-3-031-66352-9_2.

© The Author(s), under exclusive license to Springer Nature Switzerland AG 2024

G. F. Nieman, N. M. Habashi, *Applied Physiology to Reduce Ventilator Induced Lung Injury*, https://doi.org/10.1007/978-3-031-66352-9_2

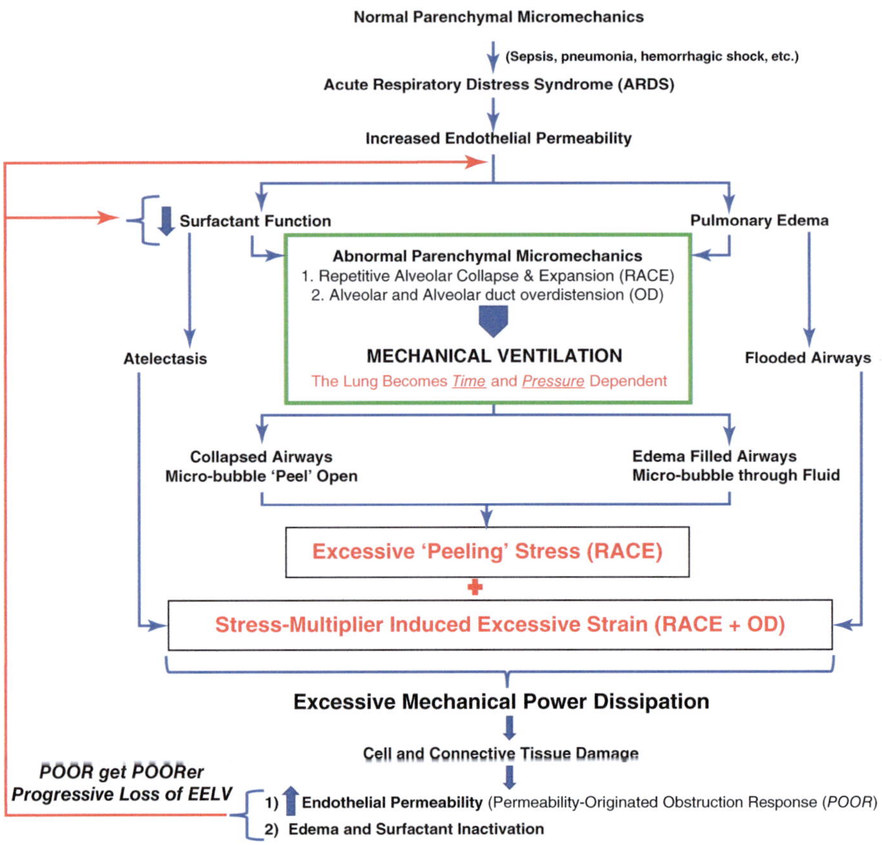

Fig. 2.1 The unifying hypothesis of how acute respiratory distress syndrome (ARDS) pathophysiology predisposes the lung to a secondary ventilator-induced lung injury (VILI). This chapter discusses Abnormal Parenchymal Micromechanics and MECHANICAL VENTILATION (green line)

research demonstrated that positive pressure ventilation could alleviate pulmonary edema in animals and humans [3]. The recognition and characterization of ARDS as a distinct clinical syndrome were notably advanced by Ashbaugh et al. in 1967. Ashbaugh et al. identified ARDS as a distinct clinical syndrome and demonstrated that positive end-expiratory pressure (PEEP) could potentially decrease ARDS-related mortality. This finding contributed to the widespread adoption of positive pressure ventilation for acute respiratory failure, both with and without PEEP [4]. However, the realization of the life-saving benefits of positive pressure ventilation and PEEP was soon accompanied by the awareness that delivering positive pressure to a severely injured lung could worsen lung damage, leading to complications such as pneumothoraces.

In 1944, research demonstrated that positive airway pressure could cause the tearing of pulmonary membranes, leading to barotrauma [5]. In 1964, Greenfield found that high airway pressures (26–32 cmH_2O) coupled with large tidal volumes

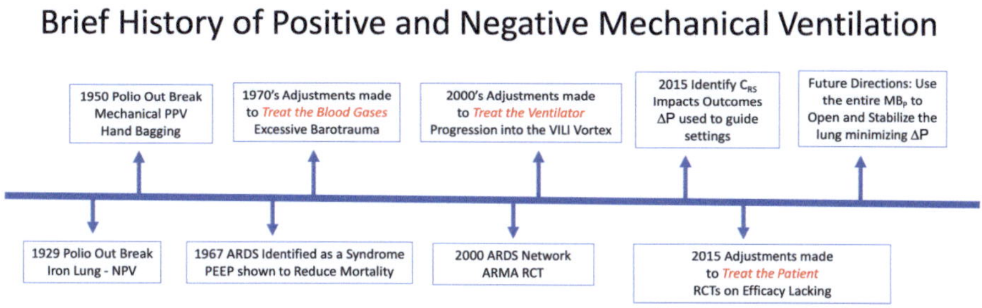

Fig. 2.2 Timeline of major developments in mechanical ventilation. Both negative pressure ventilation (NPV) using the *Iron Lung* and positive pressure ventilation (PPV) using ventilators and hand-bagging expanded rapidly in response to the polio epidemics of 1929 and 1950. Hand-bagging was a form of positive pressure ventilation that was necessary since there were more polio patients than ventilators. Acute respiratory distress syndrome (ARDS) was identified as a syndrome in 1967, and it was shown that ventilator settings (Positive end-expiratory pressure—PEEP) could be used to reduce mortality, suggesting that mechanical ventilation could be used as a *tool* to improve ARDS-related mortality. *Treating the Blood Gases*: The ventilation strategy for ARDS patients in the 1970s attempted to achieve the blood gases of a normal patient, necessitating a very large tidal volume (V_T) and high airway pressure, causing barotrauma. This ventilation strategy can be thought of *as treating the blood gases* and not the patient
The ARDS Network ARMA randomized controlled trial (RCT) showed that low V_T and airway pressure reduced mortality, ushering in lung-protective ventilation strategies. *Treating the Ventilator*: The ARMA study is a protective ventilation strategy using a one-size-fits-all low V_T and plateau pressure while setting PEEP adjusted by changes in oxygenation and is not based on the patient's lung pathophysiology. Thus, this strategy can be considered as *treating the ventilator* since the ventilator is "happy" with a V_T < **6** cc/kg and a plateau pressure <**30** cmH_2O without regard to the patient's lung pathophysiology. *Treating the Patient*: The discovery that the relationship between lung pathophysiology, measured as the respiratory system compliance (C_{RS}), and V_T was critical to patient outcomes led to using driving pressure ($\Delta P = V_T/C_{RS}$) to adjust ventilator settings. Future directions will identify the Mechanical Breath Profile (MB_P), consisting of all airway pressures, volumes, flows, rates, and the time they are applied during both inspiration and expiration that will best open and stabilize the lung, pulling it from the VILI vortex (Fig. 2.4) and improving ARDS-related mortality

(14 mL/kg) resulted in a significant loss of surfactant function, leading to severe atelectasis [6]. Despite mounting evidence that high airway pressures and volumes caused severe lung damage, physicians in the 1970s adjusted ventilator settings (V_T and PEEP) to target the blood gases of the normal patient (PaO_2 ~100 mmHg and $PaCO_2$ ~40 mmHg). This approach required tidal volumes ranging from 12 to 18 mL/kg, peak airway pressures exceeding 36 cmH_2O, and PEEP levels as high as 14 cmH_2O. Essentially, these physicians focused on treating blood gases rather than the underlying patient condition (Fig. 2.2) [7].

Furthermore, during this period, there was hesitancy among physicians to increase the fraction of inspired oxygen (FiO_2) to achieve their oxygenation goals due to concerns about oxygen toxicity. This reluctance contributed to the need for excessively high tidal volumes and airway pressures. The ventilator settings required to normalize blood gases far exceeded the currently accepted lung-protective limits of V_T of less than 6 mL/kg and plateau pressure of less than 30 cmH_2O [8]. The initial understanding that high tidal volume (HV_T) and airway pressure cause barotrauma underwent modification when it was revealed that the lung could withstand high pressures without damage if the lung volume was not increased. Consequently, lung volume, not airway pressure per se, emerged as the actual mechanism of injury, leading to the term volutrauma [9].

In addition to excessive static strain (i.e., high plateau pressure—Pplat) causing volutrauma, it was discovered that high dynamic strain represents an additional mechanism of VILI. Excessive dynamic strain can occur during tidal ventilation when a substantial cyclic volume change happens with each tidal volume when the lung is below the normal EELV. High dynamic strain is induced by repetitive alveolar collapse and expansion (RACE) and is known as atelectrauma. Muscedere et al. employed an acute respiratory distress syndrome (ARDS)-saline lavage model using isolated nonperfused rat lungs. Their study revealed that ventilation at low EELV without PEEP resulted in significant morphological tissue damage. The authors concluded that the underlying mechanism of this injury was the cyclic opening and collapse of lung tissue, termed cyclic recruitment and derecruitment (R/D) [10]. Volutrauma and atelectrauma, causing mechanical damage to lung tissue, lead to severe inflammation and the release of cytokines—a phenomenon referred to as biotrauma, which exacerbates the initial mechanical injury [11]. Gattinoni et al., in an anatomical and physiological review of VILI, asserted that "Barotrauma, volutrauma, biotrauma, and atelectrauma are considered as undisputable truth and represent the background for the development and universal acceptance of the so-called lung-protective strategy [12]. These pathophysiological mechanisms are believed to drive VILI, influencing the formulation of current lung-protective strategies.

Current Protective Ventilation Approach for ARDS Patients

The first in a series of clinical trials testing the use of lower V_T and higher PEEP to limit both volutrauma and atelectrauma was published by Amato et al. in 1998, marked the initiation of investigations into the efficacy of employing lower V_T and higher PEEP to mitigate both volutrauma and atelectrauma. This study marked the advent of lung-protective mechanical ventilation [13].

After this, two randomized controlled trials (RCT) failed to demonstrate significant improvement between low and high V_T. However, these setbacks paved the way for the pivotal ARDSNetwork Acute Respiratory Management Approach (ARMA) trial. The ARMA trial showcased a noteworthy reduction in mortality by advocating for the use of low V_T (6 cc/kg) as opposed to high V_T (12 cc/kg) [8]. This landmark trial was crucial in shaping the current standards for protective ventilation strategies in ARDS patients. Nevertheless, challenges have arisen in interpreting these findings, questioning the notion that LV_T is universally linked to reduced mortality. Instead, it is proposed that mortality is a composite outcome influenced by both tidal volume size and the severity of lung injury, as measured by respiratory system compliance (C_{RS}). Subgroup analyses have indicated that when LV_T is applied to a patient with higher C_{RS}, mortality significantly increases. Conversely, applying HV_T to a patient with a similar high C_{RS} significantly decreases mortality [14, 15].

These challenges suggest that some clinicians have prioritized adherence to ventilator settings over individual patient needs. In other words, they may have been "treating the ventilator" rather than tailoring the approach to the specific patient (Fig. 2.2). For instance, adhering to a low tidal volume strategy (i.e., V_T <6 cmH_2O and Pplat <30 cmH_2O) may not be beneficial if applied indiscriminately, irrespective of the underlying lung pathophysiology.

Deans et al. emphasized in 2005 that lung pathophysiology must be considered when adjusting V_T [14]. However, it took 15 years for this concept to be revisited. In 2020, Amato et al. conducted a comprehensive analysis using data from 3562 acute respiratory distress syndrome (ARDS) patients involved in nine randomized controlled trials (RCTs). Their findings challenged the conventional wisdom, revealing that individual adjustments in PEEP and V_T were not independently linked to mortality. Instead, changes in driving pressure ($\Delta P = V_T/C_{RS}$) were associated with survival [16].

The significance of this discovery lies in its affirmation of Deans' initial observations: it's not just the size of the V_T, but also the size of the EELV and the specific pathophysiology of the lung measured by the C_{RS}, to which the V_T is being delivered, that determines whether a ventilation strategy is harmful or protective. A more recent secondary analysis of patients from five RCTs comparing low versus high V_T reinforced this notion. It revealed that the mortality benefit of a low V_T varied with C_{RS}, suggesting that ΔP should be the primary guide to protect the lung from ventilator-induced lung injury (VILI) [17].

By employing ΔP to inform protective ventilation strategies, physicians are effectively treating the patient, as C_{RS} assesses lung pathophysiology (Fig. 2.2) by normalizing V_T to C_{RS}. The LV_T ARMA method is aptly called a "Protect the Lung Approach." The underlying hypothesis is that reducing the V_T and Pplat serves to "protect" the normal lung tissue from overdistension and rupture, allowing the injured, collapsed tissue to "rest" and remain collapsed throughout the ventilator cycle (Fig. 2.3) [8]. Positive end-expiratory pressure is adjusted based on oxygenation needs to mitigate progressive lung collapse and prevent the lung from entering the so-called VILI Vortex (Fig. 2.4) [18–20]. An adaptation of the LV_T ARMA method, known as the Open Lung Approach, seeks to initially recruit the lung over a few seconds or minutes and then adjusts PEEP to prevent the newly opened lung from re-collapsing [21]—a strategy to optimize lung function. At the other end of the spectrum, an extreme iteration of the Protect the Lung Approach involves using very low V_T or no V_T with blood gas exchange facilitated by extracorporeal membrane oxygenation (ECMO) [22].

However, despite these variations, statistical analyses and meta-analyses have indicated that the LV_T Protect the Lung Approach, regardless if it is combined with ECMO or recruitment maneuvers, has not demonstrated a significant reduction in mortality for patients with established ARDS since its implementation over 22 years ago [23–38]. Table 2.1 provides a comprehensive overview of the results from multiple RCTs and meta-analyses on ARDS-related mortality from 1998 to 2022.

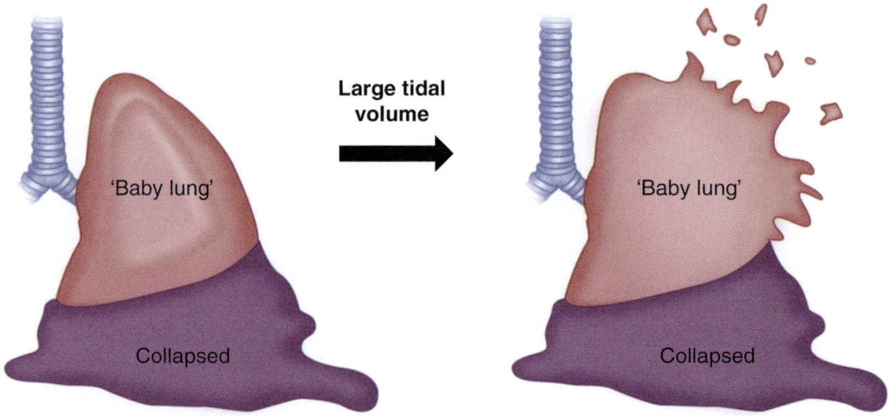

Fig. 2.3 The two-compartment model of ARDS pathophysiology, with collapsed and edema-filled tissue in the dependent compartment and a small amount of normal tissue in the nondependent compartment, known as the baby lung. This model led to the hypothesis that VILI was caused by overdistension of the baby lung if ventilated with a normal-size V_T, and it would "pop" like a balloon. The ARDS Network low V_T protective ventilation strategy was designed to minimize overdistension of the baby lung since this was the mechanism believed to be driving progressive VILI

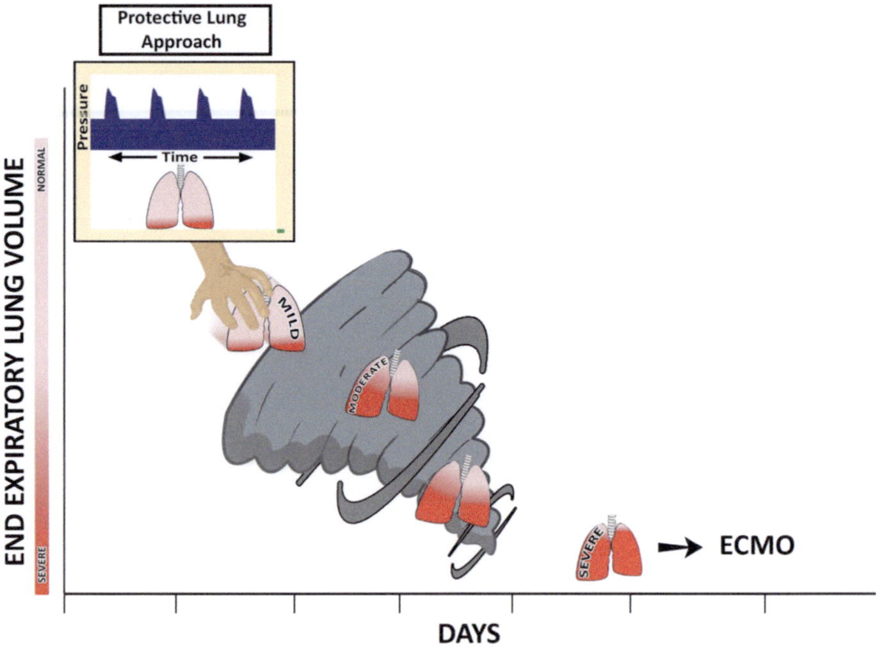

Fig. 2.4 ARDS's pathogenesis can be considered a ventilation-induced lung injury (VILI) vortex. Ventilation with low V_T and airway pressure encourages progressive lung collapse, resulting in the lung going from mild, to moderate, and finally to severe ARDS and respiratory failure, necessitating the use of extracorporeal membrane oxygenation (ECMO). With progressive lung collapse, the remaining normal tissue must withstand more stress and strain during each mechanical breath. Thus, the smaller the amount of normal lung tissue, the higher the risk of VILI

Table 2.1 Clinical trials comparing low (LV_T) and high (HV_T) tidal volume and LV_T as the control with an additional treatment on ARDS-related mortality. Also, using hospital standard-of-care treatment, statistical- and meta-analyses on mild, moderate, and severe ARDS-related in hospital, ICU, 28-, 60-, and 90-day mortality

	Mortality			
	LV_T	**HV_T**		
LV_T vs HV_T				
Amato M. NEJM 1998 (low<6 PEEP Pflex vs high V_T12 PEEP low) [13]	[a]38%	71%[d, g]		
Stewart TE. NEJM 1998 (low8 vs high Vt10-15) [100]	50%	47%[e]		
Brower R. Crit Care Med 1999;27 (low5-8 vs high10-12 V_T) [101]	50%	46%[e]		
Brochard L. AJRCCM 1998 (low<10 vs high V_T10 or >) [102]	46.6%	37.9%[h]		
ARDSnet NEJM ARMA 2000 (low 6 vs high12 V_T) [8]	[a]31.0%	39.8%[a, e]		
Villar J. Crit Care Med 2006 (V_T 5-8 vs V_T 9-11) [103]	[a]32%[a, c, f] 34%[c, e]	53%[b, f] 55%[b, e]		
Shen Y. Crit Care. 2019;23. (Low vs High P/F) [90]	[a]22.4%[o]; 37.1%[p]	39.5%[o]; 40.8%[e, p]		
	LV_T	**LV_T +Treatment**		
LV_T vs LV_T + Additional treatment				
Thompson BT. ARDSnet JAMA 2000;283 (Ketoconazole) [104]	34.1%	35.2%[e]		
Abraham E. ARDSnet Crit Care Med 2002;30 (Lisofylline) [105]	31.9%	24.7%[g]		
Brower R. ARDSnet NEJM ALVEOLI 2004;351 (low vs high PEEP) [106]	24.9%	27.5%[b, e]		
ARDSnet NEJM 2006;354 (Fluid Resuscitation) [107]	28.4% (AF)	25.9% (CF)[h]		
Talmor D. NEJM 2008;359 Vt ~7; PEEP guided by Ptp [108]	39%	17%[g]		
ARDSnet NEJM 2006;354 (Methylprednisolone) [109]	28.6%	29.2%[h]		
Meade M. ARDSnet JAMA LOV 2008;299 (High PEEP) [110]	36.4%	40.4%[e]		
Mercat A. ARDSnet JAMA EXPRESS 2008;299 (High PEEP) [111]	31.2%	27.8%[g]		
Taccone P. JAMA 2009;302Vt<8; Prone [112]	46.1%	37.8%[g]		
Papazian L. NEJM 2010;363Vt6-8 ARMA; Cisatracurium [113]	[a]40.7%	31.6%[i]		

(continued)

Table 2.1 (continued)

	Mortality			
	LV_T	**HV_T**		
Oscillate NEJM 2013;368 (HFOV) [114]	35%	47%[e]		
Oscar NEJM 2013; 368 (HFOV) [115]	41.1%	41.7%[g]		
Guerin C. ARDSnet NEJM 2013;368Vt6; Prone [116]	[a]32.8%	16.0%[g]		
Esteban AJRCCM 2013;188 (Mortality 1998 vs 2010) [117]	[a]31% (1998)	28% (2010)[e]		
Kacmarek R. Crit Care Med 2016;44 Vt4-8; RM titrate PEEP [118]	33%	29%[e]		
Cavalcanti A. JAMA 2017 Vt5.8; RM titrate PEEP [119]	[a]49.3%	55.3%[g]		
Hodgson C. AJRCCM 2019;200 V_T 4- 6; Max recruitment [120]	26.8%	24.6%[g]		
Ganesan SL. AJRCCM 2018;198. Pediatric LV_T vs APRV [121]	[a]26.9%	53.8%[g]		
Zhou Y. Inten Care Med 2017;43. LV_T vs APRV [122]	34.3%	19.7%[f]		
Statistical analyses on ARDS-induced mortality	**ARDS mortality** **Criteria of Mortality**			
Nolan S. Inten Care Med 1997;23 [123]	59%[e]	47%[f]		
Luhr OR. AJRCCM 1999;159 [124]	41.0% (ARF) 42.2% (ALI)	41.2% (ARDS)[i]		
Bersten AD. AJRCCM 2002;165 [125]	32% (ALI)	34% (ARDS)[g]		
Brun-Buisson C. Inten Care Med 2004;30 [126]	49.4%	57.9%[e]		
Rubenfeld GD NEJM 2005;353 [127]	38.5% (ALI)	41.1% (ARDS)[e]		
Manzano F. J Crit Care 2005;20 [128]	52%[g]	66%[e]		
Sakr Y. Chest 2004;128 [129]	38.9%[f]	45.5%[e]		
Linko R. Inten Care Med 2009;35 [130]	31% (ARF) 32% (MV>24hr)	47% (ARDS)[i]		
Li G. AJRCCM 2011;183 [131]	20% (2001)	16% (2008)[e]		
Villar J. Inten Care Med 2011;37 [89]	42.7%[f]	47.8%[e]		
Maca J. Resp Care 2017;62 [24]	45%[e]	38%[f]	30%[g]	32%[h]
Caser EB. Crit Care Med 2014;42 [88]	38.5%[g]	49.2%[e]		
Laffey JG. Inten Care Med 2016;42 [87]	35%[j]	40%[k]	46%[l]	

(continued)

Table 2.1 (continued)

Statistical analyses on ARDS-induced mortality	**ARDS mortality**			
	Criteria of Mortality			
Zhang Z. Crit Care Med. 2019;47 [34]	35.4%[e] (1996)	28%[e] (2013)		
Fan E. JAMA. 2018;319 [27]	27%[e, j]	32%[e, k]	45%[e, l]	
Phua J. AJRCCM. 2009;179 [26]	40%–45%[m]	35%–40%[a]		
Rezoagli E. Ann Translational Med. 2017;5 [28]	~40%[e]			
Villar J. Curr Opin Crit Care. 2016;22 [29]	>40%[e, k, l, m]			
Caser EB. Crit Care Med. 2014;42 [88]	38.5%[g]	49.2%[e]		
Bellani G. JAMA.2016;315 [25]	34.9%[e, j]; 40.3%[e, k]; 46.1%[e, l]			
Pham T. Anesthesiology 2019;130 [132]	30%[e]			
Matthay M. Inten Care Med 2020 [133]	Phenotype & mortality[n]			
Lin P. Crit Care 2021;25 [134]	[a]39.4%(Steroid)	49.1% (No Steroid)		
Qadir N. Chest 2021;160 [135]	40.7%[g, m] (16.7%–73.3%: Range between Centers)			
Beyls C. ASAIO J 2022;68 COVID on ECMO [136]	1st Wave" 43%; 2nd Wave 85%; 3rd Wave 38%			

Ptp Transpulmonary pressure, *HF* Aggressive fluid resuscitation, *CF* Conservative fluid resuscitation, *HFOV* High-frequency oscillatory ventilation, *ARF* Acute respiratory failure, *ALI* Acute lung injury, *MV* Mechanical ventilation, *ARDS* Acute respiratory distress syndrome, *Pflex* Lower infection point on the whole lung pressure/volume curve

Key:

a = Statistically significant
b = PEEP>5cmH_2O
c = PEEP set at Pflex+2cmH_2O
d = LV_T group PEEP by Pflex vs HV_T group PEEP set by oxygenation
e = In-hospital mortality
f = ICU mortality
g = 28d mortality
h = 60d mortality
i = 90d mortality
j = Mild ARDS
k = Moderate ARDS
l = Severe ARDS
m = Observational Studies
n = All ARDS patients
o = PF > 150
p = PF < 150

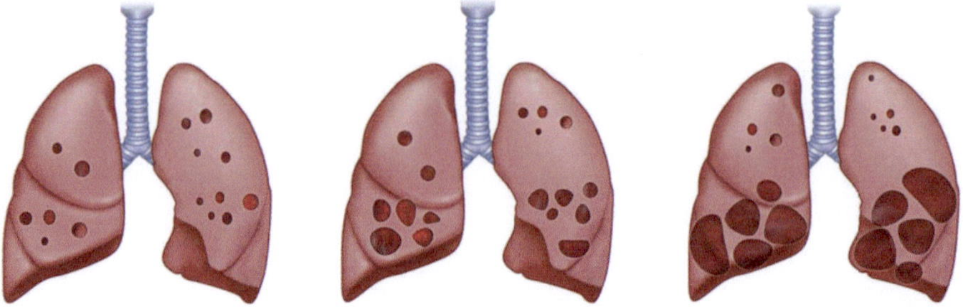

Fig. 2.5 The current concept of ARDS pathophysiology is that it begins as a heterogeneous scattering of regional alveolar instability and collapse (red dots) and that tissue damage expands radially from these lesions. These lesions originate secondary to the Permeability-Originated Obstruction Response (POOR), causing a heterogeneity of tissue stiffness between the injured POOR areas and the normal tissue surrounding these primary lesions. If exposed to nonprotective ventilation, these tissue injuries will rapidly expand concentrically from these initial lesions throughout the lung in a POOR get POORer fashion [39]

The current approach to protective mechanical ventilation has not resulted in further reductions in mortality associated with ARDS. A plausible explanation for this limited success is the potential inadequacy of the prevailing two-compartment ARDS pathology model, as discussed earlier, combined with population heterogeneity. Recent studies challenge this model, revealing a complex ARDS pathophysiology characterized by regional alveolar collapse and instability scattered throughout the lung, encompassing areas traditionally considered normal, such as the baby lung (Fig. 2.5) [40–43].

In ARDS, local and systemic inflammation from conditions like pneumonia, sepsis, or hemorrhagic shock causes leaky pulmonary capillaries, leading to alveolar flooding with edema fluid. This edema deactivates pulmonary surfactant, initiating alveolar instability, collapse, and flooding (Fig. 1.1). This cascade sets off a regional Permeability-Originated Obstruction Response (POOR) (Fig. 1.1—**Endothelial Leakage**) [39]. Consequently, a heterogeneity of tissue stiffness emerges between the injured POOR areas and the normal tissue surrounding these primary lesions (Fig. 1.1—**Alveolar Edema**, green arrow). Nonprotective ventilation in these regional lesions can result in rapid concentric expansion in a "POOR get POORer" fashion (Fig. 2.5) [39]. This refined understanding emphasizes the necessity for a more nuanced approach to ventilation strategies in ARDS, considering the complexities of regional pathophysiology and potential variations in tissue responses to mechanical stress. Alveolar instability (RACE) constitutes the primary mechanism of atelectrauma. This process not only inflicts damage on the unstable alveoli during their collapse and reopening but also affects adjacent stable alveoli due to the interconnected nature of alveolar walls (Fig. 2.6). The collateral effect is the

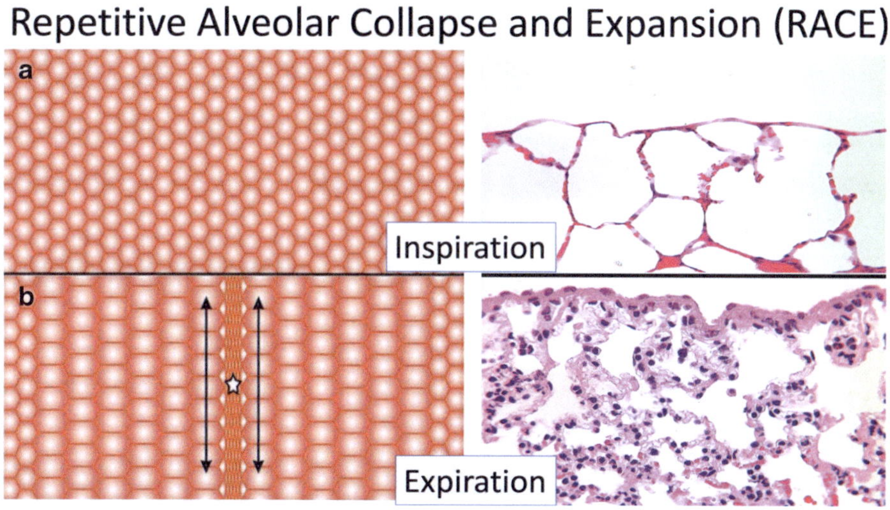

Fig. 2.6 Repetitive alveolar collapse and reopening (RACE) is the mechanism causing atelectrauma. **Left panels**: Alveoli with interconnected walls are modeled as hexagons. (**a**) At peak inspiration, fully inflated "alveoli" at peak inspiration are homogeneous and uniformly inflated. (**b**) At end-expiration with surfactant dysfunction, a hallmark of ARDS pathophysiology renders "alveoli" unstable, and they collapse (star) bordered by black arrows. Opening and re-collapse with each breath will cause mechanical damage to these unstable alveoli, much like bending a paperclip back and forth will cause it to break. In addition, since alveoli share walls, the patent alveoli adjacent to the collapsed are overdistended during each expiration. **Right panels**: Histology of a surfactant-depleted rat ARDS model with the lungs fixed at inspiration and end-expiration. Note the thin walls of the homogeneous fully inflated alveoli at inspiration and the crumpled stacked walls as the alveoli collapse, much like a crumpled paper bag during expiration

overdistension of stable alveoli during each expiratory cycle. Collapsed or edema-filled tissue amplifies the stress exerted on the lung during mechanical ventilation in the regions surrounding the collapse.

When a force is applied to a homogenous structure, the lines of force are uniformly transmitted through the structure, necessitating a substantial amount of stress before stress failure occurs. However, in a heterogeneous structure with regional defects, the lines of force concentrate around these defects, significantly amplifying the stress applied in these areas. This, in turn, requires much less force to cause stress failure and structural damage (Fig. 2.7, Video 2.1). These areas in the ARDS lung are termed "Hidden Microatelectasis" because they cannot be visualized on chest X-rays or computerized tomography (CT) scans. These hidden micro-atelectasis regions have been demonstrated to render the lung more susceptible to VILI (Fig. 2.8) [44].

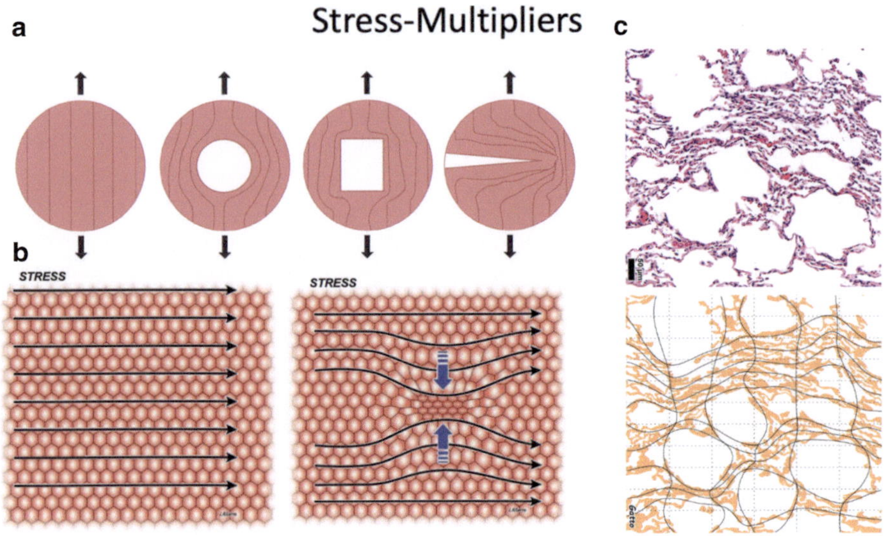

Fig. 2.7 The concept of stress multiplication by regional areas of collapsed or edema-filled tissue. (**a**) A force (arrows) is applied to a board without any defects, and the lines of force will be equally spread over the board. Defects in the board act as a stress multiplier, and the lines of force can be seen to concentrate near the defect, resulting in the board breaking (stress failure) at a much lower applied force (large arrows in each direction). (**b**) "Alveoli" with interconnected walls are depicted as hexagons. The lines of force (straight black arrows) are evenly distributed in the homogeneously inflated lung tissue, similar to that in the board without a defect (**a**). Regional alveolar collapse or edema (small dense hexagons, blue arrows) concentrates the lines of force (curved black arrows) around the lesion, resulting in overdistension of the adjacent open alveoli. (**c**) Top panel: histology of surfactant-depleted rat lung fixed at end-expiration showing the typical crumpling of collapsed alveolar walls. Bottom panel: theoretical lines of force superimposed (curved black lines) over the collapsed tissue show multiple areas of stress multiplication

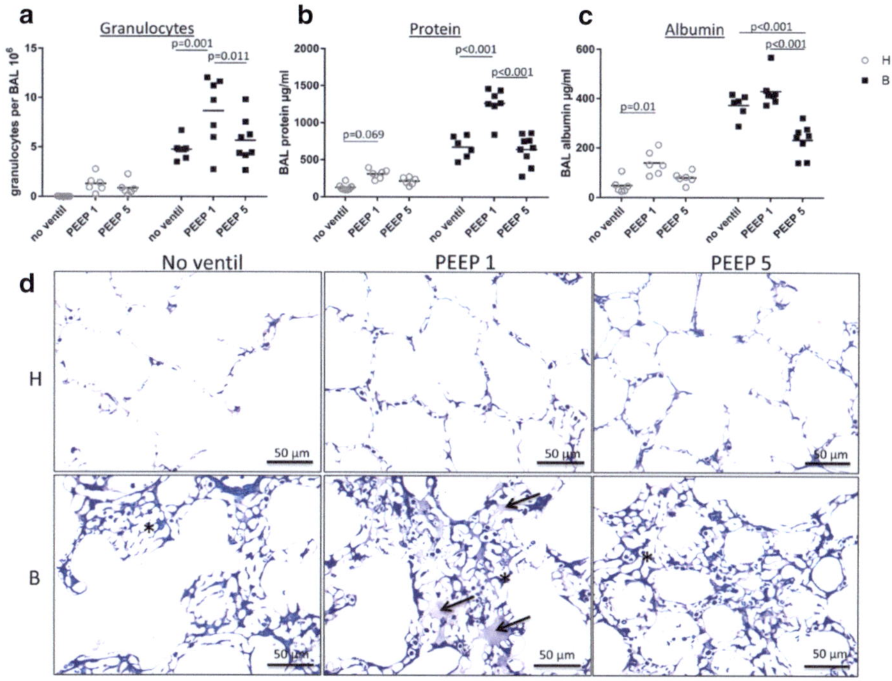

Fig. 2.8 (**a–c**) Intra-alveolar edema and bronchoalveolar lavage (BAL) data in both healthy tissue (H) and bleomycin-injured tissue (B). (**a**) A large influx of neutrophil granulocytes into the alveolar space in the bleomycin group with 1 cmH_2O PEEP (PEEP1—B). (**b**) In the PEEP1 - B, BAL protein content is significantly elevated versus the bleomycin group with 5 cmH_2O (PEEP5—B, $p < 0.001$). (**c**) The concentrations of BAL albumin are highest in group B/PEEP1 and are significantly greater than PEEP5—B but not from bleomycin with no ventilation (no ventil—B). Granulocytes, protein, and albumin were all significantly lower in healthy (H) as compared with bleomycin-injured (B) lungs. (**d**) Lung histology fixed by vascular perfusion at end-inspiratory pressure. Alveolar edema and microatelectasis are not present in healthy lungs (H). All bleomycin-treated lungs (B) contain micro-atelectatic regions (asterisk). Alveolar edema fluid can be seen adjacent to microatelectasis in the B/PEEP1 group (arrows). No intra-alveolar edema was found in PEEP5—B group

Hidden Microatelectasis

Knudsen's group used a bleomycin-induced acute respiratory distress syndrome (ARDS) model to study changes in tissue histopathology. Their study demonstrated that surfactant deactivation and microatelectasis manifested on the first day following bleomycin administration, even when oxygenation and lung function remained normal [44]. This early occurrence of surfactant dysfunction and atelectasis has been proposed as an initial trigger for the progressive pathology leading to ARDS. In this scenario, VILI is posited as the instigating mechanism of acute lung injury, resulting in the loss of surfactant function and the onset of pulmonary edema [44].

These findings suggest that regional lung injury, characterized by small areas of alveolar instability, collapse, and edema flooding, may exist before observable changes in lung function at the bedside (such as lung elastance and blood gases). When animals with "hidden microatelectasis" were ventilated with low PEEP at 1 cmH_2O, there was an increase in elastance, indicating acinar instability. This instability led to heightened interstitial edema, epithelial cell injury, and stressed endoplasmic reticulum (Fig. 2.8) [44]. These insights highlight the importance of considering regional lung injury mechanisms, even before evident changes in global lung function parameters. An additional explanation for the challenges in comprehending and addressing VILI mechanisms may lie in our incomplete understanding of the intricate biophysical mechanisms unfolding at the alveolar level. The lung is a highly complex system, featuring interconnected alveolar architectures that involve various cell types, an uninterrupted network of elastin and collagen extending from alveolar walls to the visceral pleura (serving as a load-bearing scaffolding), and a dynamic surfactant system (Fig. 2.9) [45–50]. This intricate interplay of components plays a crucial role in governing the mechanics of normal alveolar and alveolar duct (acini) volume changes in response to spontaneous or mechanical breaths.

ARDS pathophysiology significantly disrupts these alveolar mechanics, creating a predisposition for secondary VILI (Figs. 2.6 and 2.7, Video 2.1). Fully comprehending the nuanced alterations in these mechanics becomes essential for formulating effective strategies to prevent or mitigate VILI. The current body of evidence indicates that the primary mechanisms driving VILI involve regional alveolar instability, collapse, and edema leading to stress-induced multiplication [44]. This pathophysiology imposes excessive stress and strain on alveolar walls, dissipating considerable energy and leading to intercellular and intracellular stress failure of the load-bearing structures during ventilation (Figs. 2.6 and 2.7, Video 2.1) [51]. Consequently, regional stress multipliers can physically damage the surrounding normal tissue through both RACE-induced atelectrauma (Fig. 2.6) and volutrauma (2.7, Video 2.1), significantly accelerating the propagation of acute lung injury initiated by systemic or local inflammation [40–42, 52].

Additionally, the injured, unstable, or flooded acini may experience excessive shear or "peeling" stress as microbubbles "peel open" the tissue (Fig. 4.4) or push through edema-filled airways (Fig. 4.6), causing atelectrauma (2.1, green box) [53]. Tissue injury rapidly extends from the primary lesions in a "POOR get POORer" manner (Figs. 2.1 and 2.5) [39], triggering progressive loss of EELV known as the "VILI Vortex" [20] (Fig. 2.4). On the other hand, the homogeneously ventilated lung is highly resistant to injury by high static lung strain but is at risk of severe damage by high dynamic strain [54–58]. Thus, it is not so much the static peak-inspiratory and end-expiratory pressures that cause VILI but rather the dynamic changes between these two points [54–59]. Lung heterogeneity caused by surfactant deactivation generates regional areas of stress multiplication and, when combined with high dynamic and static strain, is the "perfect storm" necessary to damage lung tissue with each breath [60]. Thus, logic dictates that VILI could be prevented if the mechanical breath strategy eliminates stress multipliers (volutrauma) and reduces dynamic strain (atelectrauma). In addition, the entire

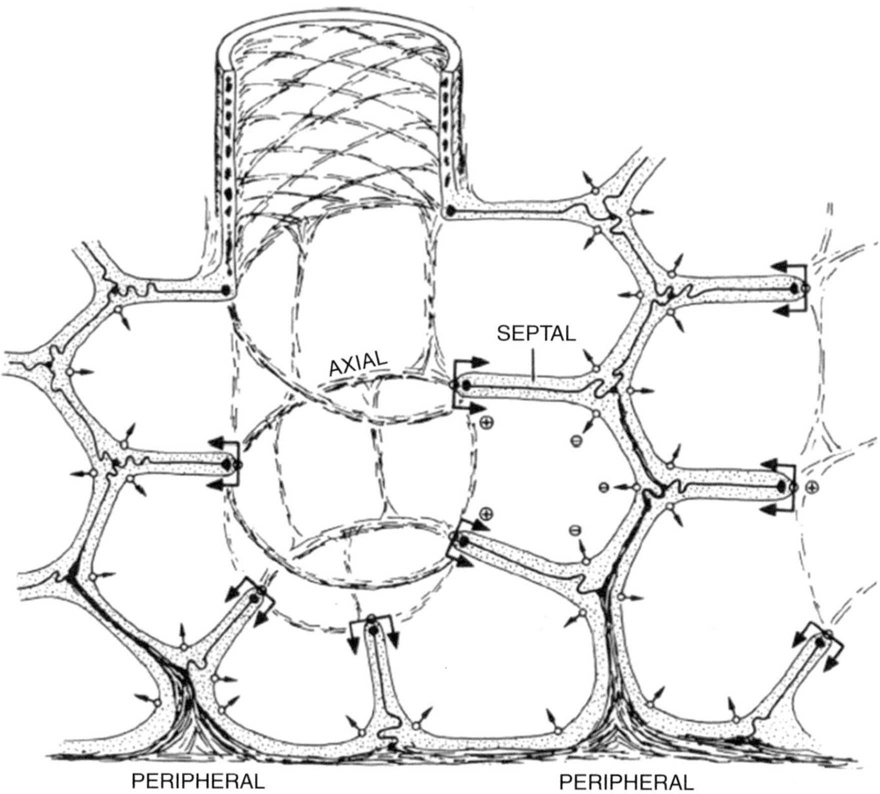

Fig. 2.9 Diagram of alveoli with a shared wall that forms a circle with the alveolar duct in the center. The alveolar duct is not an independent structure but is formed by the elastin rings surrounding each alveolar mouth that opens into the duct. Axial, septal, and peripheral connective tissue fibers form a continuum from the alveolar wall to the pleural surface. Negative surface tension is depicted by the double arrows in the alveolar corners, with positive surface tension depicted by single arrows at the edge of the alveolar septum

mechanical breath profile (MB_P), which includes all airway pressures, volumes, flows, rates, and the time they are applied during inspiration and expiration, must be analyzed for the ability to eliminate these VILI mechanisms.

Computational Models of Acinar Mechanics in the Acutely Injured Lung

In a study by Knudsen et al., computational models were employed to investigate acinar mechanics in the acutely injured lung, aiming to elucidate alveolar micromechanics with progressive acute lung injury and understand the role of these changes as mechanisms underlying atelectrauma and volutrauma [61]. Under normal conditions, alveoli in the lung remain open across a wide range of airway pressures

(1–20 cmH_2O). Consequently, in a homogeneously ventilated lung, the spatial propagation of acinar strain is uniformly distributed and thus non-injurious.

However, acute lung injury induces regional alveolar instability, collapse, and flooding with edema fluid. This alteration in acinar function leads to heterogeneous ventilation, giving rise to local areas of stress multiplication. The damage to alveoli expands concentrically from these initial lesions in a POOR get POORer fashion (Figs. 2.5 and 4.11) [62, 63]. The computational models employed in this study provide valuable insights into the dynamic micromechanics of acini in acute lung injury, shedding light on the mechanisms contributing to atelectrauma and volutrauma. In an experimental model in rats utilizing a chronic bleomycin-induced ARDS, characterized by the deactivation of pulmonary surfactant function, lung mechanics were assessed across various PEEP levels. The researchers conducted quantitative histologic analysis and integrated this data into a multi-compartmental computational model of alveolar micromechanics [45]. The study involved three groups observed over 3 days, with and without exogenous surfactant replacement therapy (SRT). The hypothesis under investigation posited that SRT would reduce the airway pressure needed to prevent alveolar collapse.

The computational model was constructed based on the contemporary understanding of intricate acinar microanatomy (Figs. 2.9 and 3.3) [64–67]. This comprehensive approach aimed to amalgamate experimental data, histologic analyses, and computational modeling, providing insights into the impact of SRT on lung mechanics and alveolar micromechanics within the context of chronic bleomycin-induced ARDS. The model comprises a single alveolar duct with 1024 parallel alveolar units. Anatomically, multiple alveoli with shared walls form a cylinder, with the elastin-rich alveolar mouths constituting the alveolar duct. The elastic and collagenous fibers that compose the alveolar mouth extend to become the alveolar duct, an integral part of the tissue continuum that connects the visceral pleura with each alveolar wall using septal, axial, and peripheral fibers (Fig. 2.9). Due to the distinct mechanical properties of alveoli and alveolar ducts, the elastance and tissue resistance properties were independently assigned and analyzed separately. In their investigation, the researchers observed a consistent number of open alveoli in the normal lung across a range of airway pressures from 1 to 20 cmH_2O. However, the impairment of surfactant function following bleomycin injury resulted in microatelectasis at all airway pressures, and the application of SRT did not prevent this tissue collapse [61]. Three days after bleomycin treatment, an increase in airway pressure failed to open approximately 40% of the alveoli, leading to increased alveolar size and heterogeneity. Simulation results highlighted that recruitment pressure was significantly higher than derecruitment pressure, indicating minimal RACE. However, there was a notable increase in alveolar strain caused by stress multipliers.

The researchers concluded that the primary micromechanical alteration in this model of ARDS was alveolar collapse, resulting in the overdistension of adjacent open tissue, rather than RACE. Furthermore, they demonstrated that an extended expiratory duration or low PEEP could induce gas maldistribution, leading to highly distended alveolar ducts (Fig. 5.8) [68–70].

Reasons for the Unacceptably High Mortality

The high mortality rates associated with the current "Protect the Lung Approach" can be attributed to two key factors: (i) allowing a significant portion of the lung to remain collapsed in an attempt to "rest" the tissue until it heals may lead to various pathologies in these tissues, as detailed in the section on *Problems Caused by Long-term Atelectasis* below and (ii) the "Protect the Lung Approach" is *confined* to ventilating a heterogeneously injured lung. As a result, regional alveolar instability caused by RACE and stress multipliers, commonly considered the primary drivers of VILI, is not eliminated. Consequently, if these VILI mechanisms persist, some degree of tissue damage will occur with each breath, regardless of the chosen ventilation strategy. The overarching physiological objective should be the elimination of RACE and stress multipliers, promoting lung healing in a fully inflated and stable state [71].

Problems Caused by Long-Term Atelectasis

The lung is a dynamic organ designed to inflate and deflate continually and is not intended to rest. "Resting" the lung in the collapsed state generates multiple pathophysiologic problems [72]. Atelectasis results in the loss of lung volume, leading to increased stress and strain on the remaining normal tissue during ventilation. This phenomenon, often called the "VILI Vortex" (see Fig. 2.4), can contribute to ventilator-induced lung injury [20]. Studies have demonstrated that high V_T combined with low PEEP can induce VILI in normal lung tissue. Although these settings would not be clinically applied, they highlight the susceptibility of normal homogeneous lung tissue to injury by high dynamic strain and strain rate, even in the absence of high static airway pressure. This underscores the importance of minimizing dynamic strain to prevent RACE, as high static airway pressure is associated with less tissue damage [54–58, 60, 73–75].

Normal homogeneous lung tissue is generally resistant to injury caused by high static airway pressure alone. However, it is crucial to acknowledge that elevated airway pressure, while less damaging than high dynamic strain, can still exacerbate initial tissue damage caused by RACE in a "POOR get POORer" fashion (see Figs. 2.1 and 4.11) [75]. Areas of atelectasis that persist in a collapsed state, called collapse induration, are known to undergo dysfunction and fibrosis, resulting in a permanent loss of lung function [76–79]. The implications of such atelectatic regions are manifold:

1. Dysfunctional and fibrotic tissue: Collapse induration can lead to dysfunctional and fibrotic tissue development, representing a permanent loss of lung function [76–79].
2. Reduction in diffusion surface area: Collapsed tissue reduces the diffusion surface area for both oxygen (O_2) and carbon dioxide (CO_2), leading to hypercapnia and hypoxemia. To address these conditions, higher fractions of inspired oxygen

(FiO_2) may be required, posing a risk of oxygen toxicity. Additionally, absorption atelectasis may exacerbate the problem [72, 80].
3. Loss of surfactant function: Atelectasis directly contributes to the loss of surfactant function, further complicating the respiratory dynamics [72, 80].
4. Patient-Ventilator Dyssynchrony: The large volume of collapsed lung tissue can lead to hypoxemia, hypercapnia, and stretch receptors, causing patient-ventilator dyssynchrony [81, 82].
5. Reduction in End-Expiratory Lung Volume (EELV): Increasing atelectasis results in a decrease in EELV, which, in turn, increases pulmonary vascular resistance (PVR) [83, 84]. Elevated PVR may necessitate higher doses of vasoactive drugs to prevent right heart failure [85].
6. Damage to remote alveoli: Atelectasis has been demonstrated to cause damage to non-atelectatic alveoli in remote regions [86].

Thus, from multiple physiological perspectives, the effectiveness of the Protect the Lung Approach is questionable. Outcome data align with these physiologically based assumptions, as numerous statistical analyses and meta-analyses indicate that this ventilation strategy has not significantly reduced mortality in patients with established Acute Respiratory Distress Syndrome (ARDS) compared to the findings of the ARMA study published 24 years ago [8] (Table 2.1) [25, 87–91]. Extensive reviews discuss pulmonary microanatomy, gas exchange, dynamic alveolar inflation physiology [45–47, 92, 93], and the mechanisms of tissue damage associated with mechanical ventilation in the acutely injured lung [19, 94–97]. This book will focus on the dynamic physical damage to pulmonary tissue caused by the regional development of atelectrauma and volutrauma. It will not address the inflammatory injury reviewed in detail elsewhere [96, 98, 99]. To use applied physiology and reduce the morbidity and mortality associated with VILI, multiple biologic systems must be analyzed and integrated into a unifying hypothesis of pathogenesis (Fig. 2.1), including:

- The microanatomy of alveoli and alveolar ducts forms the acinus, the lung's functional unit.
- The dynamic mechanism of acinar volume change in the normal and acutely injured lung.
- Altered acinar mechanics in the acutely injured lung as a mechanism of VILI.
- The role of pulmonary surfactant in dynamic acinar mechanics and dissipated energy.
- The importance of viscoelastic acinar volume change in the normal and acutely injured lung.
- Determine what components of the MB_P and in which combination will normalize altered acinar mechanics, reduce dissipated power, and minimize VILI-related tissue damage.
- The role of all MB_P components on dynamic alveolar inflation and stability, including roles of the inspiratory and expiratory time.
- Identifying the role of dissipated mechanical power at the alveolar level as the pathophysiology mechanism that causes cell and connective tissue damage.

Summary

Mechanical ventilation, both positive and negative, has been integral, particularly in the context of polio pandemics, driving its clinical adoption. Initially employed for respiratory muscle paralysis in polio, the focus has shifted to acutely injured lungs, notably in patients with ARDS. The historical progression of positive pressure ventilation strategies for ARDS initially involved adjusting settings for normal PaO_2 and $PaCO_2$, leading to challenges such as excessive barotrauma (Fig. 2.2).

Current protective ventilation strategies, including the Protect the Lung Approach and the Open Lung Approach, aim to shield the remaining normal lung from overdistension by employing LV_T and Pplat, the latter involving higher PEEP and potential recruitment maneuvers. Despite these strategies, ARDS-related mortality persists at unacceptably high levels.

Several factors contribute to this limited success. The Protect the Lung Approach confines ventilation to a heterogeneously injured lung. Evidence suggests that overdistension of the baby lung might not be the primary driver of VILI, and allowing collapsed tissue to "rest" may induce multiple pathologies. A deeper understanding of alveolar-level tissue damage mechanisms is essential to make advancements. The upcoming chapters will construct a unified hypothesis on these mechanisms, proposing an optimal protective ventilation strategy grounded in applied physiology to minimize VILI and reduce ARDS-related mortality (Fig. 2.1).

References

1. Drinker P, Shaw LA. An apparatus for the prolonged administration of artificial respiration: I. A design for adults and children. J Clin Invest. 1929;7(2):229–47.
2. Lassen HC. A preliminary report on the 1952 epidemic of poliomyelitis in Copenhagen with special reference to the treatment of acute respiratory insufficiency. Lancet. 1953;1(6749):37–41.
3. Barach AL, Martin J, Eckman M. Positive pressure respiration and its application to the treatment of acute pulmonary edema. Ann Intern Med. 1938;12(6):754–95.
4. Ashbaugh DG, Bigelow DB, Petty TL, Levine BE. Acute respiratory distress in adults. Lancet. 1967;2(7511):319–23.
5. Macklin MT, Macklin CC. Malignant interstitial emphysema of the lungs and mediastinum as an important occult complication in many respiratory diseases and other conditions: an interpretation of the clinical literature in the light of laboratory experiment. Medicine. 1944;23(4):281–358.
6. Greenfield LJ, Ebert PA, Benson DW. Effect of positive pressure ventilation on surface tension properties of lung extracts. Anesthesiology. 1964;25:312–6.
7. Kumar A, Pontoppidan H, Falke KJ, Wilson RS, Laver MB. Pulmonary barotrauma during mechanical ventilation. Crit Care Med. 1973;1(4):181–6.
8. The Acute Respiratory Distress Syndrome Network. ARDSnet: ventilation with lower tidal volumes as compared with traditional tidal volumes for acute lung injury and the acute respiratory distress syndrome. N Engl J Med. 2000;342(18):1301–8.
9. Dreyfuss D, Soler P, Basset G, Saumon G. High inflation pressure pulmonary edema. Respective effects of high airway pressure, high tidal volume, and positive end-expiratory pressure. Am Rev Respir Dis. 1988;137(5):1159–64.

10. Muscedere JG, Mullen JB, Gan K, Slutsky AS. Tidal ventilation at low airway pressures can augment lung injury. Am J Respir Crit Care Med. 1994;149(5):1327–34.
11. Tremblay L, Valenza F, Ribeiro SP, Li J, Slutsky AS. Injurious ventilatory strategies increase cytokines and c-fos m-RNA expression in an isolated rat lung model. J Clin Invest. 1997;99(5):944–52.
12. Gattinoni L, Protti A, Caironi P, Carlesso E. Ventilator-induced lung injury: the anatomical and physiological framework. Crit Care Med. 2010;38(10 Suppl):S539–48.
13. Amato MB, Barbas CS, Medeiros DM, Magaldi RB, Schettino GP, Lorenzi-Filho G, Kairalla RA, Deheinzelin D, Munoz C, Oliveira R, et al. Effect of a protective-ventilation strategy on mortality in the acute respiratory distress syndrome. N Engl J Med. 1998;338(6):347–54.
14. Deans KJ, Minneci PC, Cui X, Banks SM, Natanson C, Eichacker PQ. Mechanical ventilation in ARDS: one size does not fit all. Crit Care Med. 2005;33(5):1141–3.
15. Brower R, Thompson BT. Investigators AN: Tidal volumes in acute respiratory distress syndrome—one size does not fit all. Crit Care Med. 2006;34(1):263–4; author reply 264–267.
16. Amato MB, Meade MO, Slutsky AS, Brochard L, Costa EL, Schoenfeld DA, Stewart TE, Briel M, Talmor D, Mercat A, et al. Driving pressure and survival in the acute respiratory distress syndrome. N Engl J Med. 2015;372(8):747–55.
17. Goligher EC, Costa ELV, Yarnell CJ, Brochard LJ, Stewart TE, Tomlinson G, Brower RG, Slutsky AS, Amato MPB. Effect of lowering Vt on mortality in acute respiratory distress syndrome varies with respiratory system elastance. Am J Respir Crit Care Med. 2021;203(11):1378–85.
18. Slutsky AS. Lung injury caused by mechanical ventilation. Chest. 1999;116(1 Suppl):9S–15S.
19. Slutsky AS, Ranieri VM. Ventilator-induced lung injury. N Engl J Med. 2013;369(22):2126–36.
20. Marini JJ, Gattinoni L. Time course of evolving ventilator-induced lung injury: the "shrinking baby lung". Crit Care Med. 2020;48(8):1203–9.
21. Cui Y, Cao R, Wang Y, Li G. Lung recruitment maneuvers for ARDS patients: a systematic review and meta-analysis. Respiration. 2020;99(3):264–76.
22. Araos J, Alegria L, Garcia P, Cruces P, Soto D, Erranz B, Amthauer M, Salomon T, Medina T, Rodriguez F, et al. Near-apneic ventilation decreases lung injury and fibroproliferation in an acute respiratory distress syndrome model with extracorporeal membrane oxygenation. Am J Respir Crit Care Med. 2019;199(5):603–12.
23. Cavalcanti AB, Suzumura EA, Laranjeira LN, Paisani DM, Damiani LP, Guimaraes HP, Romano ER, Regenga MM, Taniguchi LNT, Teixeira C, et al. Effect of lung recruitment and titrated positive end-expiratory pressure (PEEP) vs low PEEP on mortality in patients with acute respiratory distress syndrome: a randomized clinical trial. JAMA. 2017;318(14):1335–45.
24. Maca J, Jor O, Holub M, Sklienka P, Bursa F, Burda M, Janout V, Sevcik P. Past and present ARDS mortality rates: a systematic review. Respir Care. 2017;62(1):113–22.
25. Bellani G, Laffey JG, Pham T, Fan E, Brochard L, Esteban A, Gattinoni L, van Haren F, Larsson A, McAuley DF, et al. Epidemiology, patterns of care, and mortality for patients with acute respiratory distress syndrome in intensive care units in 50 countries. JAMA. 2016;315(8):788–800.
26. Phua J, Badia JR, Adhikari NK, Friedrich JO, Fowler RA, Singh JM, Scales DC, Stather DR, Li A, Jones A, et al. Has mortality from acute respiratory distress syndrome decreased over time?: a systematic review. Am J Respir Crit Care Med. 2009;179(3):220–7.
27. Fan E, Brodie D, Slutsky AS. Acute respiratory distress syndrome: advances in diagnosis and treatment. JAMA. 2018;319(7):698–710.
28. Rezoagli E, Fumagalli R, Bellani G. Definition and epidemiology of acute respiratory distress syndrome. Ann Transl Med. 2017;5(14):282.
29. Villar J, Blanco J, Kacmarek RM. Current incidence and outcome of the acute respiratory distress syndrome. Curr Opin Crit Care. 2016;22(1):1–6.
30. McNicholas BA, Rooney GM, Laffey JG. Lessons to learn from epidemiologic studies in ARDS. Curr Opin Crit Care. 2018;24(1):41–8.

31. Raymondos K, Dirks T, Quintel M, Molitoris U, Ahrens J, Dieck T, Johanning K, Henzler D, Rossaint R, Putensen C, et al. Outcome of acute respiratory distress syndrome in university and non-university hospitals in Germany. Crit Care. 2017;21(1):122.
32. Cochi SE, Kempker JA, Annangi S, Kramer MR, Martin GS. Mortality trends of acute respiratory distress syndrome in the United States from 1999 to 2013. Ann Am Thorac Soc. 2016;13(10):1742–51.
33. Pham T, Serpa Neto A, Pelosi P, Laffey JG, De Haro C, Lorente JA, Bellani G, Fan E, Brochard LJ, Pesenti A, et al. Outcomes of patients presenting with mild acute respiratory distress syndrome: insights from the LUNG SAFE study. Anesthesiology. 2018;130:263.
34. Zhang Z, Spieth PM, Chiumello D, Goyal H, Torres A, Laffey JG, Hong Y. Declining mortality in patients with acute respiratory distress syndrome: an analysis of the acute respiratory distress syndrome network trials. Crit Care Med. 2019;47(3):315–23.
35. Combes A, Hajage D, Capellier G, Demoule A, Lavoue S, Guervilly C, Da Silva D, Zafrani L, Tirot P, Veber B, et al. Extracorporeal membrane oxygenation for severe acute respiratory distress syndrome. N Engl J Med. 2018;378(21):1965–75.
36. Writing C, Steering Committee for the RCG, Algera AG, Pisani L, Serpa Neto A, den Boer SS, Bosch FFH, Bruin K, Klooster PM, Van der Meer NJM, et al. Effect of a lower vs higher positive end-expiratory pressure strategy on ventilator-free days in ICU patients without ARDS: a randomized clinical trial. JAMA. 2020;
37. Abrams D, Agerstrand C, Beitler JR, Karagiannidis C, Madahar P, Yip NH, Pesenti A, Slutsky AS, Brochard L, Brodie D. Risks and benefits of ultra-lung-protective invasive mechanical ventilation strategies with a focus on extracorporeal support. Am J Respir Crit Care Med. 2022;205(8):873–82.
38. Yamamoto R, Okazaki SR, Fujita Y, Seki N, Kokei Y, Sekine S, Wada S, Norisue Y, Narita C. Usefulness of low tidal volume ventilation strategy for patients with acute respiratory distress syndrome: a systematic review and meta-analysis. Sci Rep. 2022;12(1):9331.
39. Gaver DP 3rd, Nieman GF, Gatto LA, Cereda M, Habashi NM, Bates JHT. The POOR get POORer: a hypothesis for the pathogenesis of ventilator-induced lung injury. Am J Respir Crit Care Med. 2020;202(8):1081–7.
40. Cereda M, Xin Y. Alveolar recruitment and lung injury: an issue of timing and location? Crit Care Med. 2013;41(12):2837–8.
41. Cereda M, Xin Y, Hamedani H, Bellani G, Kadlecek S, Clapp J, Guerra L, Meeder N, Rajaei J, Tustison NJ, et al. Tidal changes on CT and progression of ARDS. Thorax. 2017;72(11):981–9.
42. Cereda M, Xin Y, Hamedani H, Clapp J, Kadlecek S, Meeder N, Zeng J, Profka H, Kavanagh BP, Rizi RR. Mild loss of lung aeration augments stretch in healthy lung regions. J Appl Physiol (1985). 2016;120(4):444–54.
43. Cereda M, Xin Y, Meeder N, Zeng J, Jiang Y, Hamedani H, Profka H, Kadlecek S, Clapp J, Deshpande CG, et al. Visualizing the propagation of acute lung injury. Anesthesiology. 2016;124(1):121–31.
44. Albert K, Krischer JM, Pfaffenroth A, Wilde S, Lopez-Rodriguez E, Braun A, Smith BJ, Knudsen L. Hidden microatelectases increase vulnerability to ventilation-induced lung injury. Front Physiol. 2020;11:530485.
45. Knudsen L, Ochs M. The micromechanics of lung alveoli: structure and function of surfactant and tissue components. Histochem Cell Biol. 2018;150(6):661–76.
46. Weibel ER. Lung morphometry: the link between structure and function. Cell Tissue Res. 2017;367(3):413–26.
47. Hsia CC, Hyde DM, Weibel ER. Lung structure and the intrinsic challenges of gas exchange. Compr Physiol. 2016;6(2):827–95.
48. Toshima M, Ohtani Y, Ohtani O. Three-dimensional architecture of elastin and collagen fiber networks in the human and rat lung. Arch Histol Cytol. 2004;67(1):31–40.
49. Whimster WF. The microanatomy of the alveolar duct system. Thorax. 1970;25(2):141–9.
50. Autilio C, Perez-Gil J. Understanding the principle biophysics concepts of pulmonary surfactant in health and disease. Arch Dis Child Fetal Neonatal Ed. 2019;104(4):F443–51.

51. Suki B, Hubmayr R. Epithelial and endothelial damage induced by mechanical ventilation modes. Curr Opin Crit Care. 2014;20(1):17–24.
52. Cereda M, Xin Y, Emami K, Huang J, Rajaei J, Profka H, Han B, Mongkolwisetwara P, Kadlecek S, Kuzma NN, et al. Positive end-expiratory pressure increments during anesthesia in normal lung result in hysteresis and greater numbers of smaller aerated airspaces. Anesthesiology. 2013;119(6):1402–9.
53. Bilek AM, Dee KC, Gaver DP 3rd. Mechanisms of surface-tension-induced epithelial cell damage in a model of pulmonary airway reopening. J Appl Physiol. 2003;94(2):770–83.
54. Protti A, Andreis DT, Monti M, Santini A, Sparacino CC, Langer T, Votta E, Gatti S, Lombardi L, Leopardi O, et al. Lung stress and strain during mechanical ventilation: any difference between statics and dynamics? Crit Care Med. 2013;41(4):1046–55.
55. Protti A, Andreis DT, Iapichino GE, Monti M, Comini B, Milesi M, Zani L, Gatti S, Lombardi L, Gattinoni L. High positive end-expiratory pressure: only a dam against oedema formation? Crit Care. 2013;17(4):R131.
56. Jain SV, Kollisch-Singule M, Satalin J, Searles Q, Dombert L, Abdel-Razek O, Yepuri N, Leonard A, Gruessner A, Andrews P, et al. The role of high airway pressure and dynamic strain on ventilator-induced lung injury in a heterogeneous acute lung injury model. Intensive Care Med Exp. 2017;5(1):25.
57. Seah AS, Grant KA, Aliyeva M, Allen GB, Bates JH. Quantifying the roles of tidal volume and PEEP in the pathogenesis of ventilator-induced lung injury. Ann Biomed Eng. 2011;39(5):1505–16.
58. Wilson MR, Patel BV, Takata M. Ventilation with "clinically relevant" high tidal volumes does not promote stretch-induced injury in the lungs of healthy mice. Crit Care Med. 2012;40(10):2850–7.
59. Costa ELV, Slutsky A, Brochard LJ, Brower R, Serpa-Neto A, Cavalcanti AB, Mercat A, Meade M, Morais CCA, Goligher E, et al. Ventilatory variables and mechanical power in patients with acute respiratory distress syndrome. Am J Respir Crit Care Med. 2021;204:303.
60. Ramcharran H, Bates JHT, Satalin J, Blair S, Andrews PL, Gaver DP, Gatto LA, Wang G, Ghosh AJ, Robedee B, et al. Protective ventilation in a pig model of acute lung injury: timing is as important as pressure. J Appl Physiol (1985). 2022;133(5):1093–105.
61. Knudsen L, Lopez-Rodriguez E, Berndt L, Steffen L, Ruppert C, Bates JHT, Ochs M, Smith BJ. Alveolar micromechanics in bleomycin-induced lung injury. Am J Respir Cell Mol Biol. 2018;59(6):757–69.
62. Makiyama AM, Gibson LJ, Harris RS, Venegas JG. Stress concentration around an atelectatic region: a finite element model. Respir Physiol Neurobiol. 2014;201:101–10.
63. Mead J, Takishima T, Leith D. Stress distribution in lungs: a model of pulmonary elasticity. J Appl Physiol. 1970;28(5):596–608.
64. Bachofen H, Schurch S. Alveolar surface forces and lung architecture. Comp Biochem Physiol A Mol Integr Physiol. 2001;129(1):183–93.
65. Haefeli-Bleuer B, Weibel ER. Morphometry of the human pulmonary acinus. Anat Rec. 1988;220:401–14.
66. Wilson TA, Bachofen H. A model for mechanical structure of the alveolar duct. J Appl Physiol Respir Environ Exerc Physiol. 1982;52(4):1064–70.
67. Hajari AJ, Yablonskiy DA, Sukstanskii AL, Quirk JD, Conradi MS, Woods JC. Morphometric changes in the human pulmonary acinus during inflation. J Appl Physiol (1985). 2012;112(6):937–43.
68. Kollisch-Singule M, Emr B, Smith B, Roy S, Jain S, Satalin J, Snyder K, Andrews P, Habashi N, Bates J, et al. Mechanical breath profile of airway pressure release ventilation: the effect on alveolar recruitment and microstrain in acute lung injury. JAMA Surg. 2014;149(11):1138–45.
69. Kollisch-Singule M, Emr B, Smith B, Ruiz C, Roy S, Meng Q, Jain S, Satalin J, Snyder K, Ghosh A, et al. Airway pressure release ventilation reduces conducting airway micro-strain in lung injury. J Am Coll Surg. 2014;219(5):968–76.

70. Kollisch-Singule M, Jain S, Andrews P, Smith BJ, Hamlington-Smith KL, Roy S, DiStefano D, Nuss E, Satalin J, Meng Q, et al. Effect of airway pressure release ventilation on dynamic alveolar heterogeneity. JAMA Surg. 2016;151(1):64–72.
71. Nieman GF, Andrews P, Satalin J, Wilcox K, Kollisch-Singule M, Madden M, Aiash H, Blair SJ, Gatto LA, Habashi NM. Acute lung injury: how to stabilize a broken lung. Crit Care. 2018;22(1):136.
72. Duggan M, Kavanagh BP. Pulmonary atelectasis: a pathogenic perioperative entity. Anesthesiology. 2005;102(4):838–54.
73. Protti A, Maraffi T, Milesi M, Votta E, Santini A, Pugni P, Andreis DT, Nicosia F, Zannin E, Gatti S, et al. Role of strain rate in the pathogenesis of ventilator-induced lung edema. Crit Care Med. 2016;44(9):e838–45.
74. Syring RS, Otto CM, Spivack RE, Markstaller K, Baumgardner JE. Maintenance of end-expiratory recruitment with increased respiratory rate after saline-lavage lung injury. J Appl Physiol (1985). 2007;102(1):331–9.
75. Hamlington KL, Smith BJ, Dunn CM, Charlebois CM, Roy GS, Bates JHT. Linking lung function to structural damage of alveolar epithelium in ventilator-induced lung injury. Respir Physiol Neurobiol. 2018;255:22–9.
76. Cabrera-Benitez NE, Laffey JG, Parotto M, Spieth PM, Villar J, Zhang H, Slutsky AS. Mechanical ventilation-associated lung fibrosis in acute respiratory distress syndrome: a significant contributor to poor outcome. Anesthesiology. 2014;121(1):189–98.
77. Burkhardt A. Alveolitis and collapse in the pathogenesis of pulmonary fibrosis. Am Rev Respir Dis. 1989;140(2):513–24.
78. Knudsen L, Ruppert C, Ochs M. Tissue remodelling in pulmonary fibrosis. Cell Tissue Res. 2017;367(3):607–26.
79. Lutz D, Gazdhar A, Lopez-Rodriguez E, Ruppert C, Mahavadi P, Gunther A, Klepetko W, Bates JH, Smith B, Geiser T, et al. Alveolar derecruitment and collapse induration as crucial mechanisms in lung injury and fibrosis. Am J Respir Cell Mol Biol. 2015;52(2):232–43.
80. Albert RK. The role of ventilation-induced surfactant dysfunction and atelectasis in causing acute respiratory distress syndrome. Am J Respir Crit Care Med. 2012;185(7):702–8.
81. Spinelli E, Mauri T, Beitler JR, Pesenti A, Brodie D. Respiratory drive in the acute respiratory distress syndrome: pathophysiology, monitoring, and therapeutic interventions. Intensive Care Med. 2020;46(4):606–18.
82. Petersson J, Glenny RW. Gas exchange and ventilation-perfusion relationships in the lung. Eur Respir J. 2014;44(4):1023–41.
83. Simmons DH, Linde LM, Miller JH, O'Reilly RJ. Relation between lung volume and pulmonary vascular resistance. Circ Res. 1961;9(2):465–71.
84. Duggan M, McCaul CL, McNamara PJ, Engelberts D, Ackerley C, Kavanagh BP. Atelectasis causes vascular leak and lethal right ventricular failure in uninjured rat lungs. Am J Respir Crit Care Med. 2003;167(12):1633–40.
85. Sipmann FS, Santos A, Tusman G. Heart-lung interactions in acute respiratory distress syndrome: pathophysiology, detection and management strategies. Ann Transl Med. 2018;6(2):27.
86. Tsuchida S, Engelberts D, Peltekova V, Hopkins N, Frndova H, Babyn P, McKerlie C, Post M, McLoughlin P, Kavanagh BP. Atelectasis causes alveolar injury in nonatelectatic lung regions. Am J Respir Crit Care Med. 2006;174(3):279–89.
87. Laffey JG, Bellani G, Pham T, Fan E, Madotto F, Bajwa EK, Brochard L, Clarkson K, Esteban A, Gattinoni L, et al. Potentially modifiable factors contributing to outcome from acute respiratory distress syndrome: the LUNG SAFE study. Intensive Care Med. 2016;42(12):1865–76.
88. Caser EB, Zandonade E, Pereira E, Gama AM, Barbas CS. Impact of distinct definitions of acute lung injury on its incidence and outcomes in Brazilian ICUs: prospective evaluation of 7,133 patients*. Crit Care Med. 2014;42(3):574–82.
89. Villar J, Blanco J, Anon JM, Santos-Bouza A, Blanch L, Ambros A, Gandia F, Carriedo D, Mosteiro F, Basaldua S, et al. The ALIEN study: incidence and outcome of acute respi-

ratory distress syndrome in the era of lung protective ventilation. Intensive Care Med. 2011;37(12):1932–41.
90. Shen Y, Cai G, Gong S, Dong L, Yan J, Cai W. Interaction between low tidal volume ventilation strategy and severity of acute respiratory distress syndrome: a retrospective cohort study. Crit Care. 2019;23(1):254.
91. Parcha V, Kalra R, Bhatt SP, Berra L, Arora G, Arora P. Trends and geographic variation in acute respiratory failure and ARDS mortality in the United States. Chest. 2021;159(4):1460–72.
92. Roan E, Waters CM. What do we know about mechanical strain in lung alveoli? Am J Physiol Lung Cell Mol Physiol. 2011;301(5):L625–35.
93. Suki B, Stamenovic D, Hubmayr R. Lung parenchymal mechanics. Compr Physiol. 2011;1(3):1317–51.
94. Nieman GF, Gatto LA, Habashi NM. Impact of mechanical ventilation on the pathophysiology of progressive acute lung injury. J Appl Physiol. 2015;119(11):1245–61.
95. Cong X, Hubmayr RD, Li C, Zhao X. Plasma membrane wounding and repair in pulmonary diseases. Am J Physiol Lung Cell Mol Physiol. 2017;312(3):L371–91.
96. Uhlig U, Uhlig S. Ventilator-induced lung injury. Comprehensive. Physiology. 2011;1:635–61.
97. Reiss LK, Uhlig U, Uhlig S. Models and mechanisms of acute lung injury caused by direct insults. Eur J Cell Biol. 2012;91(6–7):590–601.
98. Curley GF, Laffey JG, Zhang H, Slutsky AS. Biotrauma and ventilator-induced lung injury: clinical implications. Chest. 2016;150(5):1109–17.
99. Wurfel MM. Microarray-based analysis of ventilator-induced lung injury. Proc Am Thorac Soc. 2007;4(1):77–84.
100. Stewart TE, Meade MO, Cook DJ, Granton JT, Hodder RV, Lapinsky SE, Mazer CD, McLean RF, Rogovein TS, Schouten BD, et al. Evaluation of a ventilation strategy to prevent barotrauma in patients at high risk for acute respiratory distress syndrome. Pressure- and Volume-Limited Ventilation Strategy Group. N Engl J Med. 1998;338(6):355–61.
101. Brower RG, Shanholtz CB, Fessler HE, Shade DM, White P Jr, Wiener CM, Teeter JG, Dodd-o JM, Almog Y, Piantadosi S. Prospective, randomized, controlled clinical trial comparing traditional versus reduced tidal volume ventilation in acute respiratory distress syndrome patients. Crit Care Med. 1999;27(8):1492–8.
102. Brochard L, Roudot-Thoraval F, Roupie E, Delclaux C, Chastre J, Fernandez-Mondejar E, Clementi E, Mancebo J, Factor P, Matamis D, et al. Tidal volume reduction for prevention of ventilator-induced lung injury in acute respiratory distress syndrome. The Multicenter Trail Group on tidal volume reduction in ARDS. Am J Respir Crit Care Med. 1998;158(6):1831–8.
103. Villar J, Kacmarek RM, Perez-Mendez L, Aguirre-Jaime A. A high positive end-expiratory pressure, low tidal volume ventilatory strategy improves outcome in persistent acute respiratory distress syndrome: a randomized, controlled trial. Crit Care Med. 2006;34(5):1311–8.
104. The ARDS Network. Ketoconazole for early treatment of acute lung injury and acute respiratory distress syndrome: a randomized controlled trial. JAMA. 2000;283(15):1995–2002.
105. Randomized, placebo-controlled trial of lisofylline for early treatment of acute lung injury and acute respiratory distress syndrome. Crit Care Med. 2002;30(1):1–6.
106. Brower RG, Lanken PN, MacIntyre N, Matthay MA, Morris A, Ancukiewicz M, Schoenfeld D, Thompson BT, National Heart L, Blood Institute ACTN. Higher versus lower positive end-expiratory pressures in patients with the acute respiratory distress syndrome. N Engl J Med. 2004;351(4):327–36.
107. National Heart L, Blood Institute Acute Respiratory Distress Syndrome Clinical Trials N, Wiedemann HP, Wheeler AP, Bernard GR, Thompson BT, Hayden D, DeBoisblanc B, Connors AF Jr, Hite RD, et al. Comparison of two fluid-management strategies in acute lung injury. N Engl J Med. 2006;354(24):2564–75.
108. Talmor D, Sarge T, Malhotra A, O'Donnell CR, Ritz R, Lisbon A, Novack V, Loring SH. Mechanical ventilation guided by esophageal pressure in acute lung injury. N Engl J Med. 2008;359(20):2095–104.
109. Steinberg KP, Hudson LD, Goodman RB, Hough CL, Lanken PN, Hyzy R, Thompson BT, Ancukiewicz M, National Heart L. Blood Institute Acute Respiratory Distress syndrome

Clinical Trials N: efficacy and safety of corticosteroids for persistent acute respiratory distress syndrome. N Engl J Med. 2006;354(16):1671–84.
110. Meade MO, Cook DJ, Guyatt GH, Slutsky AS, Arabi YM, Cooper DJ, Davies AR, Hand LE, Zhou Q, Thabane L, et al. Ventilation strategy using low tidal volumes, recruitment maneuvers, and high positive end-expiratory pressure for acute lung injury and acute respiratory distress syndrome: a randomized controlled trial. JAMA. 2008;299(6):637–45.
111. Mercat A, Richard JC, Vielle B, Jaber S, Osman D, Diehl JL, Lefrant JY, Prat G, Richecoeur J, Nieszkowska A, et al. Positive end-expiratory pressure setting in adults with acute lung injury and acute respiratory distress syndrome: a randomized controlled trial. JAMA. 2008;299(6):646–55.
112. Taccone P, Pesenti A, Latini R, Polli F, Vagginelli F, Mietto C, Caspani L, Raimondi F, Bordone G, Iapichino G, et al. Prone positioning in patients with moderate and severe acute respiratory distress syndrome: a randomized controlled trial. JAMA. 2009;302(18):1977–84.
113. Papazian L, Forel JM, Gacouin A, Penot-Ragon C, Perrin G, Loundou A, Jaber S, Arnal JM, Perez D, Seghboyan JM, et al. Neuromuscular blockers in early acute respiratory distress syndrome. N Engl J Med. 2010;363(12):1107–16.
114. Ferguson ND, Cook DJ, Guyatt GH, Mehta S, Hand L, Austin P, Zhou Q, Matte A, Walter SD, Lamontagne F, et al. High-frequency oscillation in early acute respiratory distress syndrome. N Engl J Med. 2013;368(9):795–805.
115. Young D, Lamb SE, Shah S, MacKenzie I, Tunnicliffe W, Lall R, Rowan K, Cuthbertson BH, Group OS. High-frequency oscillation for acute respiratory distress syndrome. N Engl J Med. 2013;368(9):806–13.
116. Guerin C, Reignier J, Richard JC, Beuret P, Gacouin A, Boulain T, Mercier E, Badet M, Mercat A, Baudin O, et al. Prone positioning in severe acute respiratory distress syndrome. N Engl J Med. 2013;368(23):2159–68.
117. Esteban A, Frutos-Vivar F, Muriel A, Ferguson ND, Penuelas O, Abraira V, Raymondos K, Rios F, Nin N, Apezteguia C, et al. Evolution of mortality over time in patients receiving mechanical ventilation. Am J Respir Crit Care Med. 2013;188(2):220–30.
118. Kacmarek RM, Villar J, Sulemanji D, Montiel R, Ferrando C, Blanco J, Koh Y, Soler JA, Martinez D, Hernandez M, et al. Open lung approach for the acute respiratory distress syndrome: a pilot, randomized controlled trial. Crit Care Med. 2016;44(1):32–42.
119. Writing Group for the Alveolar Recruitment for Acute Respiratory Distress Syndrome Trial I, Cavalcanti AB, Suzumura EA, Laranjeira LN, Paisani DM, Damiani LP, Guimaraes HP, Romano ER, Regenga MM, Taniguchi LNT, et al. Effect of lung recruitment and titrated positive end-expiratory pressure (PEEP) vs low PEEP on mortality in patients with acute respiratory distress syndrome: a randomized clinical trial. JAMA. 2017;318(14):1335–45.
120. Hodgson CL, Cooper DJ, Arabi Y, King V, Bersten A, Bihari S, Brickell K, Davies A, Fahey C, Fraser J, et al. Maximal recruitment open lung ventilation in acute respiratory distress syndrome (PHARLAP). A phase II, multicenter randomized controlled clinical trial. Am J Respir Crit Care Med. 2019;200(11):1363–72.
121. Lalgudi Ganesan S, Jayashree M, Chandra Singhi S, Bansal A. Airway pressure release ventilation in pediatric acute respiratory distress syndrome. A randomized controlled trial. Am J Respir Crit Care Med. 2018;198(9):1199–207.
122. Zhou Y, Jin X, Lv Y, Wang P, Yang Y, Liang G, Wang B, Kang Y. Early application of airway pressure release ventilation may reduce the duration of mechanical ventilation in acute respiratory distress syndrome. Intensive Care Med. 2017;43(11):1648–59.
123. Nolan S, Burgess K, Hopper L, Braude S. Acute respiratory distress syndrome in a community hospital ICU. Intensive Care Med. 1997;23(5):530–8.
124. Luhr OR, Antonsen K, Karlsson M, Aardal S, Thorsteinsson A, Frostell CG, Bonde J. Incidence and mortality after acute respiratory failure and acute respiratory distress syndrome in Sweden, Denmark, and Iceland. The ARF Study Group. Am J Respir Crit Care Med. 1999;159(6):1849–61.
125. Bersten AD, Edibam C, Hunt T, Moran J. Australian, New Zealand Intensive Care Society Clinical Trials G: incidence and mortality of acute lung injury and the acute respiratory distress syndrome in three Australian states. Am J Respir Crit Care Med. 2002;165(4):443–8.

126. Brun-Buisson C, Minelli C, Bertolini G, Brazzi L, Pimentel J, Lewandowski K, Bion J, Romand JA, Villar J, Thorsteinsson A, et al. Epidemiology and outcome of acute lung injury in European intensive care units. Results from the ALIVE study. Intensive Care Med. 2004;30(1):51–61.
127. Rubenfeld GD, Caldwell E, Peabody E, Weaver J, Martin DP, Neff M, Stern EJ, Hudson LD. Incidence and outcomes of acute lung injury. N Engl J Med. 2005;353(16):1685–93.
128. Manzano F, Yuste E, Colmenero M, Aranda A, Garcia-Horcajadas A, Rivera R, Fernandez-Mondejar E. Granada respiratory failure study G: incidence of acute respiratory distress syndrome and its relation to age. J Crit Care. 2005;20(3):274–80.
129. Sakr Y, Vincent JL, Reinhart K, Groeneveld J, Michalopoulos A, Sprung CL, Artigas A, Ranieri VM. Sepsis occurrence in acutely ill patients I: high tidal volume and positive fluid balance are associated with worse outcome in acute lung injury. Chest. 2005;128(5):3098–108.
130. Linko R, Okkonen M, Pettila V, Perttila J, Parviainen I, Ruokonen E, Tenhunen J, Ala-Kokko T. Varpula T, group FI-s: acute respiratory failure in intensive care units. FINNALI: a prospective cohort study. Intensive Care Med. 2009;35(8):1352–61.
131. Li G, Malinchoc M, Cartin-Ceba R, Venkata CV, Kor DJ, Peters SG, Hubmayr RD, Gajic O. Eight-year trend of acute respiratory distress syndrome: a population-based study in Olmsted County, Minnesota. Am J Respir Crit Care Med. 2011;183(1):59–66.
132. Pham T, Serpa Neto A, Pelosi P, Laffey JG, De Haro C, Lorente JA, Bellani G, Fan E, Brochard LJ, Pesenti A, et al. Outcomes of patients presenting with mild acute respiratory distress syndrome: insights from the LUNG SAFE study. Anesthesiology. 2019;130(2):263–83.
133. Matthay MA, Arabi YM, Siegel ER, Ware LB, Bos LDJ, Sinha P, Beitler JR, Wick KD, Curley MAQ, Constantin JM, et al. Phenotypes and personalized medicine in the acute respiratory distress syndrome. Intensive Care Med. 2020;46(12):2136–52.
134. Lin P, Zhao Y, Li X, Jiang F, Liang Z. Decreased mortality in acute respiratory distress syndrome patients treated with corticosteroids: an updated meta-analysis of randomized clinical trials with trial sequential analysis. Crit Care. 2021;25(1):122.
135. Qadir N, Bartz RR, Cooter ML, Hough CL, Lanspa MJ, Banner-Goodspeed VM, Chen JT, Giovanni S, Gomaa D, Sjoding MW, et al. Variation in early management practices in moderate-to-severe ARDS in the United States: the severe ARDS: generating evidence study. Chest. 2021;160(4):1304–15.
136. Beyls C, Huette P, Viart C, Mestan B, Haye G, Guilbart M, Bernasinski M, Besserve P, Leviel F, Witte Pfister A, et al. Mortality of COVID-19 patients requiring extracorporeal membrane oxygenation during the three epidemic waves. ASAIO J. 2022;68(12):1434–42.

Chapter 3
Alveolar and Alveolar Duct (Acinar) Mechanics in the Normal Lung

Introduction

A Unifying Hypothesis for Ventilator-Induced Lung Injury (VILI) hinges on a comprehensive understanding of normal alveolar micromechanics (Fig. 3.1, green box). The lung is not a singular elastic balloon or a cluster of individual elastic grapes; rather, it constitutes a complex and interdependent viscoelastic system (Figs. 2.9 and 3.2). When exposed to an applied force, such as airway pressure during mechanical ventilation, this elicits stress in the lung tissue, leading to its expansion, known as strain. Strain is defined as the change in the size of a structure in response to an applied load. The modification in the size of alveoli and alveolar ducts due to the mechanically delivered tidal volume (V_T) signifies parenchymal strain. Excessive strain poses the risk of stress failure in alveolar microstructures. In the normal lung, alveolar volume change remains minimal (low alveolar strain) during the respiratory cycle, owing to the exponential decay of pressure, flow, and volume through branching airways. Convective gas movement transforms into diffusive gas exchange beyond the terminal airways. In addition, the strain in normal homogeneous alveoli is in the alveolar duct, which consists of elastin and is designed to stretch, not the alveolar walls (Figs. 3.3 and 3.4).

Additionally, the lung's normal functioning surfactant plays a crucial role in averting airway closure, ensuring that the functional residual capacity (FRC) remains above the closing capacity of the lung. This interplay of near homogeneity and alveolar stability results in very low alveolar volume change and strain. Remarkably, even under extreme stress, such as strenuous exercise with tidal volumes surpassing 30 mL/kg and transpulmonary pressures exceeding 50 cmH_2O, the

Supplementary Information The online version contains supplementary material available at https://doi.org/10.1007/978-3-031-66352-9_3.

© The Author(s), under exclusive license to Springer Nature Switzerland AG 2024

G. F. Nieman, N. M. Habashi, *Applied Physiology to Reduce Ventilator Induced Lung Injury*, https://doi.org/10.1007/978-3-031-66352-9_3

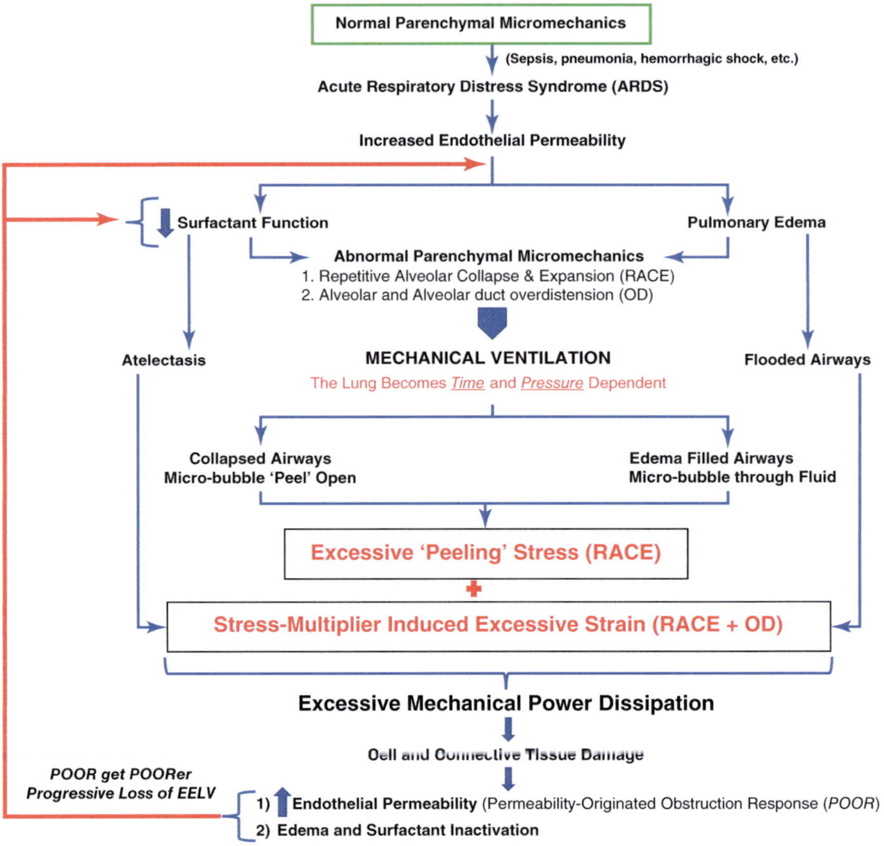

Fig. 3.1 The unifying hypothesis of the mechanisms by which the acute respiratory distress syndrome (ARDS) pathophysiology predisposes the lung to a secondary ventilator-induced lung injury (VILI). This chapter discusses normal parenchymal micromechanics (green box)

normal lung demonstrates minimal energy dissipation, other than the normal dissipation due to airway resistance. However, as alveolar instability and inhomogeneity increase with progressive lung injury, both strain and energy dissipation increase at progressively lower tidal volumes and applied airway pressure levels.

Moreover, the strain on the alveolus during ventilation is not static; rather, it constitutes a dynamic and interdependent system. Therefore, assessing the impact of any Mechanical Breath Profile (MB_P), which includes all airway pressures, volumes, flows, rates, and the time they are applied during both inspiration and

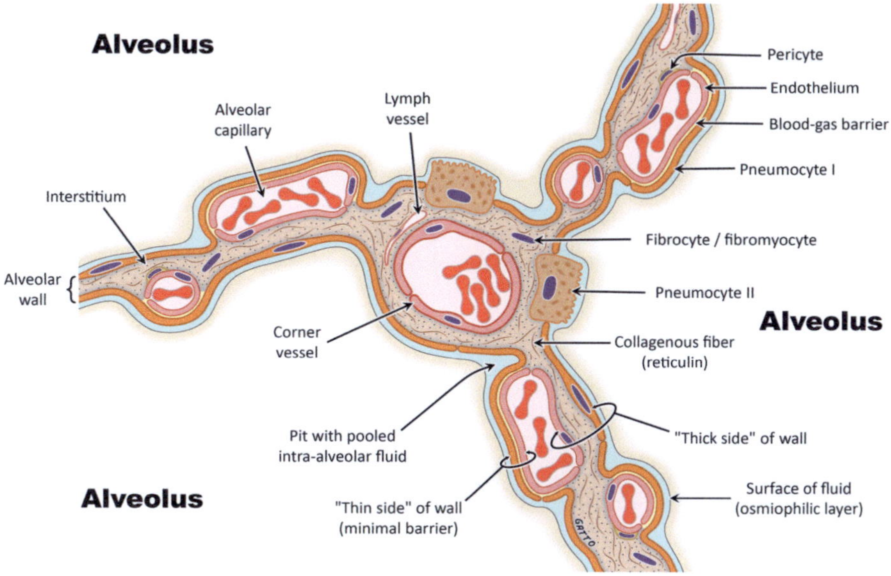

Fig. 3.2 Highly complex alveolar architectures, interconnected alveolar walls containing many cell types, and an interstitium containing elastin and collagen that runs from the alveolar walls to the visceral pleura that functions as a load-bearing scaffolding (Fig. 2.9). A dynamic surfactant system is necessary for alveoli stability and is located on the surface fluid or osmiophilic layer. An understanding of pulmonary parenchymal microanatomy is essential to logically construct a Mechanical Breath Profile (MB_P), defined as all airway pressures, volumes, flows, rates, and *time* applied during inspiration and expiration, necessary to reduce VILI. The complex microanatomy must be analyzed according to how normal alveoli change volume during tidal ventilation and how these alveolar mechanics are altered during acute lung injury, damaging the delicate alveolar walls and capillaries

expiration, on lung tissue stress failure, the dynamic nature of acinar volume change must be considered [1]. Significantly, the dynamic mechanics of normal alveolar ventilation do not induce tissue injury. However, these mechanics undergo significant changes with acute lung injury, altering ventilation biophysics substantially and predisposing lung tissue to secondary VILI. This chapter aims to analyze normal acinar anatomy and mechanics, exploring stabilizing factors such as microarchitecture (alveolar interdependence, parenchymal tethering), connective tissue scaffolding, and pulmonary surfactant.

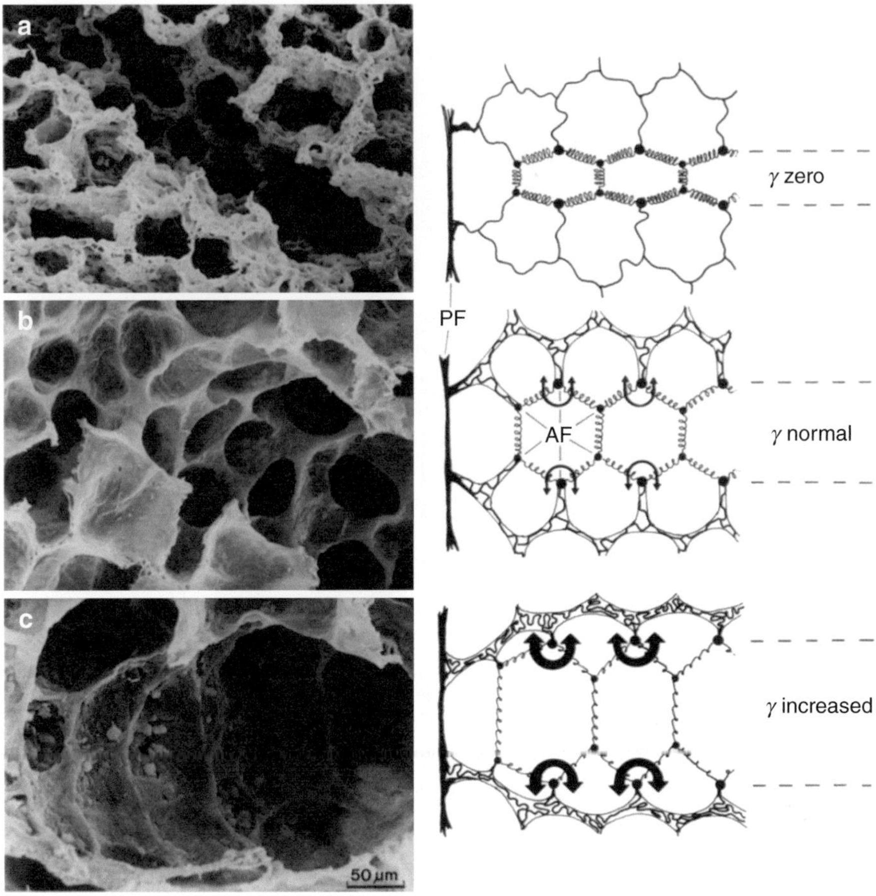

Fig. 3.3 *Left side*: scanning electron micrographs of alveoli and alveolar ducts of saline-filled (**a**), air-filled (**b**), and detergent-rinsed rabbit lungs (**c**). Note the increase in diameter of the ducts with increasing surface tension. Alveoli go from "deep cups" (γ zero) to "shallow cups" (γ increased) as the alveolar duct expands. Note that the diameter of the alveolus (horizontal wall to wall) changes little, but the depth of the alveolus into the duct changes significantly with a change in duct size. *Right side*: a corresponding model of the mechanical structure of the alveoli and alveolar duct in response to changes in surface tension
γ Surface tension, *PF* Peripheral connective tissue fibers, *AF* Axial fiber system elements that form alveolar entrance rings. All photomicrographs are at the same magnification, and the lungs were fixed by vascular perfusion at about the same lung volume. Arrows depict surface forces on the alveolar walls

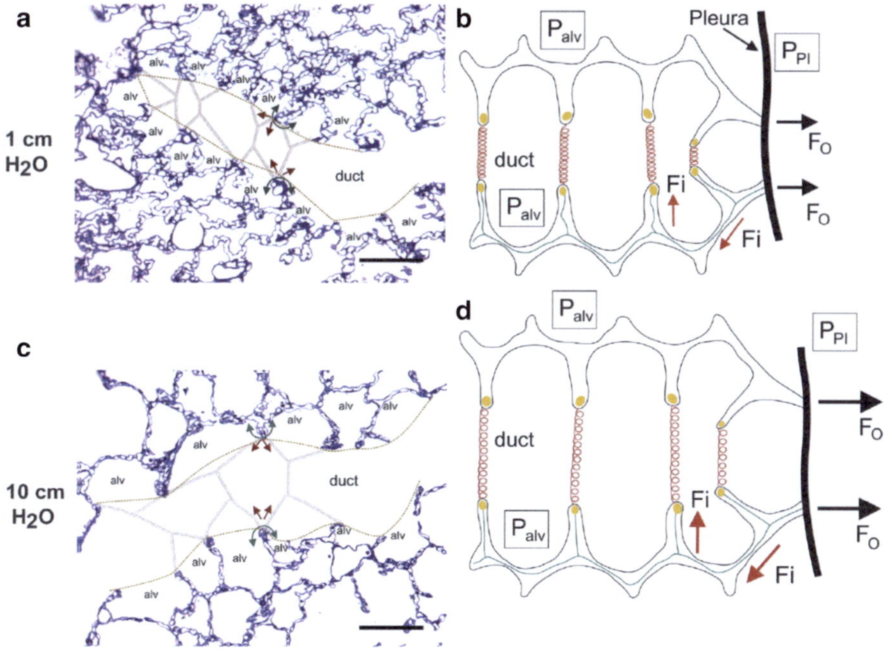

Fig. 3.4 Normal rat lungs were fixed at 1 (**a**) and 10 cm H_2O (**c**). At 1 cm, H_2O alveolar ducts are narrow, and the inter-alveolar septal walls have folds and pleats. Alveolar walls protrude and comprise the alveolar duct via the elastic (elastin) alveolar mouths. Septal walls, alveolar, and ductal airspaces were separated (fine dashed lines). The axial network of elastic and collagen fibers is illustrated as springs forming the alveolar duct (**b** red springs). At 1 cm H_2O, the elastic fibers are only stretched slightly (**a**, **b red springs**) and exert a force in the direction of the ductal lumen (**a**, red arrows **a**, **c**). This force counteracts the forces of surface tension (green arrows in **a**, **c**), which pull the septal wall away from the duct, collapsing the alveoli. At 10 cm H_2O, the axial fiber system stretched (red springs in **d**), widening the alveolar duct. The pressure gradient between the pleural space (P_{Pl}) and the alveolar space (Palv) is responsible for lung inflation. The outward forces (F_O) are transmitted to the fiber system in the septal walls and over ride the inward forces (F_i) to cause alveolar and duct expansion

Acinar Microarchitecture

Understanding the impact of an applied force on the strain of inflatable objects, particularly pulmonary acini (comprising alveoli and alveolar ducts) requires knowledge of their materials and architecture. Unlike a single elastic balloon, the acinus is a complex, interdependent structure incorporating multiple alveolar ducts (see Figs. 2.9 and 3.4). The lung is composed of viscoelastic tissues and features a dynamic pulmonary surfactant system that alters ventilation biophysics. It is crucial to recognize that the force-inducing stress failure in an elastic balloon, commonly utilized to analyze VILI [2], may not necessarily cause tissue damage leading to stress failure in a viscoelastic acinus. The human lung comprises approximately 280,000,000 alveoli [3], intricately interlocked to form a complex and interdependent structure (Fig. 2.9). Various cell types constitute the pulmonary parenchyma, including alveolar epithelial Type I and II cells, fibroblasts, vascular endothelial cells, Clara cells, and smooth muscle cells [4]. Alveolar walls exhibit a thick septal midplane containing a fibrous network and a thin section with only endothelium and epithelium fused by the basement membrane (Fig. 3.2, Video 3.1) [5]. Each alveolus shares walls with its neighboring alveoli, establishing structural interdependence, and they are arranged cylindrically to create a central alveolar duct (Fig. 2.9). An acinus, the functional unit of the lung, is formed by a collection of alveoli and alveolar ducts enveloped by peripheral connective tissue [5]. Numerous comprehensive reviews on lung function, structure, and gas exchange have been published [6, 7]. The intimate interconnection of alveoli, alveolar ducts, and small airways is crucial for maintaining alveolar patency, stability, and resistance to stress failure during ventilation [6]. This design, characterized by alveolar interdependence and the tethering of small airways by surrounding inflated alveoli, significantly contributes to a normally inflated lung's structural integrity and stability [8–12].

Analyzing the impact of applied forces, such as tidal volume (V_T) during mechanical ventilation, on the acinus involves measuring both strain (change in size from baseline) and stress (force applied per unit area, i.e., airway pressure) [13]. The pathological consequences of VILI, encompassing inflammation, edema, fibrosis, and tissue remodeling, can be attributed to the stress failure of cellular membranes alone [13]. However, it is crucial to recognize that the mechanics of alveoli and alveolar ducts differs, preventing them from being treated as a single entity for analysis. Each component will exhibit a unique stress/strain relationship in response to the applied mechanical breath [14, 15].

Connective Tissue Scaffolding

Excessive strain induced during ventilation can lead to cellular damage involving mechanical and molecular mechanisms [16–19]. In the normal lung, the interdependent connective tissue scaffolding system and the presence of pulmonary surfactant collaborate to mitigate excessive stress and strain on endothelial cells [5]. The primary contributors to lung mechanical properties are the extracellular matrix scaffolding (Fig. 2.9), with the cellular component (Fig. 3.2) playing a minor role in lung stiffness or elastic recoil [20, 21].

During tidal ventilation, the normal deformation of cellular components occurs without reaching excessive strain, thanks to the combined effects of a stabilizing connective tissue system acting as a stress-bearing scaffold and pulmonary surfactant reducing alveolar surface tension at low lung volumes [22]. However, it's important to note that endothelial and epithelial cells are linked to the basal lamina (Fig. 3.2, Video 3.1), making them susceptible to excessive cellular stress, even in the normal lung, especially at high lung volumes [23]. The stabilizing connective tissue system establishes a continuum of septal, axial, and peripheral fibers that unite the visceral pleura with each alveolar wall, as illustrated in Fig. 2.9. The functional unit of the lung is the acinus, formed by multiple alveoli and alveolar ducts [5, 24]. The alveolar duct features axial elastin fibers, constituting the entrance or mouth of the alveoli (Fig. 2.9). Peripheral fibers, serving as force-bearing line elements, connect the pleura to the lobules, creating an interdependent system unaffected by surface forces but subject to strain variations with changes in lung volume. The central system consists of axial fibers surrounding arteries and bronchi, encircling the alveolar mouths. Surface tension influences the central scaffold system, with higher surface tension resulting in increased expansion of the alveolar duct (Fig. 3.3) [14]. Comprehensive reviews have delved into lung soft tissue and matrix biomechanics, exploring the roles of viscoelasticity, the elastic fiber system, proteoglycans, and surfactant function in shaping the static and dynamic stability of the pulmonary parenchyma [12].

Pulmonary Surfactant

Besides the intricate interdependence of acinar architecture and connective tissue scaffolding, a dynamic pulmonary surfactant system plays a pivotal role in acinar mechanics during tidal ventilation. Surfactant serves multiple functions, including:

(i) Molding Effect: It molds acinar structures, influencing lung recoil pressure, capillary configuration, and pulmonary microcirculation [5].
(ii) Strain Reduction: Surfactant reduces strain on alveolar epithelial cells at low lung volumes, with the matrix scaffolding acting as the stress-bearing structure [22].
(iii) Edema Prevention: It protects the lung from edema formation by decreasing interstitial pressure around pulmonary capillaries [25–28].
(iv) Stabilization: Surfactant stabilizes alveoli and alveolar ducts at low lung volumes [29].
(v) Anti-Glue Properties: Acting as an anti-glue between alveolar walls, it prevents their collapse into apposition, significantly lowering the force required to "peel" these walls apart (Fig. 4.4) [30].

Before delving into the pathophysiology of VILI, it is imperative to grasp the stabilizing characteristics of the healthy lung that shield it from damage despite its intricate and delicate nature (Fig. 3.3, "Normal"). Despite the micron-scale separation between atmospheric air in the lungs and blood flowing through capillary networks, the air is in direct contact with a thin lining of liquid covering the interior surfaces of airways and alveoli (Fig. 3.2). This system's flow occurs in two phases: gases flow within the airways and alveoli, while fluids flow within the liquid lining layer. The pressures governing these multiphase flows and the interactions between fluid and tissue are critical determinants of lung function and the work of breathing.

This importance is underscored by von Neergaard's groundbreaking experiments, revealing a significant alteration in lung compliance when the air–liquid interface is eliminated by filling the lung with saline, thereby removing any surface tension-related distortions of the tissues (Fig. 3.3, "Zero") [31]. During tidal ventilation, stresses arising from surface tension can mechanically disrupt the delicate cellular components of the blood–gas barrier (Fig. 3.2). However, surfactant crucially mitigates this in the normal lung, which reduces surface tension at low lung volumes [22]. The network of connective tissue serves as a stress-bearing scaffold, countering excessive cellular deformation. As previously discussed, the healthy lung at high volume may experience excessive cellular stress due to the connection of endothelial and epithelial cells to the basal lamina (Fig. 3.2, Video 3.1) [23].

Models of alveolar mechanics, which are based on a collection of balloons, suggest that surface tension must vary according to the law of LaPlace in individual alveoli to prevent pendelluft (air movement) from small alveoli into larger ones [32]. However, this hypothesis contradicts our current understanding of pulmonary microanatomy and physiology [5, 33]. Alveoli are not independent "balloons"; they share walls, and the interconnected fibrous arrangement linking alveolar walls to the pleura indicates that alveoli are not independent structures (see Figs. 2.9, 3.3, and 3.4). Furthermore, surface tension remains the same in all alveoli, irrespective of size, at multiple lung volumes [34].

Although the mechanisms of surfactant function are not entirely understood, an operational surfactant system is crucial for normal lung mechanics. Without it, the lung becomes highly susceptible to instability, collapse, and VILI. In acute respiratory distress syndrome (ARDS), a low lung volume with altered surfactant function can result in extensive folding of alveolar walls and overdistension of alveolar ducts (Figs. 3.3 and 3.4), leading to significant cell and tissue injury. However, even in the absence of normal surfactant function, if a ventilation strategy with an MB_P could prevent regional alveolar instability and collapse and maintain an end-expiratory lung volume (EELV) at or near-normal functional residual capacity (FRC), the stabilizing function of the fibrous network would be re-established [5].

Despite the acutely injured lung remaining time- and pressure-dependent (meaning alveoli would take more time to open and less time to collapse for any given airway pressure), if held open with an appropriately set mechanical breath, it would function mechanically similar to a healthy lung. This ability of the MB_P to "cast the broken lung" into a stable and open position [35] is akin to putting a cast on a broken arm—a concept that will be further discussed in Chap. 8.

Despite its structural complexity (Figs. 2.9, 3.2, 3.3, and 3.4, Video 3.1), the healthy homogeneously inflated lung is remarkably stable because of two interacting bio-mechanical processes:

(a) Pulmonary surfactant reduces and dynamically modifies the surface tension (γ) of the lining fluid during respiration. The importance of surfactant is conventionally explained by the inverse relationship between the pressure drop (ΔP) across a surface with a radius of curvature (R) expressed as the Law of Laplace $\left(\Delta P = \frac{2\gamma}{R}\right)$. This explains how small radii challenge alveolar stability and that reducing γ is crucial to meeting this challenge. This simple relationship thus demonstrates the critical importance of the ultra-low surface tensions afforded by pulmonary surfactant. Surfactant deactivation in the ARDS lung (Fig. 1.1—Surfactant Deactivation) increases surface tension dramatically, which causes deranged micromechanical behavior, leading to an overdistension of alveolar ducts and alveolar wall folding (Figs. 3.3 δ increased, 3.4, and 5.8). Experimental evidence is incontrovertible that surfactant counteracts the interfacial instabilities that can lead to the collapse of airways and alveoli, as well as their accompanying effects of impaired gas exchange and generation of excessive mechanical stresses that can damage lung tissue. Loss of surfactant function also causes repetitive alveolar collapse and expansion (RACE), which is the mechanism of atelectrauma (Fig. 1.1—RACE, Video 4.3).

(b) The mechanical interdependency between alveoli and airways allows the parenchyma to function as a supportive foam material, tethering compliant airways and contributing to maintaining patent alveoli (Fig. 3.3 δ Normal) [36–38]. Alveolar walls are intricately linked to the visceral pleura and, consequently, pleural pressure through a continuum of septal, axial, and peripheral connective tissue fibers (Fig. 2.9). From a mechanical standpoint, the functional unit of the lung is either an alveolar duct or multiple ducts forming an acinus, surrounded by its peripheral connective tissue [5, 24]. As the force-bearing line elements of the peripheral fibers connect to the pleura and the axial fibers forming the entrance rings of alveoli, any alterations in alveolar geometry and changes in surface tension (γ) affect the entire connective tissue system (Fig. 3.4). Therefore, heterogeneous alveolar closure can impact regional parenchymal tethering, potentially compromising lung stability [11].

(c) Hence, the normally functioning acinus represents a complex amalgamation of microarchitecture, connective tissue scaffolding, and pulmonary surfactant. Together, these elements dictate the typical dynamic mechanics of the acinus during both spontaneous and mechanical ventilation. This intricate system facilitates substantial changes in lung volume without subjecting the constituent cells of the acinus to excessive strain (Fig. 3.5, Videos 3.2 and 3.3). As a result, the normal lung demonstrates high resistance to injury during ventilation.

(d) Despite decades of study, the mechanism of lung volume change at the alveolar level still needs to be better understood [22, 41]. Interdependent alveoli, integral components of larger structures like alveolar ducts and acini, do not behave as individual elastic balloons, expanding and contracting independently. The delicate structures forming the alveolar-capillary membrane (Fig. 3.2) cannot endure excessive stretching with each breath without risking catastrophic injury. The thin side of the alveolar-capillary barrier consists of a single epithelial and endothelial cell attached by the basement membrane, lacking a supporting connective tissue matrix (Fig. 3.2, Video 3.1).

(e) Proposed mechanisms for alveolar volume change during ventilation include: (i) alveolar wall folding and unfolding, akin to a paper bag, (ii) alterations in alveolar shape, (iii) balloon-like isotropic stretching, and (iv) alveolar opening and collapse [41, 42]. To analyze the impact of a given MB_P on alveolar mechan-

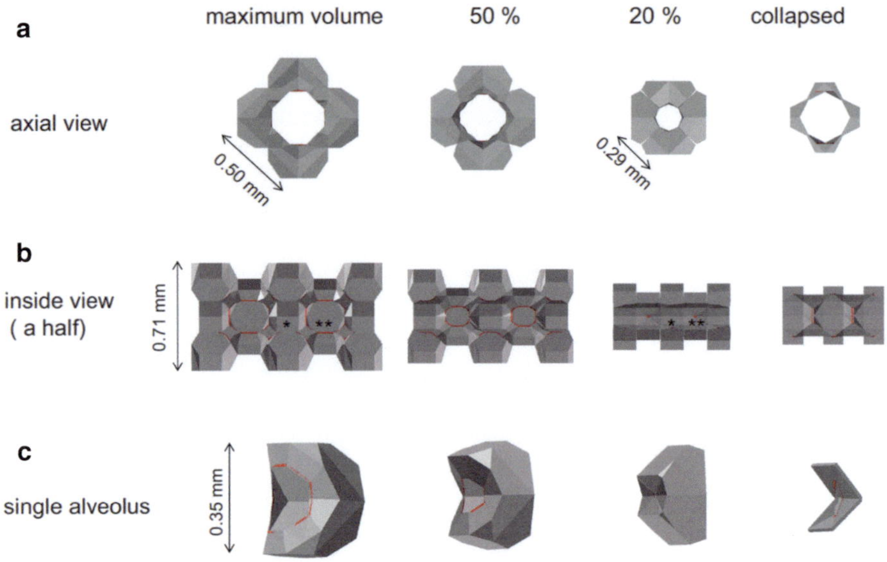

Fig. 3.5 Alveoli forming an alveolar duct are seen in both axial (**a**) and inside views (**b**) and a single alveolus (**c**). Four-dimensional model of the mechanism by which alveoli and alveolar ducts change volume from total lung capacity (TLC) (**maximum volume**) to below functional residual capacity (FRC) (**collapsed**) [39]. Shallow (*) and deep (**) alveoli are arranged alternately (**b**). The model was constructed with interdependent alveoli arranged to form a central cylinder, which becomes the alveolar duct, simulating the anatomical design of the acinus (**a**, **b**) (Figs. 2.9, 3.3, and 3.4) [40]. The alveolar mouths (Red) open into and form the alveolar duct (**a–c**). With increasing lung volume (**20% maximum volume**), the mouth of a single alveolus (**c**, Red) progressively opens, which expands the alveolar duct (**a**, **b**). As airway pressure decreases and acinar volume falls (**50%** and **20%** of **maximum volume**), the alveolar mouth contraction (**c**) decreases the size of the duct (**a**, **b**). Alveolar size (other than the mouth) only changes dramatically at very low volumes when the walls fold together in apposition (**collapsed**, **c**) [5]. Animation of changes in alveolar and alveolar duct volume is shown in Videos 3.2, 3.3, and 3.4

ics, understanding how the normal acini change volume, and more crucially, how acute lung injury alters acinar mechanics, is essential, as it predisposes the tissue to VILI. Using this knowledge to identify the optimal MB_P becomes crucial for minimizing tissue injury during mechanical ventilation.

The force exerted on the lung through positive pressure tidal ventilation induces enough stress (i.e., the ratio of the applied force divided by the resisting area) to cause strain in the alveoli and alveolar ducts. Alveolar walls do not stretch significantly during ventilation; instead, they unfold at the septal pleats within the tidal volume range [42]. Since epithelial cells are connected to the basal lamina (Fig. 3.2), they may function as stress-bearing structures and experience slight stretching during mechanical ventilation at high lung volumes, spontaneous deep sighs, or strenuous exercise [17, 18, 23, 41–45]. However, even at high lung volumes, the thin side of alveolar walls (Fig. 3.2) does not become distended but maintains folds, suggesting potential protection of endothelial cells from overdistension injury in these regions [43].

Type I cells appear more susceptible to stress failure at high lung volumes than Type II cells [46]. Endothelial cells are shielded from stress failure by unfolding plasma membrane pleats to reduce lateral stresses. Shear stress on epithelial cells, as the folded walls “peel” apart, is minimized by a functioning pulmonary surfactant system, acting as an anti-glue and significantly reducing the shear or “peeling” stress that could lead to energy dissipation-induced tissue damage (Fig. 4.4) [30]. The most robust evidence supports the mechanism of normal acinar volume changes as a combination of alveolar duct expansion and the folding and unfolding of alveolar walls, as this combination is deemed most economical from an energy dissipation perspective [14, 22, 42].

In the normal lung, fixed at an airway opening pressure of 1 and 10 cmH_2O, most lung expansion occurs in the alveolar ducts, with only a slight stretch in the alveolar walls (Fig. 3.4) [22, 47, 48]. At low lung volumes (1 cmH_2O), alveolar size is reduced by folding and pleating alveolar walls. As lung volume increases (10 cmH_2O), alveolar walls unfold, and the alveolar duct expands due to a widening of the alveolar mouths (Fig. 3.4, red springs). Crucially, maintaining tidal volume within the normal range (40%–80% of total lung capacity) significantly reduces the stress applied to cellular components (predominantly epithelial and endothelial cells) due to the load-bearing components of alveolar surface forces and the fibrinous network of elastic and collagenous connective tissues [22].

Knudsen et al. established a link between data from macro- and micro-scales through a multi-compartment computational model of alveolar micromechanics. This model incorporated the viscoelastic properties of lung tissue and considered the dependence of both time and pressure on alveolar opening and collapse. Notably, the model was constructed based on the microanatomical design of intra-acinar conducting airways and alveolar ducts, characterized by the absence of well-defined walls. Instead, the duct is formed by elastic and collagen fibers, creating the alveolar mouth or entrance ring (Fig. 2.9) [49]. This anatomical design is supported by the work of others as well [14, 40]. According to this microanatomical structure, changes in lung volume were accommodated by a modification in the width of the alveolar duct, aligning with the findings of Kitaoka (Fig. 3.5, Videos 3.2, 3.3, and 3.4) [39]. Kitaoka et al. developed a 4-dimensional (4D) model of lung parenchymal volume change during ventilation, supporting the hypothesis that the majority of lung volume change occurs in the ducts (Fig. 3.5) [39]. Duct volume change is achieved through the expansion or contraction of alveolar mouths in response to alterations in transpulmonary pressure. Little change is observed in alveolar volume throughout the lung volume range from total lung capacity (TLC—maximum volume) to 20% TLC (Fig. 3.5 Maximum volume—20% TLC), consistent with histological observations (Fig. 3.4). Individual alveoli decrease in size only at very low lung volumes (Fig. 3.5—Collapsed).

The axial and inside views of an alveolar duct surrounded by alveoli and a single alveolus are constructed using a 4-dimensional alveolar model that combines springs and hinges, corresponding to the elastin forming the alveolar mouth (which becomes the alveolar duct) and the alveolar septa junctions, respectively (Fig. 3.5 axial view). In the axial view, most of the volume changes occur in the alveolar ducts (from Maximum Volume (TLC) to 20% TLC) with little change in alveolar size (Videos 3.3 and 3.4). However, in this 4D model, when "alveoli" collapse, the "alveolar duct" significantly expands (Figs. 3.3 γ increased, 3.5 collapsed) [39]. At this point, the alveolar walls are in apposition, stacked onto each other like an accordion (see Fig. 3.4—1 cmH_2O purple alveolar walls). In response to changes in airway pressure, the alveolar mouth widens or closes (Video 3.2). Given that the alveolar duct is not a separate organ but is composed of all interconnected alveolar mouths, any change in the size of the alveolar mouth necessitates a corresponding change in the alveolar duct (Videos 3.3 and 3.4).

This system allows the lung to alter volume by stretching or contracting the elastin in the alveolar mouth, thereby minimizing strain on the epithelial cells in the alveolar walls during ventilation within the tidal volume range. The load-bearing structures in this process are the surfactant system and the continuous framework of the interstitial connective tissue system, not the endothelial cells [22]. This suggests that if a protective mechanical ventilation strategy maintains a normal EELV, the anatomical load-bearing components would be preserved, thereby reducing mechanical damage to parenchymal cells [35]. As discussed earlier, the acinus is a highly complex and interdependent structure that cannot be modeled as an individual elastic entity exhibiting an immediate linear strain, akin to a stretching spring, in response to the applied force of airway pressure. Physiologically, the lung undergoes volume changes as a viscoelastic system, demonstrating time-dependent strain with the application or removal of the force (i.e., airway pressure). This behavior can be analyzed using a spring and dashpot model (Fig. 3.6, Videos 3.5, 3.6, and 3.7) [50]. In this model, viscoelastic behavior is represented as a spring (indicating elastic strain) in parallel with a dashpot (indicating viscous strain), providing a framework for analyzing acinar volume change during mechanical ventilation (Fig. 3.6, Video 3.5) [51].

(a) *Elastic behavior*—results in a rapid strain to the distensible limits of the spring, at which point the strain ends regardless of how long the force (red arrows) is applied (Fig. 3.6 Elastic Behavior, red curve). The reverse occurs during exhalation.
(b) *Viscous behavior*—a continual gradual strain over time follows an initial time lag without increased applied force (red arrows). The movement rate depends on the fluid's viscosity in the pot and the force applied (Fig. 3.6 Viscous BEHAVIOR, red curve). The reverse occurs during exhalation.
(c) *Viscoelastic behavior*—with the application or removal of a force (red arrows) there is an initial rapid strain as the spring portion fully expands (Inspiration) or contracts (Expiration), followed by a gradual, continual opening or closing over an extended period (2–5 s) as the dash moves slowly through the pot (Fig. 3.6 Viscoelastic behavior, red curve). Because alveoli recruit as a viscoelastic system, the longer the inspiratory time is held, the more lung tissue will open with each breath Fig. 3.6—Viscoelastic behavior—Inspiration, Red HOLD, Video 3.6), and the shorter the expiratory time, the less lung tissue that will collapse with each breath (Fig. 3.5—Viscoelastic Behavior—Expiration, Red RELEASE, Video 3.7) [52–56].

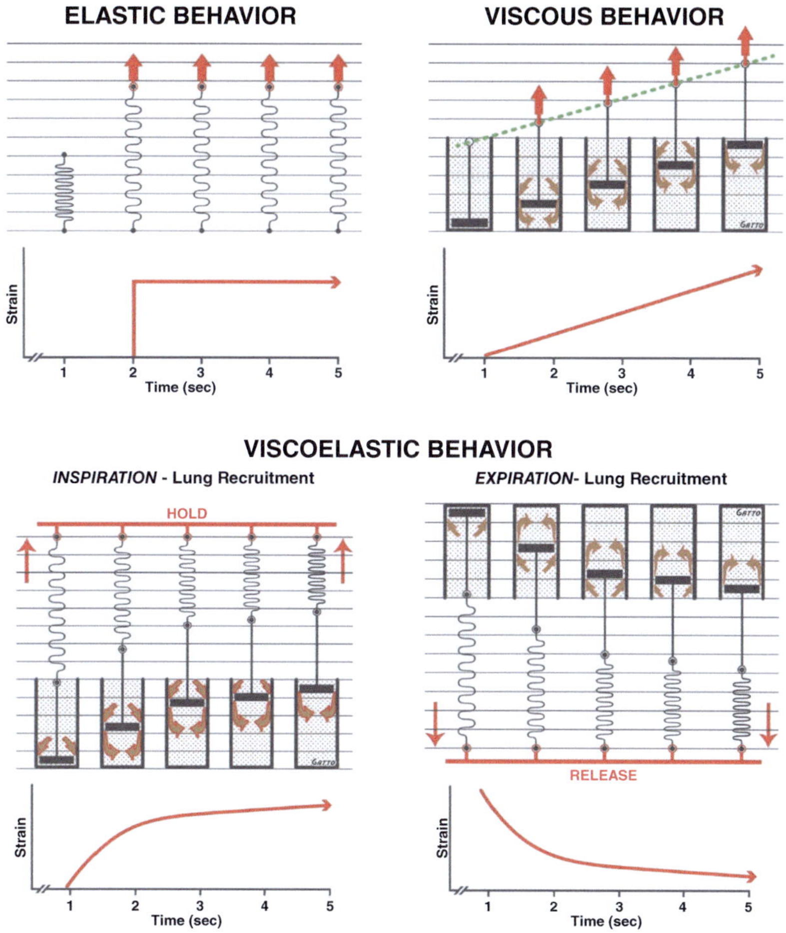

Fig. 3.6 Spring and dashpot model to illustrate the viscoelastic change in size (strain). Strain/time curves for elastic (spring), viscous (dash in pot), and viscoelastic (spring and dashpot) systems. *Elastic Behavior*: The red arrows simulate an applied force generating stress that causes a yield or strain once the force reaches critical yield pressure. The spring strains rapidly to the applied force and will not increase or decrease in length as long as the force doesn't change. *Viscous Behavior*: The dashpot is used to model viscous strain. There is a linear and continuous strain with the applied force (red arrows) such that the dash in the pot continues to move for some time without a change in the applied force (green dashed line). The amount of time it takes the dash to reach the top of the pot with any given applied force is modeled by the viscosity of the fluid in the pot (brown arrows). *Viscoelastic Behavior*: A spring attached to a dash in a pot is used to model viscoelastic behavior *INSPIRATION—Lung Recruitment*: Simulation of viscoelastic lung recruitment with an applied force that is held for some time during inspiratory duration (HOLD red bar). There is a time-dependent but rapid initial strain as the spring stretches (Strain/Time curve 1–2 s). This is followed by gradual and continual strain over time (2–5 s) as the dash moves up the pot. *Expiration—Lung Derecruitment*: Simulation of viscoelastic lung derecruitment with removing an applied force (expiratory duration) (RELEASE red bar). There is a time-dependent but rapid initial collapse as the spring retracts (Strain/Time curve 1–2 s). This is followed by gradual and continual collapse over time (2–5 s) as the dash moves down the pot. These time constants are altered in ARDS causing the lung to be time- and pressure-dependent (Fig. 5.1) (green box). Lung viscoelastic inflation and deflation behavior suggest that the longer the inspiratory duration, the more lung recruitment; the shorter the expiratory duration, the less derecruitment

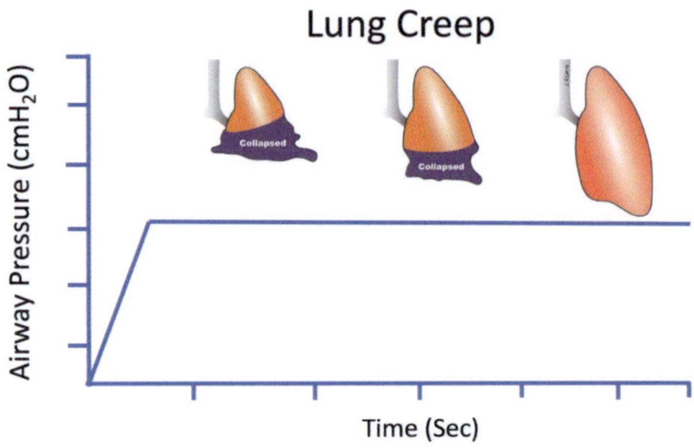

Fig. 3.7 Example of the viscoelastic component of creep in which the lung will continue to open over time without an increase in airway pressure. The lung can be recruited at lower airway pressures without an additional "cost" in dissipated mechanical energy using inspiratory time

In a viscoelastic system, both creep (a progressive increase in volume without an increase in force) and stress relaxation (not returning to the initial volume following the removal of the force) can occur [57]. Lung creep leads to a gradual increase in volume without a concurrent rise in airway pressure (Fig. 3.7, Video 3.6) [58, 59]. In a rat, acute respiratory distress syndrome (ARDS) model subjected to three recruitment pressures of 40 cmH_2O for 40 s, both in vivo microscope and gross lung recruitment measurements were taken in real-time, showing that the alveolar recruitment/time curve exhibited viscoelastic characteristics (see Fig. 3.6—Viscoelastic Behavior) and closely resembled opening and collapse time constant curves (Fig. 5.2) [60].

The lung recruitment process exhibited three stages.

1. A ~2-s delay without any recruitment.
2. Rapid initial recruitment.
3. Continual gradual recruitment over the 40 s without an increase in airway pressure (Fig. 5.3, Video 5.1) [60].

Video 5.1 compares the amount of lung tissue recruited during a 1-s inspiratory time, typical in conventional ventilation modes, and a 5-s inspiratory time, typical in the Airway Pressure Release Ventilation (APRV) mode set by the Time-Controlled Adaptive Ventilation (TCAV) method. No lung tissue was recruited during a 1-s inspiratory time (red collapsed tissue turning pink), while much of the lung was recruited with the 5-s inspiratory hold. Therefore, there was continuous lung inflation throughout the entire 5-s inspiratory hold without an additional "cost" in driving pressure or mechanical energy, simply by extending the inspiratory time. In a study exploring the impact of inspiratory and expiratory duration on gas distribution in alveoli and alveolar ducts in a rat ARDS model, creep was observed as an intriguing phenomenon. By maintaining lung inflation with a combination of long inspiratory and very short expiratory durations, gas had sufficient time to redistribute (creep) from the ducts into the alveoli resulting in homogeneous ventilation similar to normal lungs [48].

In conventional mechanical ventilation with a low tidal volume and standard inspiratory:expiratory (I:E) ratio, it was demonstrated that using either PEEP 5 or PEEP 16 cmH_2O resulted in the overdistension of alveolar ducts (Fig. 5.8 PEEP 5, 16). However, when employing APRV with an extended inspiratory time combined with a very brief expiratory time (Fig. 5.8, APRV 75%), the size of both alveoli and alveolar ducts normalized. These findings suggest that both inspiratory and expiratory time may play a more crucial role than airway pressure alone in normalizing gas distribution and preventing excessive strain in the microenvironment [48]. Stress relaxation is a phenomenon where the tension in a material, held stretched for some time, reduces such that after the removal of the force, the material no longer returns to its original shape [57]. This process has been demonstrated in both animal [61] and human lungs [62]. In the lung, if alveoli are inflated in response to a force (airway pressure) and held open for a period, they will remain partially inflated after exhalation due to stress relaxation combined with pulmonary surfactant lowering surface tension. Stress relaxation becomes evident only when the force is removed.

For instance, the deflation limb of the lung pressure/volume curve reveals stress relaxation as the airway pressure is reduced, resulting in hysteresis between the inflation and deflation limbs [63]. Both creep and stress relaxation hold clinical significance as high airway pressures and volumes are associated with lung injury. Applied physiology suggests that using lower airway pressure and volume but holding them longer could effectively recruit lung tissue without an additional energy cost [64]. Therefore, adjusting inspiratory and expiratory times may offer a potential strategy to open and stabilize the lung using lower driving pressure and dissipating mechanical energy.

In summary, alveoli are intricate structures composed of diverse cell types and connective tissue (Fig. 3.2, Video 3.1), interconnected and sharing walls (Figs. 3.3 and 3.4) with a continuous network extending from the pleural surface to each alveolar wall (Fig. 2.9). While the diameter of the alveolus remains relatively stable, the size of the alveolar mouth, forming the alveolar duct and composed of elastin, changes in response to applied force rather than changes in surface tension (Fig. 3.3) or airway pressure (Fig. 3.4). Most lung volume changes occur in the microenvironment (Fig. 3.5) (i.e., alveoli and alveolar duct), demonstrating non-linear, viscoelastic behavior in acinar volume change (Fig. 3.6, Video 3.5). Understanding this viscoelastic nature is crucial when determining the optimal MB_P for opening and maintaining acini. Both airway pressure and the duration of pressure application during inspiration and expiration play a role. Prolonged inspiratory durations recruit more alveoli, and brief expiratory durations continually recruit and limit alveolar collapse, respectively (Fig. 3.6, Videos 3.6 and 3.7). This knowledge is essential for deciding on an MB_P to prevent acinar collapse. Chap. 4 will explore how these acinar mechanics are altered in the acutely injured lung, predisposing it to secondary ventilator-induced lung injury (VILI).

References

1. Kollisch-Singule M, Emr B, Smith B, Roy S, Jain S, Satalin J, Snyder K, Andrews P, Habashi N, Bates J, et al. Mechanical breath profile of airway pressure release ventilation: the effect on alveolar recruitment and microstrain in acute lung injury. JAMA Surg. 2014;149(11):1138–45.
2. Beitler J, Malhotra A, Thompson B. Ventilator-induced lung injury. Clin Chest Med. 2019:37.
3. Ochs M, Nyengaard JR, Jung A, Knudsen L, Voigt M, Wahlers T, Richter J, Gundersen HJ. The number of alveoli in the human lung. Am J Respir Crit Care Med. 2004;169(1):120–4.
4. Franks TJ, Colby TV, Travis WD, Tuder RM, Reynolds HY, Brody AR, Cardoso WV, Crystal RG, Drake CJ, Engelhardt J, et al. Resident cellular components of the human lung: current knowledge and goals for research on cell phenotyping and function. Proc Am Thorac Soc. 2008;5(7):763–6.
5. Bachofen H, Schurch S. Alveolar surface forces and lung architecture. Comp Biochem Physiol A Mol Integr Physiol. 2001;129(1):183–93.
6. Hsia CC, Hyde DM, Weibel ER. Lung structure and the intrinsic challenges of gas exchange. Compr Physiol. 2016;6(2):827–95.
7. Weibel ER. Lung morphometry: the link between structure and function. Cell Tissue Res. 2017;367(3):413–26.
8. Fujioka H, Halpern D, Gaver DP 3rd. A model of surfactant-induced surface tension effects on the parenchymal tethering of pulmonary airways. J Biomech. 2013;46(2):319–28.
9. Mead J, Takishima T, Leith D. Stress distribution in lungs: a model of pulmonary elasticity. J Appl Physiol. 1970;28(5):596–608.
10. Paré PD, Mitzner W. Airway-parenchymal interdependence. Compr Physiol. 2012;2:1921–35.
11. Ryans JM, Fujioka H, Gaver DP 3rd. Microscale to mesoscale analysis of parenchymal tethering: the effect of heterogeneous alveolar pressures on the pulmonary mechanics of compliant airways. J Appl Physiol (1985). 2019;126(5):1204–13.
12. Suki B, Stamenovic D, Hubmayr R. Lung parenchymal mechanics. Compr Physiol. 2011;1(3):1317–51.
13. Vlahakis NE, Hubmayr RD. Cellular stress failure in ventilator-injured lungs. Am J Respir Crit Care Med. 2005;171(12):1328–42.
14. Wilson TA, Bachofen H. A model for mechanical structure of the alveolar duct. J Appl Physiol Respir Environ Exerc Physiol. 1982;52(4):1064–70.
15. Hajari AJ, Yablonskiy DA, Sukstanskii AL, Quirk JD, Conradi MS, Woods JC. Morphometric changes in the human pulmonary acinus during inflation. J Appl Physiol (1985). 2012;112(6):937–43.
16. Dolinay T, Himes BE, Shumyatcher M, Lawrence GG, Margulies SS. Integrated stress response mediates epithelial injury in mechanical ventilation. Am J Respir Cell Mol Biol. 2017;57(2):193–203.
17. Tschumperlin DJ, Oswari J, Margulies AS. Deformation-induced injury of alveolar epithelial cells. Effect of frequency, duration, and amplitude. Am J Respir Crit Care Med. 2000;162(2 Pt 1):357–62.
18. Cong X, Hubmayr RD, Li C, Zhao X. Plasma membrane wounding and repair in pulmonary diseases. Am J Physiol Lung Cell Mol Physiol. 2017;312(3):L371–91.
19. Wurfel MM. Microarray-based analysis of ventilator-induced lung injury. Proc Am Thorac Soc. 2007;4(1):77–84.
20. Nonaka PN, Uriarte JJ, Campillo N, Melo E, Navajas D, Farre R, Oliveira LV. Mechanical properties of mouse lungs along organ decellularization by sodium dodecyl sulfate. Respir Physiol Neurobiol. 2014;200:1–5.
21. Oeckler RA, Hubmayr RD. Cell wounding and repair in ventilator injured lungs. Respir Physiol Neurobiol. 2008;163(1–3):44–53.
22. Knudsen L, Ochs M. The micromechanics of lung alveoli: structure and function of surfactant and tissue components. Histochem Cell Biol. 2018;150(6):661–76.

23. Tschumperlin DJ, Margulies SS. Alveolar epithelial surface area-volume relationship in isolated rat lungs. J Appl Physiol (1985). 1999;86(6):2026–33.
24. Weibel ER. Lung biology in health and disease. In: Bioengineering aspects of the lung, vol. 3. New York: M Dekker. p. 1–81.
25. Nieman GF, Bredenberg CE. High surface tension pulmonary edema induced by detergent aerosol. J Appl Physiol. 1985;58(1):129–36.
26. Nieman GF. Current concepts of lung-fluid balance. Respir Care. 1985;30(12):1062–76.
27. Bredenberg CE, Paskanik AM, Nieman GF. High surface tension pulmonary edema. J Surg Res. 1983;34(6):515–23.
28. Bredenberg CE, Nieman GF, Paskanik AM, Hart AK. Microvascular membrane permeability in high surface tension pulmonary edema. J Appl Physiol. 1986;60(1):253–9.
29. Mead J. Mechanical properties of lungs. Physiol Rev. 1961;41(2):281–330.
30. Hills BA. The role of lung surfactant. Br J Anaesth. 1990;65(1):13–29.
31. Neergaard KV. Neue Auffassungen uber einen Grundbegriff der Atemmechanik. Die Retraktionskraft der Lunge, abhaenging von der Oberflaechenspannung in den Alveolen. Z Gesant Exp Med. 1929;66:373–94.
32. Clements JA, Hustead RF, Johnson RP, Gribetz I. Pulmonary surface tension and alveolar stability. J Appl Physiol. 1961;16:444–50.
33. Prange HD. Laplace's law and the alveolus: a misconception of anatomy and a misapplication of physics. Adv Physiol Educ. 2003;27(1–4):34–40.
34. Schurch S. Surface tension at low lung volumes: dependence on time and alveolar size. Respir Physiol. 1982;48(3):339–55.
35. Nieman GF, Andrews P, Satalin J, Wilcox K, Kollisch-Singule M, Madden M, Aiash H, Blair SJ, Gatto LA, Habashi NM. Acute lung injury: how to stabilize a broken lung. Crit Care. 2018;22(1):136.
36. Perun ML, Gaver DP III. Interaction between airway lining fluid forces and parenchymal tethering during pulmonary airway reopening. J Appl Physiol. 1995;79(5):1717–28.
37. Yap DY, Liebkemann WD, Solway J, Gaver DP III. Influences of parenchymal tethering on the reopening of closed pulmonary airways. J Appl Physiol. 1994;76(5):2095–105.
38. Douville NJ, Zamankhan P, Tung YC, Li R, Vaughan BL, Tai CF, White J, Christensen PJ, Grotberg JB, Takayama S. Combination of fluid and solid mechanical stresses contribute to cell death and detachment in a microfluidic alveolar model. Lab Chip. 2011;11(4):609–19.
39. Kitaoka H, Nieman GF, Fujino Y, Carney D, DiRocco J, Kawase I. A 4-dimensional model of the alveolar structure. J Physiol Sci. 2007;57(3):175–85.
40. Haefeli-Bleuer B, Weibel ER. Morphometry of the human pulmonary acinus. Anat Rec. 1988;220:401–14.
41. Roan E, Waters CM. What do we know about mechanical strain in lung alveoli? Am J Physiol Lung Cell Mol Physiol. 2011;301(5):L625–35.
42. Gil J, Bachofen H, Gehr P, Weibel ER. Alveolar volume-surface area relation in air- and saline-filled lungs fixed by vascular perfusion. J Appl Physiol Respir Environ Exerc Physiol. 1979;47(5):990–1001.
43. Bachofen H, Schurch S, Urbinelli M, Weibel ER. Relations among alveolar surface tension, surface area, volume, and recoil pressure. J Appl Physiol. 1987;62(5):1878–87.
44. Sera T, Yokota H, Tanaka G, Uesugi K, Yagi N, Schroter RC. Murine pulmonary acinar mechanics during quasi-static inflation using synchrotron refraction-enhanced computed tomography. J Appl Physiol (1985). 2013;115(2):219–28.
45. Maina JN, West JB. Thin and strong! The bioengineering dilemma in the structural and functional design of the blood-gas barrier. Physiol Rev. 2005;85(3):811–44.
46. Dreyfuss D, Saumon G. Ventilator-induced lung injury: lessons from experimental studies. Am J Respir Crit Care Med. 1998;157(1):294–323.
47. Knudsen L, Weibel ER, Gundersen HJ, Weinstein FV, Ochs M. Assessment of air space size characteristics by intercept (chord) measurement: an accurate and efficient stereological approach. J Appl Physiol (1985). 2010;108(2):412–21.

48. Kollisch-Singule M, Emr B, Smith B, Ruiz C, Roy S, Meng Q, Jain S, Satalin J, Snyder K, Ghosh A, et al. Airway pressure release ventilation reduces conducting airway micro-strain in lung injury. J Am Coll Surg. 2014;219(5):9.
49. Knudsen L, Lopez-Rodriguez E, Berndt L, Steffen L, Ruppert C, Bates JHT, Ochs M, Smith BJ. Alveolar micromechanics in bleomycin-induced lung injury. Am J Respir Cell Mol Biol. 2018;59(6):757–69.
50. Nieman GF, Satalin J, Kollisch-Singule M, Andrews P, Aiash H, Habashi NM, Gatto LA. Physiology in medicine: understanding dynamic alveolar physiology to minimize ventilator-induced lung injury. J Appl Physiol (1985). 2017;122(6):1516–22.
51. Nieman GF, Gatto LA, Andrews P, Satalin J, Camporota L, Daxon B, Blair SJ, Al-Khalisy H, Madden M, Kollisch-Singule M, et al. Prevention and treatment of acute lung injury with time-controlled adaptive ventilation: physiologically informed modification of airway pressure release ventilation. Ann Intensive Care. 2020;10(1):3.
52. D'Angelo E, Calderini E, Torri G, Robatto FM, Bono D, Milic-Emili J. Respiratory mechanics in anesthetized paralyzed humans: effects of flow, volume, and time. J Appl Physiol. 1989;67(6):2556–64.
53. Suki B, Barabasi AL, Lutchen KR. Lung tissue viscoelasticity: a mathematical framework and its molecular basis. J Appl Physiol (1985). 1994;76(6):2749–59.
54. Johnson BD, Sieck GC. Differential susceptibility of diaphragm muscle fibers to neuromuscular transmission failure. J Appl Physiol (1985). 1993;75(1):341–8.
55. Bates JHT. Lung mechanics. An Inverse Modeling Approach. Cambridge: Cambridge University Press; 2009.
56. Lumb AB. Nunn's applied respiratory physiology. 8th ed. Edinburgh; New York: Elsevier; 2017.
57. Marshall R, Widdicombe JG. Stress relaxation of the human lung. Clin Sci. 1960;20:19–31.
58. Coughlin MF, Suki B, Stamenovic D. Dynamic behavior of lung parenchyma in shear. J Appl Physiol (1985). 1996;80(6):1880–90.
59. Van de Woestijne KP. Influence of forced inflations on the creep of lungs and thorax in the dog. Respir Physiol. 1967;3(1):78–89.
60. Albert SP, DiRocco J, Allen GB, Bates JH, Lafollette R, Kubiak BD, Fischer J, Maroney S, Nieman GF. The role of time and pressure on alveolar recruitment. J Appl Physiol. 2009;106(3):757–65.
61. Hughes R, May AJ, Widdicombe JG. Stress relaxation in rabbits' lungs. J Physiol. 1959;146(1):85–97.
62. Butler J, White HC, Arnott WM. The pulmonary compliance in normal subjects. Clin Sci. 1957;16(4):709–29.
63. Hildebrandt J. Pressure-volume data of the cat determined by a plastoelastic, linear viscoelastic model. J Appl Physiol. 1970;28(3):365–72.
64. The Acute Respiratory Distress Syndrome Network. ARDSnet: ventilation with lower tidal volumes as compared with traditional tidal volumes for acute lung injury and the acute respiratory distress syndrome. N Engl J Med. 2000;342(18):1301–8.

Chapter 4
Alveolar and Alveolar Duct Mechanics in the Acutely Injured Lung: Peeling Stress and Stress Multiplication

Introduction

In the healthy lung, acini comprising alveoli and alveolar ducts maintain inflation at end-expiration, resulting in a uniformly inflated state throughout most of the lung. However, ARDS renders the lung time- and pressure-dependent resulting in excessive stress as the walls of collapse alveoli in apposition are 'peeled' open and stress-multiplication in the open alveoli adjacent to those that are collapsed (Fig. 4.1) (green box). Through direct observation, we have demonstrated that subpleural alveoli, uniformly inflated with normal surfactant function, undergo size changes of approximately 2% with tidal ventilation, as observed using our in vivo microscope (Video 4.1). To model normal homogeneous inflation, we employed interconnected hexagons to symbolize alveoli with shared walls (Fig. 4.2, Video 4.2).

However, in progressive acute lung injury marked by pulmonary edema and surfactant deactivation (Fig. 1.1 Surfactant Deactivation and Alveolar Edema), the alveoli become time- and pressure-dependent. This means that they require more time to open and less time to collapse at any given airway pressure. Consequently, this results in widespread atelectasis, collapse, and instability, characterized by repetitive alveolar collapse and expansion (RACE) (Fig. 1.1 RACE). The consequence is a highly heterogeneous inflation pattern, with adjacent alveoli exhibiting atelectasis, edema-filled conditions, and instability, juxtaposed with patent normal alveoli.

Supplementary Information The online version contains supplementary material available at https://doi.org/10.1007/978-3-031-66352-9_4.

© The Author(s), under exclusive license to Springer Nature Switzerland AG 2024

G. F. Nieman, N. M. Habashi, *Applied Physiology to Reduce Ventilator Induced Lung Injury*, https://doi.org/10.1007/978-3-031-66352-9_4

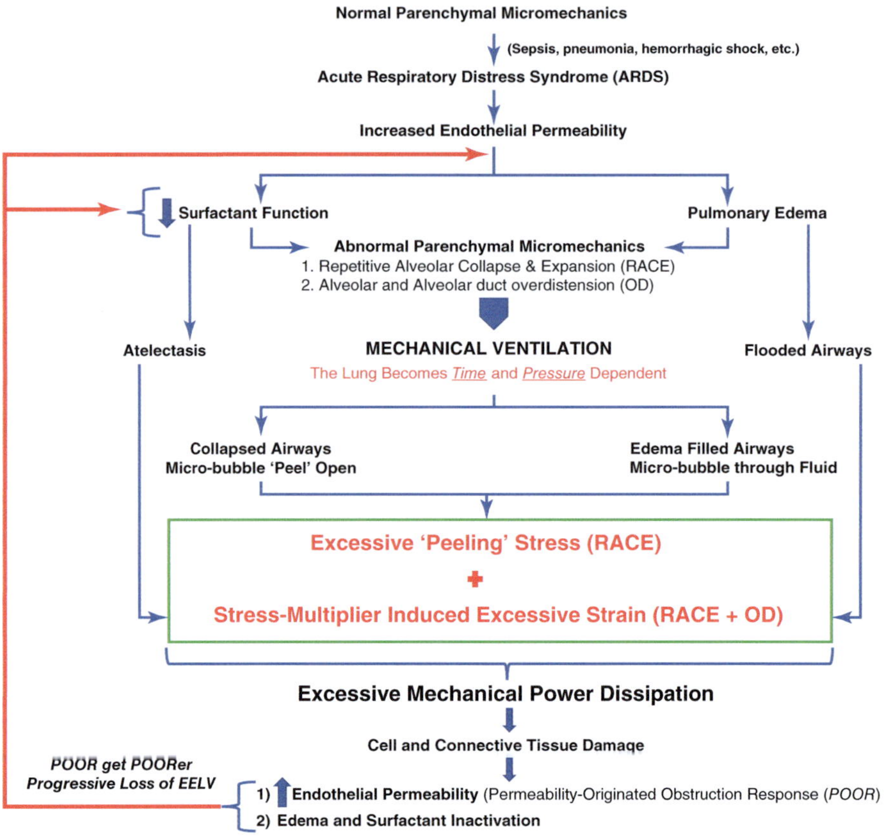

Fig. 4.1 The unifying hypothesis of the mechanisms by which acute respiratory distress syndrome (ARDS) pathophysiology predisposes the lung to a secondary ventilator-induced lung injury (VILI). This chapter discusses *Excessive "Peeling" Stress* during repetitive alveolar collapse and expansion (RACE) and *Stress Multipliers Induced Excessive Strain* that cause both RACE and alveolar and alveolar duct overdistension (OD) *(RACE + OD)* (purple dotted line). RACE and OD occur with each breath in focused regional lesions caused by increased pulmonary capillary permeability (Fig. 1.1 Endothelial Leakage), driving progressive VILI in a *POOR get POORer* mechanism (Fig. 4.11)

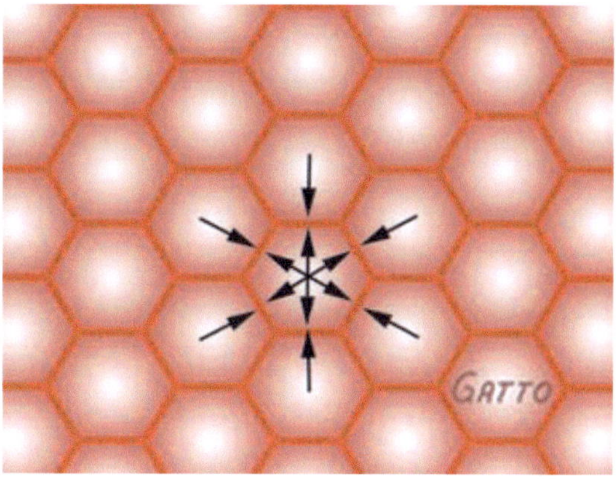

Fig. 4.2 Individual "alveoli" are modeled as a hexagon so that all walls are interconnected. A uniformly inflated lung is highly resistant to over-inflation injury since the airway pressure in all alveoli would be equal (arrows). Thus, there would be no driving pressure between adjacent alveoli to over-distend alveolar walls [100]

Atelectrauma

This pronounced heterogeneity predisposes the acutely injured lung to secondary VILI. Atelectrauma is the damage to parenchymal tissues resulting from the collapse and subsequent re-expansion occurring with each breath, known as RACE (Figs. 1.1 RACE, 2.6, Video 4.3). An illustration of RACE is evident in an excised rat lung Acute Respiratory Distress Syndrome (ARDS) model (Video 4.3). In this instance, conventional volume control ventilation is employed (tidal volume—V_T, 6 cc/kg, positive end-expiratory pressure—PEEP 5 cmH_2O) with a very short inspiratory time and an extended expiratory time. The lungs nearly collapse entirely at end-expiration, displaying a regionally varied reinflation during inspiration, indicative of extreme RACE. Subpleural alveoli are observed opening and collapsing with each breath.

To draw a comparison in the whole lung and alveolar mechanics, consider a rat lung with a similar injury but subjected to airway pressure release ventilation (APRV) in Video 5.3. In this case, an extended time at inspiration and a brief expiratory time are utilized. Unlike the previous example, the lungs do not collapse during the brief expiratory time. Alveoli remain stable without RACE, and they are homogeneously inflated during inspiration, appearing uniformly pink with no signs of red atelectasis.

Experimental evidence supporting the significance of atelectrauma as a mechanism of VILI is derived from studies demonstrating a significant worsening of injury when the lungs are ventilated at very low or zero levels of PEEP, allowing derecruitment to occur with each breath [1, 2]. While the damage induced by RACE is not as immediately apparent as overdistension, it plays a crucial role. The mechanism of atelectrauma is often attributed to the detrimental mechanical stresses applied to the epithelial surfaces of the airways and alveoli, particularly as they are peeled apart during lung inflation. To model the heterogeneous inflation pattern characteristic of

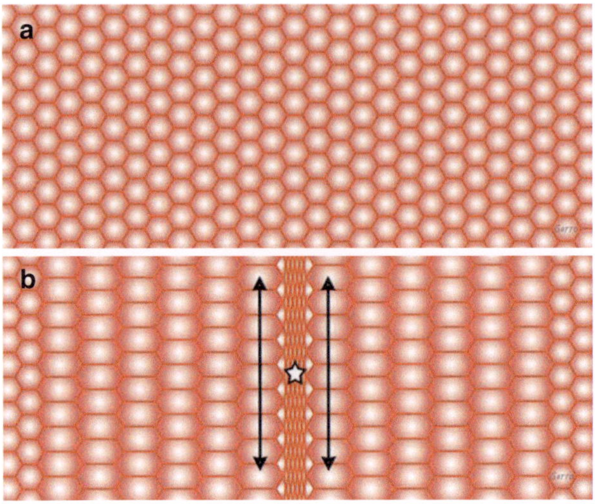

Fig. 4.3 Repetitive alveolar collapse and expansion (RACE) with "alveoli" modeled as hexagons so that all walls are interconnected. (**a**) During inflation, all alveoli are open with homogenous inflation. (**b**) During exhalation, "alveoli" with dysfunctional surfactant collapse (star), and more importantly, this collapse acts as a stress multiplier over distending adjacent "alveoli" (arrows) since their walls are connected to the walls of the collapsing "alveoli." [100]

RACE, we employed a hexagon alveolar model like the one used for homogeneous normal alveolar inflation (Fig. 4.2). This model, depicted in Fig. 4.3 and Video 4.4, illustrates that not only are the alveoli experiencing RACE, in the center of the figure and video, being damaged by excessive dynamic strain, but also the alveoli walls connected to those undergoing collapse are subjected to significant overdistension with each tidal breath.

Mechanisms of RACE-induced tissue damage at the cellular level: In the normal lung, functional surfactant functions as an anti-glue, facilitating the separation of alveolar and small airway walls that collapse with minimal shear stress or dissipated energy upon reinflation. This serves to minimize tissue damage, as depicted in Fig. 4.4 [3]. However, increased pulmonary capillary permeability is a hallmark of ARDS pathophysiology, leading to protein-rich edema fluid filling alveoli and small airways (Fig. 1.1 Surfactant Deactivation & Alveolar Edema). The presence of plasma proteins deactivates surfactant, resulting in unstable alveoli that collapse with their walls, forming a pleated configuration, as seen in Fig. 1.1 RACE Expiration [4, 5].

In a porcine sepsis-induced ARDS model, Fig. 4.5 shows two collapsed alveolar walls (ac) in apposition with a sliver of air between them. Additionally, the loss of the anti-glue function of surfactant, combined with plasma proteins on the endothelial surface, makes these surfaces "sticky," requiring excessive airway pressure to reinflate these tissues [6]. As mechanical breath forces these alveolar walls in apposition to separate, there is substantial cellular distortion, dissipating significant energy into these cells with each breath. This process, illustrated in Fig. 4.6, results

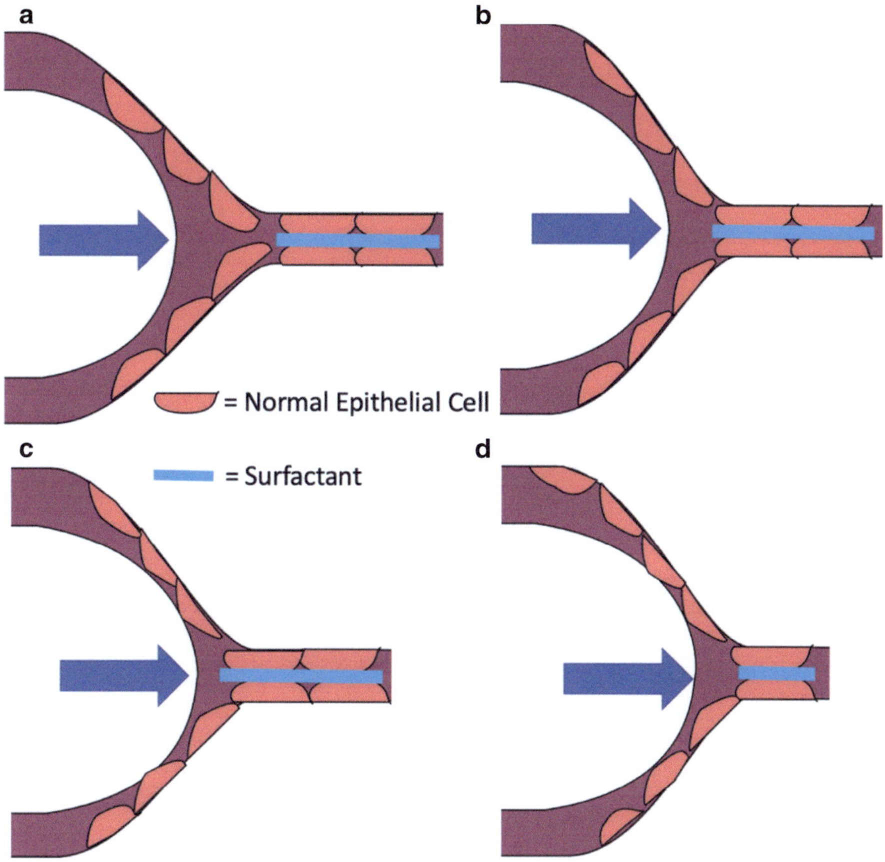

Fig. 4.4 With normal surfactant function (blue line), the endothelial cells are not injured as the air bubble (arrows) progressively recruits the small airway (**a–d**). One of surfactant's multiple functions is an "anti-glue" that would enable the endothelial cells in apposition to separate with little cellular distortion, mechanical energy dissipation, or friction-induced heat generation, thus minimizing any cellular damage (Normal Epithelial Cell)

in cellular damage due to the mechanical forces associated with RACE-induced alveolar collapse and re-expansion. The epithelial cellular lining of collapsed alveoli and alveolar ducts in apposition undergoes pressure differences and friction when a mechanical breath forces an air bubble into the collapsed airways (Fig. 4.6, blue arrow), compelling the walls to separate. In the absence of a functional surfactant layer lining the alveolar and alveolar ducts, there is pronounced cellular deformation as they are forced apart, causing excessive shear or peeling stress. This results in excessive cellular strain and energy dissipation, ultimately leading to cellular damage and death, as illustrated in Fig. 4.6 Red Damaged Epithelial Cell. If this "peeling open" of small airways and alveoli is repeated a sufficient number of times, it exacerbates surfactant deactivation, alveolar collapse, and alveolar edema (Fig. 1.1). This sequence leads to a rapid spread of tissue damage throughout the

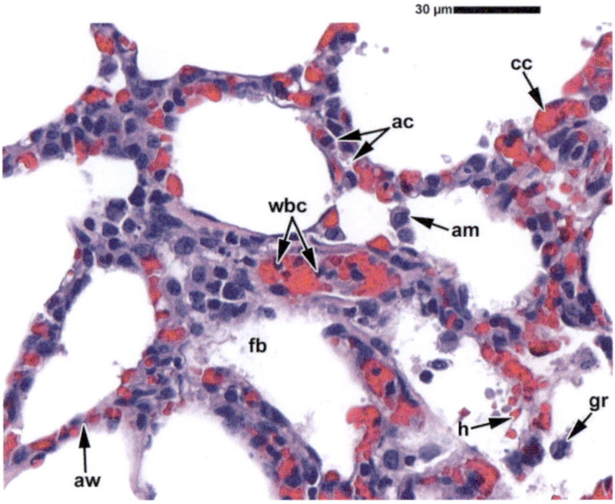

Fig. 4.5 Lung tissue from a pig with sepsis and trauma-induced ARDS analyzed by L.A. Gatto. High magnification shows histological detail at the alveolar level, where the air compartment exhibits alveolar macrophages (***am***) as well as hematogenous granulocytes (***gr***) and occasional evidence of intra-alveolar hemorrhage (***h***). The passage of blood into the air compartment contributes to the infiltration of proteinaceous edematous materials into the alveolar lumen, which in histological preparations appears as amorphous fibrinous deposition (***fb***). The blood compartment shows an occasional intravascular aggregation of leukocytes (***wbc***) in small parenchymal vessels, and congested capillaries (***cc***) within the alveolar wall (***aw***). The detail revealed at this higher magnification allows the identification of alveolar collapse (***ac***) whenever the collapse is incomplete, and there is a slender remnant of air space separating the abutting alveolar walls. Note that when alveoli collapse, the wall folds together, similar to crumpling a paper bag, and the endothelial cells lining the alveolar walls are in direct apposition

entire lung (Figs. 2.5 and 4.1 green box) [7]. This cumulative effect underscores how the mechanical forces associated with repetitive alveolar collapse and re-expansion contribute to a cascading and widespread lung tissue damage pattern.

When incorrect ventilator settings are applied to a lung undergoing acute injury, a notable reduction in end-expiratory lung volume (EELV) and the development of RACE (Videos 4.3) occur, leading to substantial damage to lung tissue (Figs. 8.14 and 8.15), pulmonary edema (Fig. 4.8a, b), and inflammation (Fig. 4.8c, d) [8]. The intricate interplay among acinar architecture, connective tissue scaffolding, and a dynamic pulmonary surfactant system is pivotal in acinar mechanics during tidal ventilation. Surfactant serves various functions, such as (i) shaping acinar structures, influencing lung recoil pressure, capillary configuration, and pulmonary microcirculation (Fig. 3.3) [9] (ii) diminishing strain on alveolar epithelial cells at low lung volumes, with matrix scaffolding serving as the stress-bearing structure [10] (iii) shielding the lung from edema formation by reducing interstitial pressure around pulmonary capillaries [11–14] (iv) stabilizing alveoli and alveolar ducts at low lung volumes [15] and (v) functioning as an “anti-glue” between collapsing alveolar walls, significantly reducing the force needed to separate these walls (Fig. 4.4) [3].

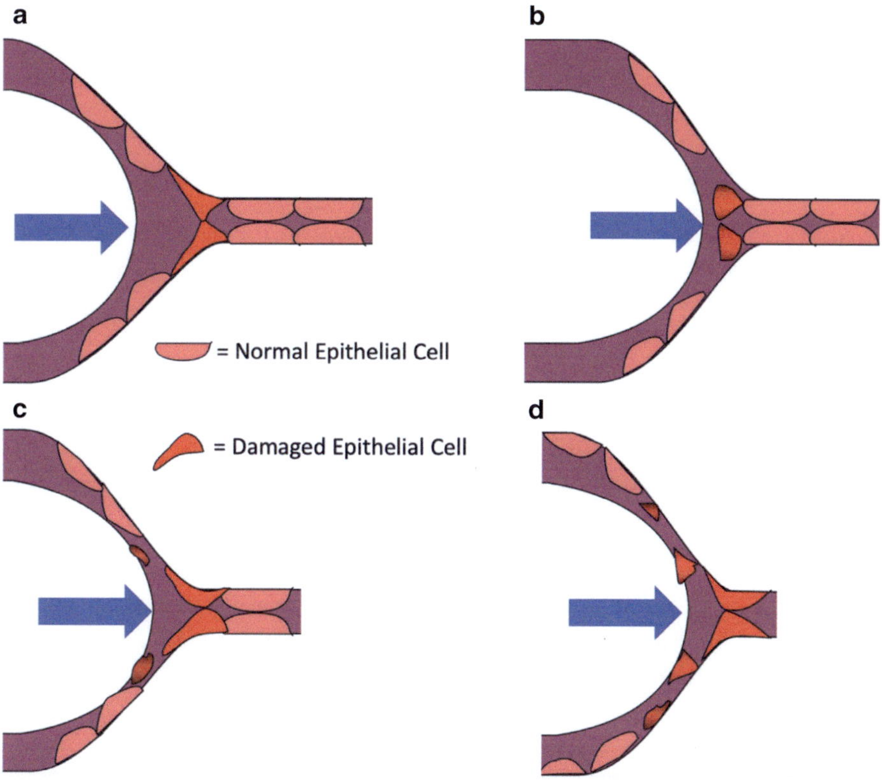

Fig. 4.6 Peeling-stress model of an air bubble being moved through and recruiting a small collapsed airway. (**a**) The air bubble has just reached the collapsed tissue with normal endothelial cells (tan) in direct apposition. (**b**) The air bubble begins to open the collapsed airway with "sticky" endothelial cells due to loss of surfactant function. This results in a great deal of cellular distortion, causing dissipation of mechanical energy and tissue injury due to friction-induced heat loss. (**c**, **d**) Endothelial damage progresses down the airway as the air bubble moves deeper into the lung. If opening during inspiration and re-collapse during expiration occur a sufficient number of times, there will be a loss of barrier function, exacerbating microvascular permeability, and edema formation

The Significance of Surfactant in the Context of an Acutely Injured Lung

Pulmonary surfactant assumes a multi-layer formation, regulated by surfactant protein B, crucial for the proper biophysical behavior of the surface film [16]. In ARDS, the surfactant's ability to reduce surface tension is compromised by the presence of high-protein pulmonary edema [17, 18], amplifying lung recoil through an increased propensity for the surface film to collapse. Surface tension is most evident at low lung volumes when surfactant concentrations on the surface of the hypophase lining the alveolar walls are high. Effective reduction in surface tension stabilizes the surface film, while dysfunction in surfactant leads to alveolar destabilization, resulting in RACE [19–21]. The contrast between normal low and pathologically high surface tensions drives edema fluid into areas affected by surfactant dysfunction [22–24].

Surfactant deactivation induced by high-protein pulmonary edema not only causes the collapse of alveolar and alveolar duct walls but also leads to the inundation of small airways and alveoli with edema fluid (Fig. 1.1 Surfactant Deactivation & Alveolar Edema). In the normal lung, alveoli and small airways frequently collapse, and a deep sigh serves to reopen these airspaces. Why do epithelial cells remain undamaged when small airways and alveoli reopen in the normal lung with a sigh? Two fundamental explanations, both related to a functional surfactant system, are proposed:

1. When small airways are reopened with a sigh, they stay open due to the surface tension-lowering ability of a functioning surfactant system. This prevents repetitive collapse and reopening, eliminating the occurrence of RACE.
2. Surfactant acts as an anti-glue [3], allowing epithelial cells in apposition to separate with minimal cellular distortion during reopening, preventing friction-induced energy dissipation as heat and subsequent injury (Fig. 4.4) [25]. This stands in stark contrast to the extreme cellular distortion experienced by "sticky" endothelial cells lacking functional surfactant when forced apart during recruitment (Fig. 4.6) [25].

Excessive cellular distortion and strain are imposed on epithelial cells during mechanical ventilation, especially as the air bubble moves edema deeper into the lungs. In the case of edema-filled alveolar and alveolar ducts, as the air bubble traverses the edema fluid, epithelial cells encounter substantial strain, akin to pushing a rolling pin across the cellular surface (Fig. 4.7) [25].

Surfactant dysfunction plays a pivotal role in generating damaging fluid stresses at the air–liquid interface in the injured lung [25–30]. The intricate fluid dynamic processes involved in the formation and dissipation of liquid plugs, along with the role played by surfactant are complex and extend beyond the scope of this chapter [24, 31–34]. Despite numerous clinical trials, there is a lack of evidence supporting the clinical benefits of increasing surfactant concentration in the lung for reducing VILI in patients with ARDS [35].

An intriguing possibility for this discrepancy revolves around surfactant dosing [35, 36]. Computational modeling studies suggest that the doses (volume of material) utilized in surfactant replacement therapy (SRT) clinical trials may have been insufficient to allow the instilled material to reach the distal lung in quantities necessary to restore normal surfactant function [35, 36] effectively. Whether surfactant therapy would prove effective in ARDS with a larger dose volume remains an open question.

The prevailing hypothesis for the ineffectiveness of SRT in ARDS patients revolves around the in situ deactivation of surfactant. Pulmonary edema, rich in

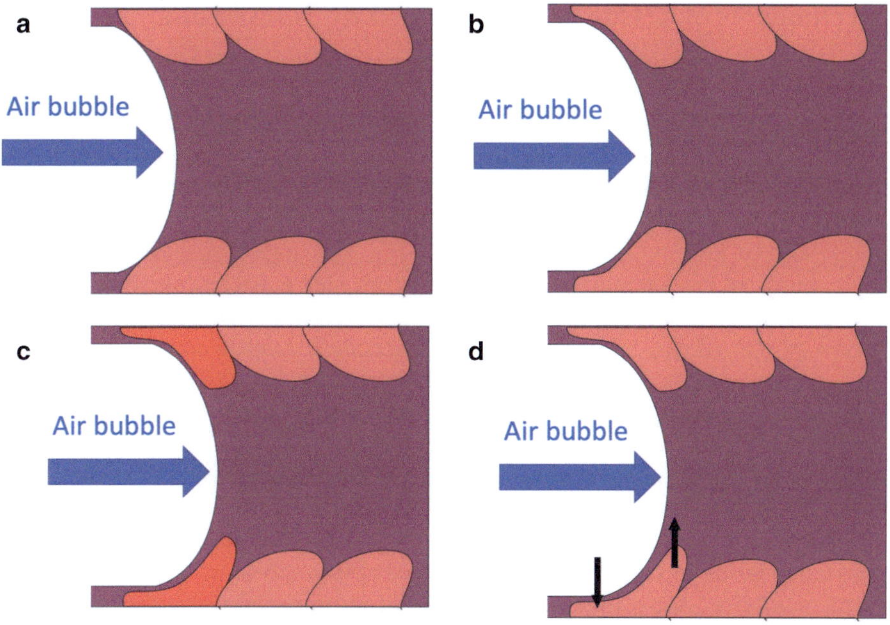

Fig. 4.7 Similar epithelial cell distortion is seen when the mechanical ventilator progressively forces an air bubble (blue arrow) into an edema-filled small airway (**a**–**d**). The epithelial cells are flattened, like a roller pin pushed over them. If this process is repeated a sufficient number of times, it will result in cellular damage and death

plasma proteins, floods the airspaces and competes with surfactant's adsorption to the liquid hypophase coating the alveolar surface, as illustrated in Fig. 1.1 Surfactant Deactivation & Edema [37]. If this hypothesis holds, these plasma proteins would similarly compete with exogenous surfactant, significantly diminishing its ability to lower surface tension. Consequently, a larger dose of surfactant during SRT might not be effective, as it could rapidly deactivate upon reaching the alveolus [18].

Mechanical ventilation could alleviate this issue by inducing surfactant release by stretching epithelial cells [38]. Additionally, when employed appropriately, mechanical ventilation may promote the reincorporation of sub-surface surfactant molecules into the air–liquid interface [39, 40]. Conversely, improper mechanical ventilation practices can lead to surfactant deactivation. Notably, a proposition suggests that the initial step in ARDS development is atelectasis due to surfactant abnormalities induced by spontaneous or mechanical ventilation, rather than primary (pneumonia, aspiration) or secondary (sepsis, hemorrhagic shock, burns) inflammation. If this postulate holds, VILI could precede and cause ARDS rather than ARDS predisposing to VILI [41].

Mechanisms of Tissue Injury Induced by Volutrauma

Elevated airway pressure during tidal ventilation can lead to a high static strain, causing stress failure in normal lung parenchyma, a condition defined as volutrauma. The "baby lung" hypothesis conceptualizes ARDS pathology as two distinct compartments. One comprises flooded or collapsed tissue in independent regions, while the other involves the ventilated open, normal lung, often located in nondependent lung regions (Fig. 2.3) [42–44]. This hypothesis originated from early computed tomography (CT) studies that unveiled a macroscopic maldistribution of aeration. The concern that excessive inspiratory volume forced into the remaining normal lung tissue could lead to mechanical damage prompted the adoption of a protective ventilation strategy with low-tidal volume (LV_T) [45]. Positron-emission tomography (PET) further supported this hypothesis by revealing strain-dependent neutrophil activity in ventilated regions of human ARDS lungs [46].

However, recent studies challenge the notion that overdistension of normal lung tissue is the primary mechanism behind VILI. Instead, the focus has shifted to regional alveolar instability and overdistension of alveolar walls in normal alveoli adjacent to unstable, collapsed, or edema-filled alveoli. These normal alveoli act as stress multipliers, the primary mechanism causing regional tissue overdistension (Figs. 2.6 and 2.7, Videos 2.1, 4.3, 4.4, and 4.5) [47–49].

Tschumperlin and Margulies have demonstrated that below 80% total lung capacity (TLC), micromechanics is primarily characterized by the unfolding of septal walls or changes in alveolar shape. Beyond this threshold, alveolar stretching becomes prominent, occurring between 80% and 100% TLC [50]. The overall strain due to stretch below 80% TLC was 35%, but it escalated to 80% with lung inflation to 80%–100% TLC, leading to endothelial damage measured in cell cultures [51]. Ventilating a normal lung at TLC (static strain 2.5) while minimizing dynamic strain by adding PEEP did not induce VILI-related ARDS over a 54-h ventilation period. However, when dynamic strain was increased by reducing PEEP, the lungs suffered severe injury, resulting in pulmonary edema and death [52]. A recent study by Seah et al. found that ventilating normal mice for up to 4 h with a tidal volume equal to TLC (high static strain) but minimizing dynamic strain by adding 3 cmH_2O PEEP did not cause lung injury [2].

Our laboratory established a heterogeneous porcine lung injury model ventilated at a peak airway pressure of 40 cmH_2O, representing a sizeable static strain, with and without a high dynamic strain (large tidal volume) [53]. This model introduces Tween via a bronchoscope into the right and left lower lung lobes to deactivate surfactant, causing regional acute lung injury (ALI). The remaining lung lobes, considered the "baby lung," were normal, and we analyzed the impact on the normal and acutely injured lung tissue separately. Two groups were examined: one with a high dynamic strain and the other with a low dynamic strain. Both groups were subjected to high static strain (40 cmH_2O peak airway pressure). Notably, the normal tissue (N_T) (i.e., the "baby lung") did not show significant injury in either group. The acutely injured lung tissue (ALI_T) was not further damaged in the low dynamic strain group. However, the ALI_T tissue in the Tween-injured group exhibited severe damage (Fig. 8.15) [53]. This study implies that if the "baby lung" in humans is indeed normal tissue, as has been previously hypothesized [42]., Thus, overdistension (volutruama) injury should not occur in normal tissue, which the N_T supports in this study [42] and in the normal lung with high peak airway pressure and static strain ventilated for 54 h [53]. Importantly, these studies indicate that overdistension of the "baby lung" by high tidal volume and airway pressure may not be a primary mechanism for VILI.

In a more recent study using the same heterogeneous porcine lung injury model, we explored four mechanical breath combinations delivered with the APRV mode. The mechanical breath settings were designed to induce lung overdistension (OD↑) or not (OD↓) and lung recruitment/derecruitment (RD↑) or not (RD↓) (Fig. 4.8) [8]. Remarkably, in the normal lung tissue, none of the mechanical breath combinations, including OD↑RD↑, resulted in pulmonary edema or increased bronchoalveolar

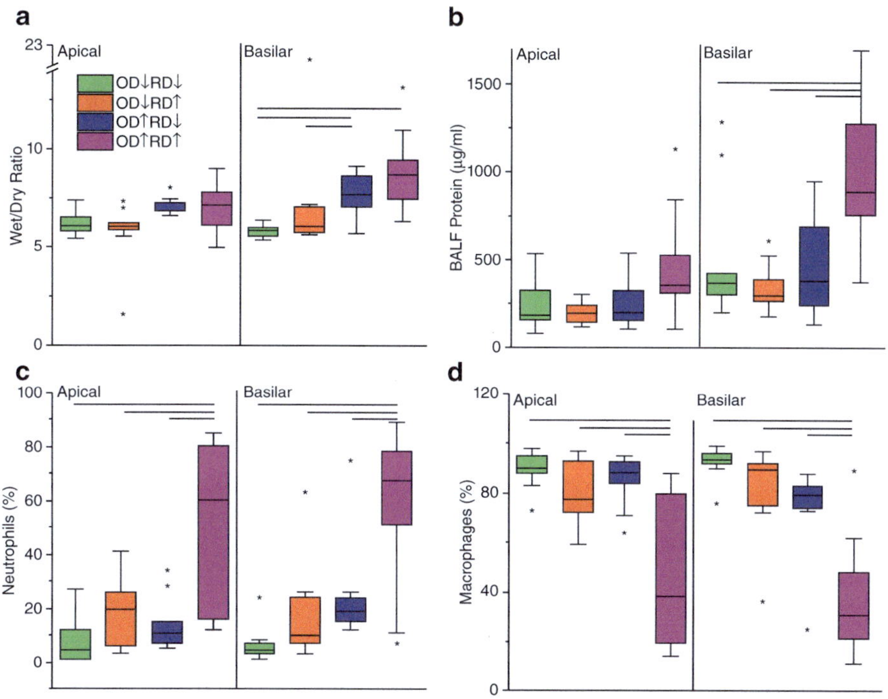

Fig. 4.8 Lung edema assessed as a lung tissue wet-to-dry weight ratio (wet/dry ratio; **a**), total protein in bronchoalveolar lavage fluid (BALF; **b**), neutrophil counts (**c**), and macrophage counts measured using Cytospin (**d**). Groups ($n = 10$ pigs per group) were ventilated with a combination of higher ↑ or lower ↓ overdistension (OD) and recruitment/derecruitment (RD) for 6 h. Measurements were made in normal (apical) and surfactant dysfunctional (basal) tissues. Black dots indicate outliers. Horizontal lines represent $P < 0.05$ between groups (ANOVA) [8]

fluid (BALF) concentration of total protein, indicating heightened microvascular permeability. However, OD↑RD↑ and OD↑RD↓ led to increased edema in the Tween-injured tissue, while only OD↑RD↑ caused a rise in BALF protein. The OD↓RD↓ was most lung protective.

Furthermore, assessments of inflammation, including increased neutrophils and decreased macrophages, were observed exclusively in response to OD↑RD↑ and occurred in both normal and Tween-injured tissues. These findings reinforce the notion that normal lung tissue (i.e., the "baby lung") is highly resilient to damage from mechanical breath, even when adjusted to induce both overdistension (OD↑) and recruitment/derecruitment (RD↑). Notably, in the presence of surfactant deactivation by Tween without the "anti-glue" function of surfactant, the OD↑RD↑ group suffered severe injury. In contrast, the OD↓RD↓ group exhibited significant protection (Fig. 4.8).

Regional Volutrauma

Regional volutrauma can be experimentally induced in the normal lung when exposed to a very high dynamic strain of 2.5 (tidal volume divided by end-expiratory lung volume) for a sufficiently extended period. In studies conducted on normal piglets subjected to high static and dynamic strain, lesions initially manifested adjacent to the pleural surface, bronchi, and large blood vessels, which function as anatomical stress multipliers [54]. Consequently, normal lung lesions tended to spread inward from the pleural surface. This observation suggests that if the "baby lung" was the primary site of Ventilator-Induced Lung Injury (VILI) in humans, the strain must be exceptionally high, and the lesions would propagate from the pleural surface inward. However, this does not align with the observed pattern of VILI, providing further evidence that damage to the "baby lung" is not the driving mechanism behind VILI [54].

Volutrauma can manifest in normal alveoli near regional alveolar instability, flooding, or collapse, leading to atelectasis (Figs. 2.6, 2.7, 4.3, 4.9, and 4.10, Videos 2.1, 4.4, and 4.5). This phenomenon may occur during general anesthesia, resulting in lung deflation below EELV. For instance, ventilation of anesthetized rats for 1 h with zero PEEP (ZEEP) resulted in a 10% loss of aeration without macroscopic atelectasis but increased airspace dimensions and ventilation heterogeneity [55]. This suggests that even a mild loss of aeration may act as a stress multiplier in an otherwise uninjured lung and cause overdistension in the surrounding open alveoli [56].

A different pattern of injury spread is observed in the acutely injured lung. Tissue damage in the injured lung propagates concentrically around areas of regional alveolar instability, collapse, or flooding that act as stress multipliers (Figs. 2.5 and 4.11). These occur throughout the lung, including what appears to be normal lung tissue on chest X-ray or CT scan ("Hidden Microatelectasis"') (Fig. 2.8). Atelectatic

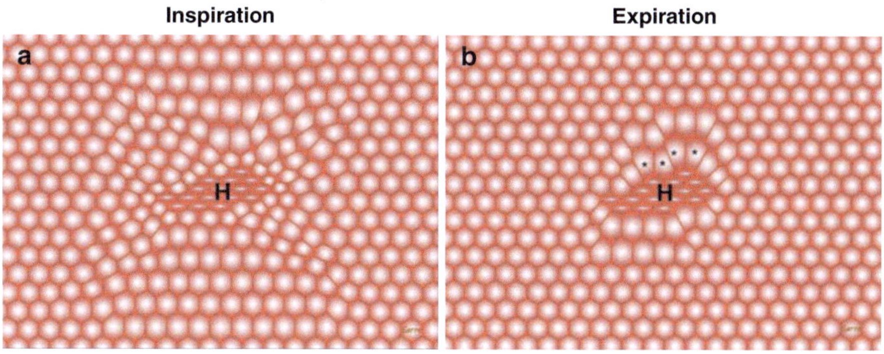

Fig. 4.9 Alveoli are modeled as hexagons with a regional heterogenous group of "alveoli" (H) showing the impact of Inspiration (**a**) and Expiration (**b**) on the inflated alveoli adjacent to the collapsed area. These collapsed areas act as stress multipliers, greatly amplifying the size of alveolar strain in the adjacent open alveoli. Note the overdistension of "alveoli" above and below the collapse alveoli during Inspiration (**a**) and the significant change in the volume of the "alveoli" directly adjacent to the collapse during Expiration (**b**, asterisk) [100]

and unstable lung tissue renders the surrounding normal tissue more susceptible to VILI, which correlates with the degree of strain [57].

The development of regional parenchymal overdistension results from the intricate relationship between heterogeneous injury (e.g., RACE or stress multiplier) and the mechanical breath profile (MB_P), which encompasses all airway pressures, volumes, rates, flows, and the *time* they are applied during both inspiration and expiration of the ventilation strategy being used to ventilate the heterogeneously damaged lung [58–64]. Consequently, the impact of applying positive airway pressure on parenchymal mechanics is complex and unpredictable. For instance, increasing PEEP has been shown to recruit alveoli and reduce atelectasis, decreasing acinar size [47, 65]. Cereda et al. demonstrated that applying PEEP to a normal or surfactant-deactivated lung caused an increase in airway size. However, surfactant deactivation also caused atelectasis, leading to two lung unit populations: (i) collapsed units and (ii) volume-expanded airspaces adjacent to the atelectatic areas, even with moderate tidal volume (Figs. 4.10 and 5.8). The volume-expanded tissue was found in areas of atelectasis, suggesting a mechanism involving interdependent tractive forces from surrounding collapsed alveoli causing reciprocal expansion of open airspaces and gas redistribution. They also showed that if PEEP or surfactant replacement recruits atelectatic tissue, the size of alveoli and alveolar ducts is not overdistended but is actually reduced, concluding that atelectasis causes VILI through a reciprocal increase in volume-expanded normal tissue surrounding the primary lesion [66]. Our data aligns with this work, showing the volume expansion of airspaces adjacent to atelectatic areas (Fig. 5.8) [67].

Stress Multipliers

In a normal, homogeneously inflated lung, resilience to overdistension injury is high unless the strain is dynamic and exceptionally high [54]. However, this resilience is compromised in an injured lung due to the forces of parenchymal interdependence at interfaces between unstable, collapsed, or edema-filled regions and the surrounding normal acini. When these regions fail to expand during lung inflation, they act as stress multipliers, substantially enhancing damaging forces (Figs. 2.7, 4.9, 4.10, and 4.11, Videos 2.1 and 4.5) [47–49].

Computed tomography (CT) images from patients with ARDS and animal models reveal that inflation heterogeneity is notable at interfaces between aerated and non-aerated tissue [54, 68]. Atelectatic regions become stress multipliers, and surrounding areas of open lung can be exposed to damaging stresses during mechanical ventilation, even when the lung is subjected to safe strain levels and appears normal on chest X-ray [59, 69–72]. Additionally, the apparent diffusion coefficient of hyperpolarized gas on magnetic resonance imaging, providing a measure of local airspace dimension [73], is elevated around regions of microatelectasis but can be normalized by recruitment maneuvers [47, 48] and PEEP, if sufficient airway

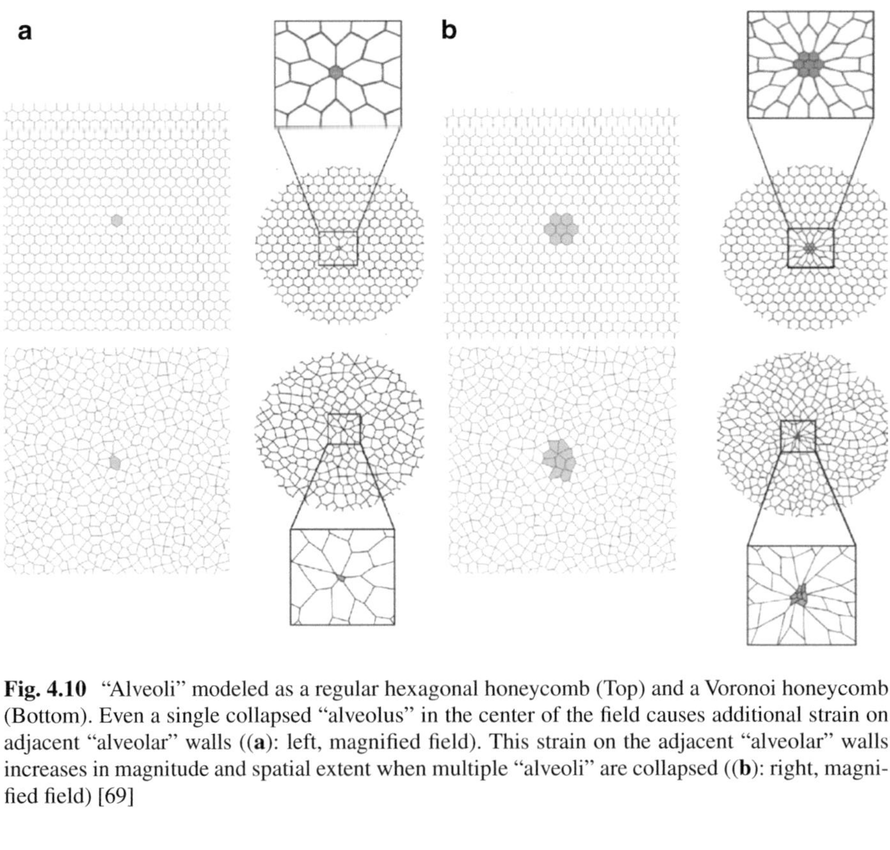

Fig. 4.10 "Alveoli" modeled as a regular hexagonal honeycomb (Top) and a Voronoi honeycomb (Bottom). Even a single collapsed "alveolus" in the center of the field causes additional strain on adjacent "alveolar" walls ((**a**): left, magnified field). This strain on the adjacent "alveolar" walls increases in magnitude and spatial extent when multiple "alveoli" are collapsed ((**b**): right, magnified field) [69]

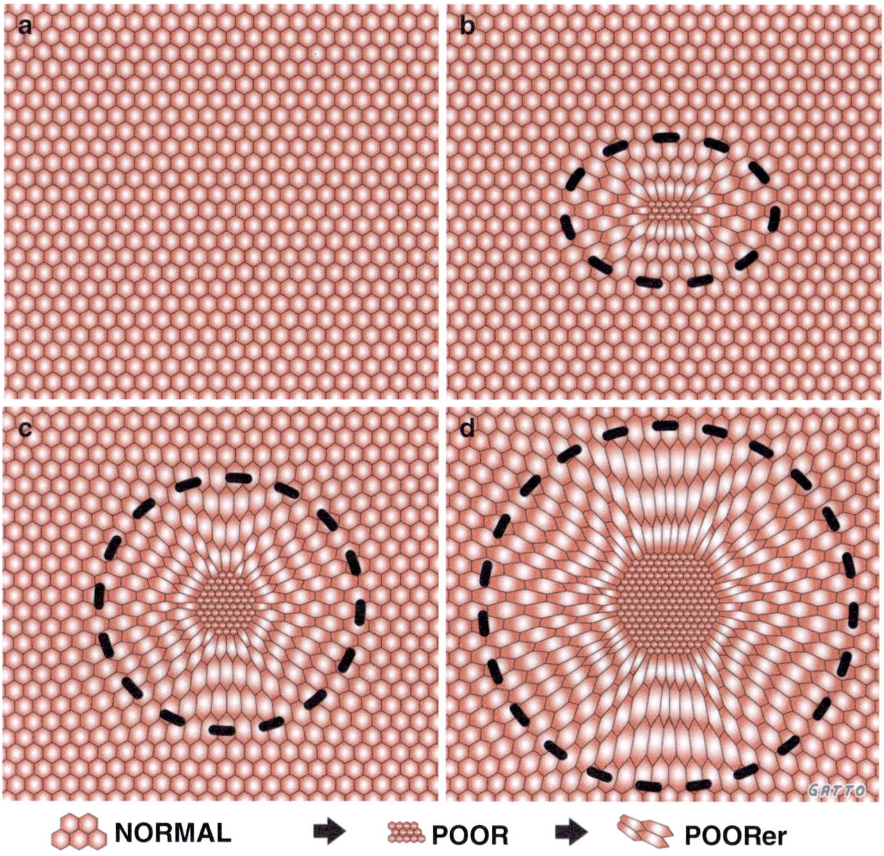

Fig. 4.11 "Alveoli"' modeled as hexagons in normal homogeneous tissue (**a**). ARDS-induced increased microvascular permeability initiates a permeability-originated obstructive response (*POOR*) with heterogeneous areas of collapsed or edema-filled tissue that acts as a stress multiplier during ventilation (**b**). Note the distortion of the adjacent open alveoli surrounding the collapse (black dotted circle). As the initial POOR lesion expands, many open alveoli are subjected to distortion and injury in the area of stress multiplication surrounding the collapse (**c**, **d** black dotted circles). Thus, not just the collapsed tissue is subject to injury but also the patent alveoli adjacent to the collapse. If these lesions are not corrected, tissue damage will progress rapidly in a POOR get POORer fashion

pressure and time necessary to recruit the collapsed tissue is applied [66]. Finite element modeling suggests that stress multiplication can be about three times larger than average lung stress, and individual cell filaments sustain stresses 16 times higher than average (Fig. 4.10) [69].

Stress multipliers are prevalent in the lung affected by ARDS, characterized by spatially heterogeneous atelectasis and edema [74–76]. These stress multipliers play a crucial role in the rapid propagation of VILI throughout the lung (Figs. 2.5 and 4.11). Morphometric studies have demonstrated that injurious mechanical ventilation increases pulmonary edema in rat lung tissues adjacent to atelectatic regions [77]. Heterogeneous inflation also correlates with neutrophil activity in animals [78] and the severity of ARDS in humans [68], establishing a link between mechanical stress and inflammation associated with ventilation defects. This connection has been observed in a sheep model of septic lung injury, even with low-stretch ventilation [79]. VILI can evolve from stress multipliers that are nearly undetectable ("Hidden Microatelectasis"') in regions where inflation is suboptimal [80] or unstable (Fig. 2.8) [81, 82].

As discussed earlier, the spatial propagation of VILI in ARDS occurs concentrically from pre-existing lesions (Figs. 2.5 and 4.11), which has been confirmed in computed tomography (CT) scans [82]. In contrast, lung tissue damage progresses from the pleural surface to the hilum in a normal lung exposed to very high dynamic strain [54]. The pleural surface in the normal lung acts as a stress multiplier, damaging the surrounding tissue, like regional stress multipliers in the acutely injured lung [74–76]. Stress multipliers are initially caused by an inflammation-induced increase in microvascular permeability, initiating a Permeability-Originated Obstructive Response (POOR). The regional POOR areas act as foci from which VILI propagates to previously normal lung regions in a "POOR get POORer" fashion, analogous to how cracks fracture solid materials. This mechanism plays a vital role in the progressive worsening of VILI (Fig. 4.11) [49].

It's crucial to highlight that the "baby lung" model cannot explain the topographic propagation of VILI from stress multipliers. According to this model, uniform tissue damage should originate de novo in open lung regions hyperinflated by mechanical ventilation, which contradicts the observed progression of VILI [54]. If overdistension of the "baby lung" was the primary mechanism of VILI, tissue injury would initiate at anatomical stress multipliers [54]. However, as described earlier, VILI progresses from focal POOR areas of injury (Figs. 2.5 and 4.11) [47, 48, 54, 66, 68, 74–78]. Lung expansion can recruit closed lung regions in sufficient quantities to reduce tensile forces in the areas of stress multipliers. This desirable effect is further enhanced by exogenous surfactant administration [71]. If stress multipliers are not eliminated, volutrauma cannot be prevented solely based on what seems to be a safe level of expansion of the so-called baby lung.

Ventilating a surfactant-deactivated rat lung using the low V_T (6 cc/kg) demonstrates that the tidal volume is not overexpanding the normal (pink) tissues on the edges of the baby lung but rather opening collapsed tissue that re-collapses with each breath (R/D or RACE) (Video 4.3). Thus, in this rat ARDS model, the mechanism of VILI using the standard-of-care low V_T method is not the overdistension of the baby lung but instead increased RACE-induced atelectrauma in the adjacent injured tissue.

Retamal et al. conducted an experiment where focal atelectasis was induced in rat lungs subjected to two ventilation strategies: Control (V_T 10 mL/kg + PEEP 3 cmH_2O) and Injurious (V_T 20 mL/kg + PEEP 0 cmH_2O). They observed alveolar disruption and neutrophil infiltration in both groups' tissue adjacent to the collapsed area. Injurious ventilation significantly increased pulmonary edema compared to the control group. Morphometric analysis revealed an increased volume-to-surface (V/S) ratio in the tissue adjacent to the atelectasis, indicating heightened parenchymal tissue strain. The conclusion drawn from the study was that atelectasis was acting as a stress multiplier [77].

Interestingly, there was no significant difference in the inflammatory mediators measured in any of the tissue regions of interest (i.e., normal, atelectatic, and peri-atelectatic tissues). This lack of difference suggested that the mechanism of tissue injury was mechanical (volutrauma and atelectrauma) rather than inflammatory (biotrauma). Mechanical tissue damage was also observed in unstable parenchymal tissue that collapsed and reopened with each breath [83].

Makiyama et al. developed a two-dimensional finite element model of 500 cells to investigate the impact of stress multipliers and parenchymal lung strain [69]. A non-linear stress–strain relationship characterized the filaments forming the cell walls. Hexagon and Voronoi honeycomb structures were employed to represent interdependent alveoli, and uniform strains between 15% and 45% were applied. "Atelectasis"'(stress multiplier) was simulated by increasing the stiffness of the filaments in either a single cell or in all connected cells, thus altering the size of the "atelectatic" area. The hexagon honeycomb model had little impact on the filaments attached to the "atelectasis"; however, in the Voronoi honeycomb model, the filaments were subjected to a substantial stress multiplier. Extrapolating this two-dimensional model to three dimensions revealed an average stress multiplier of ~62%, surpassing the 50% calculated by Mead [71]. The average maximum stress was approximately three times the 62% value, while the average stress on a single filament could experience a stress multiplication as high as 16 times. This suggests that airway pressures that would not induce VILI in a normal lung may cause regional high-stress injury in a heterogeneously injured lung, particularly in areas adjacent to collapsed tissue. Makiyama et al. calculated that the average stress concentration would be 1.62, which, when added to an airway pressure of 30 cmH_2O, would amplify the local stress-bearing components to a stress of approximately ~48 cmH_2O (1.62 × 30 cmH_2O) (Fig. 4.10) [69].

Knudsen et al. conducted a study investigating changes in alveolar micromechanics in a bleomycin-induced ARDS rat model subjected to mechanical ventilation and SRT [70]. They linked macro-lung mechanics with histologic micromechanics and employed a computational model of a viscoelastic alveolus to understand the impact of time and pressure on alveolar stability. The model predicted a significant increase in alveolar strain, attributed to interdependence and stress multipliers generated by alveolar collapse, causing increased distension of adjacent open alveoli. Design-based stereology was utilized to determine structure–function relationships, revealing that in the acutely injured lung, as airway pressure decreased, alveolar walls formed pleats and folded, bringing epithelial cells into direct contact with each other (Figs. 2.8 and 4.5) [70]. Reinflation of pleated and folded airway walls would necessitate a micro-bubble being forced through these directly opposed tissues. Without pulmonary surfactant, this process would cause epithelial cell injury (Fig. 4.6) [25, 84].

Furthermore, Knudsen et al. demonstrated that RACE played a secondary role and that static and dynamic stretch caused by stress multipliers was the primary alteration in alveolar micromechanics [70]. Additionally, their findings indicated that surfactant replacement therapy was associated with less atelectasis, leading to reduced alveolar tidal volumes. This reduction in dynamic strain on the alveolar walls normalized acinar micromechanics. Recruiting and stabilizing alveoli were linked to less alveolar edema, effectively addressing two components of the pathological tetrad associated with ARDS (Fig. 1.1 Alveolar Edema & RACE). Derecruitment primarily occurred in smaller alveoli, serving as stress multipliers that increased tethering forces and overdistended the walls of the surrounding open alveoli (Figs. 2.7, 4.9, and 4.11, Videos 2.1 and 4.5).

Contrastingly, different results were obtained in a rat surfactant deactivation ARDS model, where alveolar collapse did not over-distend adjacent open alveoli but overdistended the alveolar ducts (Fig. 5.8) [67]. This discrepancy could be attributed to lung injury model variations or the methodology used to measure histologic changes. Nonetheless, both studies underscore that stress multipliers result in overdistension of adjacent open tissue, raising the question of whether the excessive strain is on the alveolar walls or the alveolar ducts.

Motta-Ribeiro et al. proposed the hypothesis that the low V_T strategy might not shield against regional strain in early acute lung injury, as minimizing V_T without achieving a homogenous distribution of aeration has been demonstrated to exacerbate the spatial distribution of strain [79]. Xin et al. similarly demonstrated that heterogeneous unstable inflation and stress multipliers were the mechanisms of VILI [81]. Both studies indicated early prone positioning improved homogeneous ventilation and reduced lung damage [79, 81].

In summary, alveolar interdependence and parenchymal tethering significantly protect the lung from overdistension and collapse [71, 85–89]. It is very difficult to cause injury to the normal lung even when ventilated with a high static strain level [52]. Homogeneous parenchymal inflation, which adds structural support using a septal, axial, and peripheral connective tissue fiber system, establishes alveolar interdependence and parenchymal tethering, which is crucial for preventing VILI (Fig. 2.9) [71, 85, 87, 88]. ARDS induces heterogeneous alveolar instability, atelectasis, and edema [74–76], resulting in a tractive force on adjacent open tissue that significantly increases stress in the surrounding normal tissue (Figs. 2.6, 2.7, 4.9, 4.10, and 4.11, Videos 2.1, 4.3, 4.4, and 4.5) [47–49]. These stress multipliers are insidious as they can cause regional excessive strain-induced tissue injury even when the whole lung strain measurement is within the safe range [59, 69–72].

Interactions Between Volutrauma and Atelectrauma

Although volutrauma and atelectrauma are typically considered distinct mechanisms of VILI, they do not act independently, as both overdistension and RACE must be present to injure a normal lung [2]. One potential explanation for this apparent synergy is the excessive parenchymal strain occurring at the interface between collapsed lung and open regions (Fig. 4.9, Video 4.5) [47–49]. While this might explain how volutrauma and atelectrauma act in concert to advance existing damage, it does not clarify why both are required initially to damage a lung that is initially perfectly normal.

A plausible explanation for the initial genesis of injury is provided by the findings of Hamlington et al. [90] in mice injected intravenously with FITC-labelled dextran molecules of different sizes after receiving periods of injurious mechanical ventilation. The relative abundances of the dextran molecules in bronchoalveolar lavage fluid reflected the size distribution of holes in the blood–gas barrier resulting from VILI. It is unclear whether these holes (or barrier disruption) were created predominantly between the epithelial and endothelial cells [91] or through the cell membranes [92]; nevertheless, their size distribution resembled a power law. This was interpreted as evidence that the barrier disruption was generated by a "rich-get-richer" mechanism in which atelectrauma caused initial barrier disruption. Volutrauma exacerbates this initial barrier damage by causing the holes to increase in size, favoring larger over smaller holes [93]. The rich-get-richer theory suggests that if atelectrauma is avoided, robust ventilation of the lung in the pursuit of adequate gas exchange is relatively safe.

Progressive Alveolar Collapse

The VILI Vortex: In the healthy lung, the parenchymal tissue is an interdependent structure in which a fibrous matrix connects alveolar walls to the pleura (Fig. 2.9) [71, 87]. This fibrous skeleton is a tether on small airways to keep them open [85, 88] critical for normal micromechanical function. In the acutely injured lung, the increased permeability of endothelium and epithelium allows plasma-derived fluid and proteins to flood into the alveoli and small airways (Fig. 1.1 Endothelial Leakage & Alveolar Edema), resulting in patchy defects in acinar inflation, reducing interdependence and parenchyma tethering. If applied inappropriately, mechanical ventilation can exacerbate this injury through a synergistic combination of atelectrauma and volutrauma (Figs. 2.6, 2.7, 4.9, 4.10, and 4.11, Videos 2.1, 4.2, 4.3, and 4.4). The synergy arises through a combination of focused damage at sites of stress multipliers, together with diffuse damage arising through a rich-get-richer mechanism in which overdistension builds on initial cell injury caused by RACE.

However, the net result of these complex processes is that the lung gets progressively poorer (more damaged) rather than richer. Marini and Gattinoni describe the progressive collapse of lung tissue in the ARDS patient as a "VILI Vortex" and that this "Shrinking Baby Lung" drives VILI pathogenesis (Fig. 2.4) [94]. The "VILI Vortex" is caused by focal areas of acutely injured lungs manifest as a POOR (Figs. 2.5 and 4.11) [49]. In this sense, the pathogenic mechanisms described above conspire to induce a POOR get POORer scenario in the lung, pushing it further into the VILI vortex that will inevitably lead to respiratory failure unless a protective mechanical ventilation strategy can interrupt this pathogenesis. The cyclic sequence of events involved in the POOR get POORer progression lung pathogenesis is as follows (Fig. 4.1 green box): [49]

1. Alveoli in the normal lung are homogeneously inflated and stabile and thus have no RACE or stress multipliers (Fig. 4.2, Videos 4.1 and 4.2).
2. An initial injurious insult increases endothelial and epithelial permeability, causing local leakage of surfactant-deactivating proteinaceous fluid into the alveoli and airways. Loss of surfactant function leads to regional acinar instability (RACE), collapse, and filling with edema fluid (Fig. 1.1), creating POOR regions of the lung (Figs. 4.9, 4.10, and 4.11, Video 4.5).
3. The POOR regions proliferate, and thus become POORer, by a variety of mechanisms (Fig. 4.11b–d):

   (a) Proteins within the POOR region deactivate surfactant (Fig. 1.1—Surfactant Deactivation), which increases surface tension and the pressure and time needed to re-recruit.
   (b) Gas trapped downstream of obstructed airways becomes absorbed, and surfactant deactivation causes alveoli to collapse, leading to distal atelectasis. Collapsed or edema-filled tissue adjacent to open parenchyma creates a stress multiplier (Fig. 4.9, Video 4.5) that results in damage to the alveolar and alveolar duct epithelial cells during mechanical ventilation (Figs. 4.6 and 4.7), further expanding the POOR regions (Fig. 4.11b–d).
   (c) Tissue damage grows radially outward from the core of POOR areas (Figs. 2.5 and 4.11b–d) distorted alveoli surrounding the POOR area outlined by the dashed line that act as stress multipliers (Fig. 2.7), causing the adjacent normal tissue to become progressively POORer by a mechanism of overdistension and excessive dynamic strain.

4. Without intervention, the initial POOR regions expand rapidly into POORer areas and expand in a power-law fashion until the lung loses all life-sustaining functionality.

Summary. It is currently believed that the mechanisms driving VILI are heterogeneous regional alveolar instability and collapse, causing both atelectrauma and volutrauma to the surrounding normal tissue. The current standard-of-care low V_T Protect the Lung approach does not attempt to address these problems, and thus, it is *constrained* to ventilating a heterogeneous lung without causing VILI. Minimizing regional alveolar collapse, instability, and flooding would eliminate the POOR lesions from which progressive tissue injury spreads (Fig. 2.5). The central goal of the protective ventilation strategy known as the open lung approach (OLA) is to rapidly inflate (over seconds or minutes) the entire lung with a recruitment maneuver and then prevent re-collapse of the newly opened tissue with a titrated PEEP. Multiple randomized controlled trials (RCT) testing various OLA protocols have failed to show significant benefits compared to standard-of-care low-tidal volume ventilation, with some showing an increase in mortality [95–99]. Applied physiology suggests that the OLA should be highly lung protective, yet the RCTs have all failed to improve outcomes. The likely explanation is that rapid lung inflation (over seconds or minutes) followed by increased PEEP does yield durable recruitment and thus does not effectively eliminate atelectrauma and volutrauma. So, what are we missing? In Chap. 3, we discussed the physiologic mechanism of alveolar volume changes is viscoelastic in nature, and thus the *time* of the applied breath at both inspiration and expiration plays a role in recruitment and collapse (Figs. 3.6, 3.7, 5.3, 5.4, 5.6, 5.7, and 5.8, Videos 3.6, 3.7, 5.1, 5.2, and 5.3). More importantly, the acutely injured lung becomes *time*- and *pressure*-dependent, meaning it will take more time for alveoli to open and less time to re-collapse at any given airway pressure. Thus, the "trick" to successfully open and stabilize the acutely injured lung, eliminating the constraints of heterogeneous ventilation, is a longer inspiratory and brief expiratory time. In Chap. 5, we will discuss the role of ventilation time and pressure as mechanisms of alveolar opening and collapse in the acutely injured lung.

References

1. Webb HH, Tierney DF. Experimental pulmonary edema due to intermittent positive pressure ventilation with high inflation pressures. Protection by positive end-expiratory pressure. Am Rev Respir Dis. 1974;110(5):556–65.
2. Seah AS, Grant KA, Aliyeva M, Allen GB, Bates JHT. Quantifying the roles of tidal volume and PEEP in the pathogenesis of ventilator-induced lung injury. Ann Biomed Eng. 2011;39(5):1505–16.
3. Hills BA. The role of lung surfactant. Br J Anaesth. 1990;65(1):13–29. https://doi.org/10.1093/bja/65.1.13.
4. Zheng Y, Fujioka H, Grotberg JB. Effects of gravity, inertia, and surfactant on steady plug propagation in a two-dimensional channel. Phys Fluids. 2007;19(8):082107. https://doi.org/10.1063/1.2762256.
5. Whang J, Faulman C, Itin TA, Gaver DP III. The influence of tethering and gravity on the stability of compliant liquid-lined airways. J Biomech. 2016;50:228. https://doi.org/10.1016/j.jbiomech.2016.11.030.
6. Gattinoni L, Vagginelli F, Chiumello D, Taccone P, Carlesso E. Physiologic rationale for ventilator setting in acute lung injury/acute respiratory distress syndrome patients. Crit Care Med. 2003;31(4 Suppl):S300–4. https://doi.org/10.1097/01.CCM.0000057907.46502.7B.
7. Yamaguchi E, Yao J, Aymond A, et al. Electric cell-substrate impedance sensing (ECIS) as a platform for evaluating barrier-function susceptibility and damage from pulmonary atelectrauma. Biosensors (Basel). 2022;12(6) https://doi.org/10.3390/bios12060390.
8. Ramcharran H, Bates JHT, Satalin J, et al. Protective ventilation in a pig model of acute lung injury: timing is as important as pressure. J Appl Physiol (1985). 2022;133(5):1093–105. https://doi.org/10.1152/japplphysiol.00312.2022.
9. Bachofen H, Schurch S. Alveolar surface forces and lung architecture. Comp Biochem Physiol A Mol Integr Physiol. 2001;129(1):183–93.
10. Knudsen L, Ochs M. The micromechanics of lung alveoli: structure and function of surfactant and tissue components. Histochem Cell Biol. 2018;150(26):661–76. https://doi.org/10.1007/s00418-018-1747-9.
11. Nieman GF, Bredenberg CE. High surface tension pulmonary edema induced by detergent aerosol. J Appl Physiol. 1985;58(1):129–36.
12. Nieman GF. Current concepts of lung-fluid balance. Respir Care. 1985;30(12):1062–76.
13. Bredenberg CE, Paskanik AM, Nieman GF. High surface tension pulmonary edema. J Surg Res. 1983;34(6):515–23.

14. Bredenberg CE, Nieman GF, Paskanik AM, Hart AK. Microvascular membrane permeability in high surface tension pulmonary edema. J Appl Physiol. 1986;60(1):253–9.
15. Mead J. Mechanical properties of lungs. Physiol Rev. 1961;41(2):281–330.
16. Takamoto DY, Lipp MM, von Nahmen A, Lee KY, Waring AJ, Zasadzinski JA. Interaction of lung surfactant proteins with anionic phospholipids. Biophys J. 2001;81(1):153–69.
17. Zasadzinski JA, Ding J, Warriner HE, Bringezu F, Waring AJ. The physics and physiology of lung surfactants. Curr Opin Colloid Interface Sci. 2001;6(5–6):506–13.
18. Zasadzinski JA, Stenger PC, Shieh I, Dhar P. Overcoming rapid inactivation of lung surfactant: analogies between competitive adsorption and colloid stability. Biochim Biophys Acta. 2010;1798(4):801–28. https://doi.org/10.1016/j.bbamem.2009.12.010.
19. Smith JC, Stamenovic D. Surface forces in lungs. I. Alveolar surface tension-lung volume relationships. J Appl Physiol. 1986;60(4):1341–50.
20. Krueger MA, Gaver DP III. A theoretical model of pulmonary surfactant multilayer collapse under oscillating area conditions. J Colloid Interface Sci. 2000;229(2):353–64.
21. Notter RH. Lung surfactants—basic science and clinical applications. In: Lung Biology in Health and Disease, vol. 149. 1st ed. Marcel Dekker; 2000. p. 444.
22. Halpern D, Jensen OE, Grotberg JB. A theoretical study of surfactant and liquid delivery into the lung. J Appl Physiol (1985). 1998;85(1):333–52.
23. Waters SL, Grotberg JB. The propagation of a surfactant laden liquid plug in a capillary tube. Phys Fluids. 2002;14(2):471–80.
24. Grotberg JB, Jensen OE. Biofluid mechanics in flexible tubes. Annu Rev Fluid Mech. 2004;36:121–47. https://doi.org/10.1146/annurev.fluid.36.050802.121918.
25. Bilek AM, Dee KC, Gaver DP 3rd. Mechanisms of surface-tension-induced epithelial cell damage in a model of pulmonary airway reopening. J Appl Physiol (1985). 2003;94(2):770–83. https://doi.org/10.1152/japplphysiol.00764.2002.
26. Kay SS, Bilek AM, Dee KC, Gaver DP. Pressure gradient, not exposure duration, determines the extent of epithelial cell damage in a model of pulmonary airway reopening. J Appl Physiol. 2004;97:269–76.
27. Jacob AM, Gaver DP 3rd. Atelectrauma disrupts pulmonary epithelial barrier integrity and alters the distribution of tight junction proteins ZO-1 and claudin 4. Research support, N.I.H., extramural research support, U.S. Gov't, non-P.H.S. J Appl Physiol. 2012;113(9):1377–87. https://doi.org/10.1152/japplphysiol.01432.2011.
28. Dailey HL, Ricles LM, Yalcin HC, Ghadiali SN. Image-based finite element modeling of alveolar epithelial cell injury during airway reopening. J Appl Physiol. 2009;106(1):221–32. https://doi.org/10.1152/japplphysiol.90688.2008.
29. Yalcin HC, Hallow KM, Wang J, Wei MT, Ou-Yang HD, Ghadiali SN. Influence of cytoskeletal structure and mechanics on epithelial cell injury during cyclic airway reopening. Am J Physiol Lung Cell Mol Physiol. 2009;297(5):L881–91. https://doi.org/10.1152/ajplung.90562.2008.
30. Yalcin HC, Perry SF, Ghadiali SN. Influence of airway diameter and cell confluence on epithelial cell injury in an in-vitro model of airway reopening. J Appl Physiol. 2007;103:1796–807.
31. Gaver DP III, Halpern D, Jensen OE. Surfactant and airway liquid flows. In: Nag K, editor. Molecular mechanisms in lung surfactant (dys)function. Marcel Dekker; 2005. p. 187–223. Lung biology in health and disease.
32. Gaver DP III, Jacob AM, Bilek AM, Dee KC. The significance of air-liquid interfacial stresses on low-volume ventilator-induced lung injury. In: Dreyfuss D, Saumon G, Hubmayr RD, editors. Ventilator-induced lung injury. Taylor & Francis; 2006. p. 157–203. Lung biology in health and disease.
33. Martin D, Jacob AM, Gaver DP III. Surfactant transport and fluid-structure interactions during pulmonary airway reopening. In: Peattie R, Fisher R, Bronzino J, Peterson D, editors. Transport phenomena in biomedical engineering—principles and practices. CRC Press; 2013. p. 1–15; chap 10.

34. Muradoglu M, Romanò F, Fujioka H, Grotberg JB. Effects of surfactant on propagation and rupture of a liquid plug in a tube. J Fluid Mech. 2019;872:407–37. https://doi.org/10.1017/jfm.2019.333.
35. Raghavendran K, Willson D, Notter RH. Surfactant therapy for acute lung injury and acute respiratory distress syndrome. Crit Care Clin. 2011;27(3):525–59. https://doi.org/10.1016/j.ccc.2011.04.005.
36. Kazemi A, Louis B, Isabey D, et al. Surfactant delivery in rat lungs: comparing 3D geometrical simulation model with experimental instillation. PLoS Comput Biol. 2019;15(10):e1007408. https://doi.org/10.1371/journal.pcbi.1007408.
37. Seeger W, Gunther A, Walmrath HD, Grimminger F, Lasch HG. Alveolar surfactant and adult respiratory distress syndrome. Pathogenetic role and therapeutic prospects. Clin Investig. 1993;71(3):177–90. https://doi.org/10.1007/BF00180100.
38. Arold SP, Suki B, Alencar AM, Lutchen KR, Ingenito EP. Variable ventilation induces endogenous surfactant release in normal Guinea pigs. Am J Phys Lung Cell Mol Phys. 2003;285(2):L370–5.
39. Glindmeyer HW 4th, Smith BJ, Gaver DP 3rd. In situ enhancement of pulmonary surfactant function using temporary flow reversal. Research support, N.I.H., extramural research support, U.S. Gov't, non-P.H.S. J Appl Physiol. 2012;112(1):149–58. https://doi.org/10.1152/japplphysiol.00643.2011.
40. Smith BJ, Lukens S, Yamaguchi E, Gaver DP. Lagrangian transport properties of pulmonary interfacial flows. J Fluid Mech. 2012;25(705):234–57.
41. Albert RK. The role of ventilation-induced surfactant dysfunction and atelectasis in causing acute respiratory distress syndrome. Am J Respir Crit Care Med. 2012;185(7):702–8. https://doi.org/10.1164/rccm.201109-1667PP.
42. Gattinoni L, Pesenti A. The concept of "baby lung". Intensive Care Med. 2005;31(6):776–84. https://doi.org/10.1007/s00134-005-2627-z.
43. Gattinoni L, Pesenti A, Avalli L, Rossi F, Bombino M. Pressure-volume curve of total respiratory system in acute respiratory failure. Computed tomographic scan study. Am Rev Respir Dis. 1987;136(3):730–6.
44. Beitler JR, Malhotra A, Thompson BT. Ventilator-induced lung injury. Clin Chest Med. 2016;37(4):633–46. https://doi.org/10.1016/j.ccm.2016.07.004.
45. Acute Respiratory Distress Syndrome N, Brower RG, Matthay MA, et al. Ventilation with lower tidal volumes as compared with traditional tidal volumes for acute lung injury and the acute respiratory distress syndrome. N Engl J Med. 2000;342(18):1301–8. https://doi.org/10.1056/NEJM200005043421801.
46. Bellani G, Guerra L, Musch G, et al. Lung regional metabolic activity and gas volume changes induced by tidal ventilation in patients with acute lung injury. Am J Respir Crit Care Med. 2011;183(9):1193–9. https://doi.org/10.1164/rccm.201008-1318OC.
47. Cereda M, Emami K, Kadlecek S, et al. Quantitative imaging of alveolar recruitment with hyperpolarized gas MRI during mechanical ventilation. J Appl Physiol (1985). 2011;110(2):499–511. https://doi.org/10.1152/japplphysiol.00841.2010.
48. Cereda M, Xin Y, Emami K, et al. Positive end-expiratory pressure increments during anesthesia in normal lung result in hysteresis and greater numbers of smaller aerated airspaces. Anesthesiology. 2013;119(6):1402–9. https://doi.org/10.1097/ALN.0b013e3182a9b0c1yyy.
49. Gaver DP 3rd, Nieman GF, Gatto LA, Cereda M, Habashi NM, Bates JHT. The POOR get POORer: a hypothesis for the pathogenesis of ventilator-induced lung injury. Am J Respir Crit Care Med. 2020;202(8):1081–7. https://doi.org/10.1164/rccm.202002-0453CP.
50. Tschumperlin DJ, Margulies SS. Alveolar epithelial surface area-volume relationship in isolated rat lungs. J Appl Physiol (1985). 1999;86(6):2026–33.
51. Dolinay T, Himes BE, Shumyatcher M, Lawrence GG, Margulies SS. Integrated stress response mediates epithelial injury in mechanical ventilation. Am J Respir Cell Mol Biol. 2017;57(2):193–203. https://doi.org/10.1165/rcmb.2016-0404OC.

52. Protti A, Andreis DT, Monti M, et al. Lung stress and strain during mechanical ventilation: any difference between statics and dynamics? Crit Care Med. 2013;41(4):1046–55. https://doi.org/10.1097/CCM.0b013e31827417a6.
53. Jain SV, Kollisch-Singule M, Satalin J, et al. The role of high airway pressure and dynamic strain on ventilator-induced lung injury in a heterogeneous acute lung injury model. Intensive Care Med Exp. 2017;5(1):25. https://doi.org/10.1186/s40635-017-0138-1.
54. Cressoni M, Chiurazzi C, Gotti M, et al. Lung inhomogeneities and time course of ventilator-induced mechanical injuries. Anesthesiology. 2015;123(3):618–27. https://doi.org/10.1097/ALN.0000000000000727.
55. Cereda M, Xin Y, Hamedani H, et al. Mild loss of lung aeration augments stretch in healthy lung regions. J Appl Physiol (1985). 2016;120(4):444–54. https://doi.org/10.1152/japplphysiol.00734.2015.
56. Wu Y, Kharge AB, Perlman CE. Lung ventilation injures areas with discrete alveolar flooding, in a surface tension-dependent fashion. J Appl Physiol (1985). 2014;117(7):788–96. https://doi.org/10.1152/japplphysiol.00569.2014.
57. Cereda M, Xin Y, Meeder N, et al. Visualizing the propagation of acute lung injury. Anesthesiology. 2016;124(1):121–31. https://doi.org/10.1097/ALN.0000000000000916.
58. Kollisch-Singule M, Emr B, Smith B, et al. Mechanical breath profile of airway pressure release ventilation: the effect on alveolar recruitment and microstrain in acute lung injury. JAMA Surg. 2014;149(11):1138–45. https://doi.org/10.1001/jamasurg.2014.1829.
59. Nieman GF, Gatto LA, Habashi NM. Impact of mechanical ventilation on the pathophysiology of progressive acute lung injury. J Appl Physiol. 2015;119(11):1245–61. https://doi.org/10.1152/japplphysiol.00659.2015.
60. Nieman GF, Satalin J, Andrews P, Aiash H, Habashi NM, Gatto LA. Personalizing mechanical ventilation according to physiologic parameters to stabilize alveoli and minimize ventilator induced lung injury (VILI). Intensive Care Med Exp. 2017;5(1):8. https://doi.org/10.1186/s40635-017-0121-x.
61. Nieman G, Satalin J, Andrews P, et al. Preemptive mechanical ventilation based on dynamic physiology in the alveolar microenvironment: novel considerations of time-dependent properties of the respiratory system. J Trauma Acute Care Surg. 2018;85(6):1081–91. https://doi.org/10.1097/TA.0000000000002050.
62. Nieman GF, Al-Khalisy H, Kollisch-Singule M, et al. A physiologically informed strategy to effectively open, stabilize, and protect the acutely injured lung. Front Physiol. 2020;11:227. https://doi.org/10.3389/fphys.2020.00227.
63. Nieman GF, Gatto LA, Andrews P, et al. Prevention and treatment of acute lung injury with time-controlled adaptive ventilation: physiologically informed modification of airway pressure release ventilation. Ann Intensive Care. 2020;10(1):3. https://doi.org/10.1186/s13613-019-0619-3.
64. Kollisch-Singule M, Satalin J, Blair SJ, et al. Mechanical ventilation lessons learned from alveolar micromechanics. Front Physiol. 2020;11:233. https://doi.org/10.3389/fphys.2020.00233.
65. Cereda M, Xin Y. Alveolar recruitment and lung injury: an issue of timing and location? Comment editorial research support, non-U.S. Gov't. Crit Care Med. 2013;41(12):2837–8. https://doi.org/10.1097/CCM.0b013e31829cb083.
66. Cereda M, Emami K, Xin Y, et al. Imaging the interaction of atelectasis and overdistension in surfactant-depleted lungs. Crit Care Med. 2013;41(2):527–35. https://doi.org/10.1097/CCM.0b013e31826ab1f2.
67. Kollisch-Singule M, Emr B, Smith B, et al. Airway pressure release ventilation reduces conducting airway micro-strain in lung injury. J Am Coll Surg. 2014;219(5):968–76. https://doi.org/10.1016/j.jamcollsurg.2014.09.011.
68. Koniukhov SG. Results of combined treatment of patients with acute thrombosis of the major deep veins of the lower extremities and pelvis (Rezul'taty kombinirovannogo lecheniia

bol'nykh ostrym trombozom glubokikh magistral'nykh ven nizhnikh konechnostei i taza). Vestn Khir Im I I Grek. 1972;108(6):81–5.
69. Makiyama AM, Gibson LJ, Harris RS, Venegas JG. Stress concentration around an atelectatic region: a finite element model. Respir Physiol Neurobiol. 2014;201:101–10. https://doi.org/10.1016/j.resp.2014.06.017.
70. Knudsen L, Lopez-Rodriguez E, Berndt L, et al. Alveolar micromechanics in bleomycin-induced lung injury. Am J Respir Cell Mol Biol. 2018;59(6):757–69. https://doi.org/10.1165/rcmb.2018-0044OC.
71. Mead J, Takishima T, Leith D. Stress distribution in lungs: a model of pulmonary elasticity. J Appl Physiol. 1970;28(5):596–608.
72. Grasso S, Stripoli T, Sacchi M, et al. Inhomogeneity of lung parenchyma during the open lung strategy: a computed tomography scan study. Am J Respir Crit Care Med. 2009;180(5):415–23. https://doi.org/10.1164/rccm.200901-0156OC.
73. Emami K, Chia E, Kadlecek S, et al. Regional correlation of emphysematous changes in lung function and structure: a comparison between pulmonary function testing and hyperpolarized MRI metrics. J Appl Physiol (1985). 2011;110(1):225–35. https://doi.org/10.1152/japplphysiol.00269.2010.
74. Gattinoni L, Mascheroni D, Torresin A, et al. Morphological response to positive end expiratory pressure in acute respiratory failure. Computerized tomography study. Intensive Care Med. 1986;12(3):137–42.
75. Gattinoni L, Presenti A, Torresin A, et al. Adult respiratory distress syndrome profiles by computed tomography. J Thorac Imaging. 1986;1(3):25–30.
76. Pelosi P, D'Andrea L, Vitale G, Pesenti A, Gattinoni L. Vertical gradient of regional lung inflation in adult respiratory distress syndrome. Am J Respir Crit Care Med. 1994;149(1):8–13. https://doi.org/10.1164/ajrccm.149.1.8111603.
77. Retamal J, Bergamini BC, Carvalho AR, et al. Non-lobar atelectasis generates inflammation and structural alveolar injury in the surrounding healthy tissue during mechanical ventilation. Crit Care. 2014;18(5):505. https://doi.org/10.1186/s13054-014-0505-1.
78. Cressoni M, Chiumello D, Chiurazzi C, et al. Lung inhomogeneities, inflation and [18F]2-fluoro-2-deoxy-D-glucose uptake rate in acute respiratory distress syndrome. Eur Respir J. 2016;47(1):233–42. https://doi.org/10.1183/13993003.00885-2015.
79. Motta-Ribeiro GC, Hashimoto S, Winkler T, et al. Deterioration of regional lung strain and inflammation during early lung injury. Am J Respir Crit Care Med. 2018;198(7):891–902. https://doi.org/10.1164/rccm.201710-2038OC.
80. Borges JB, Costa EL, Bergquist M, et al. Lung inflammation persists after 27 hours of protective acute respiratory distress syndrome network strategy and is concentrated in the nondependent lung. Crit Care Med. 2015;43(5):e123–32. https://doi.org/10.1097/CCM.0000000000000926.
81. Xin Y, Cereda M, Hamedani H, et al. Unstable inflation causing injury. Insight from prone position and paired computed tomography scans. Am J Respir Crit Care Med. 2018;198(2):197–207. https://doi.org/10.1164/rccm.201708-1728OC.
82. Cereda M, Xin Y, Hamedani H, et al. Tidal changes on CT and progression of ARDS. Thorax. 2017;72(11):981–9. https://doi.org/10.1136/thoraxjnl-2016-209833.
83. Steinberg JM, Schiller HJ, Halter JM, et al. Alveolar instability causes early ventilator-induced lung injury independent of neutrophils. Am J Respir Crit Care Med. 2004;169(1):57–63. https://doi.org/10.1164/rccm.200304-544OC.
84. Ghadiali SN, Gaver DP. Biomechanics of liquid-epithelium interactions in pulmonary airways. Respir Physiol Neurobiol. 2008;163(1–3):232–43. https://doi.org/10.1016/j.resp.2008.04.008.
85. Fujioka H, Halpern D, Gaver DP 3rd. A model of surfactant-induced surface tension effects on the parenchymal tethering of pulmonary airways. J Biomech. 2013;46(2):319–28. https://doi.org/10.1016/j.jbiomech.2012.11.031.

86. Hsia CC, Hyde DM, Weibel ER. Lung structure and the intrinsic challenges of gas exchange. Compr Physiol. 2016;6(2):827–95. https://doi.org/10.1002/cphy.c150028.
87. Paré PD, Mitzner W. Airway-parenchymal interdependence. Compr Physiol. 2012;2:1921–35.
88. Ryans JM, Fujioka H, Gaver DP 3rd. Microscale to mesoscale analysis of parenchymal tethering: the effect of heterogeneous alveolar pressures on the pulmonary mechanics of compliant airways. J Appl Physiol (1985). 2019;126(5):1204–13. https://doi.org/10.1152/japplphysiol.00178.2018.
89. Suki B, Stamenovic D, Hubmayr R. Lung parenchymal mechanics. Compr Physiol. 2011;1(3):1317–51. https://doi.org/10.1002/cphy.c100033.
90. Hamlington KL, Bates JHT, Roy GS, et al. Alveolar leak develops by a rich-get-richer process in ventilator-induced lung injury. PLoS One. 2018;13(3):e0193934. https://doi.org/10.1371/journal.pone.0193934.
91. Hamlington KL, Ma B, Smith BJ, Bates JH. Modeling the progression of epithelial leak caused by overdistension. Cell Mol Bioeng. 2016;9(1):151–61. https://doi.org/10.1007/s12195-015-0426-3.
92. Hamlington KL, Smith BJ, Dunn CM, Charlebois CM, Roy GS, Bates JHT. Linking lung function to structural damage of alveolar epithelium in ventilator-induced lung injury. Respir Physiol Neurobiol. 2018;255:22–9. https://doi.org/10.1016/j.resp.2018.05.004.
93. Mori V, Smith BJ, Suki B, Bates JHT. Linking physiological biomarkers of ventilator-induced lung injury to a rich-get-richer mechanism of injury progression. Ann Biomed Eng. 2019;47(2):638–45. https://doi.org/10.1007/s10439-018-02165-1.
94. Marini JJ, Gattinoni L. Time course of evolving ventilator-induced lung injury: the "shrinking baby lung". Crit Care Med. 2020;48(8):1203–9. https://doi.org/10.1097/CCM.0000000000004416.
95. Brower RG, Lanken PN, MacIntyre N, et al. Higher versus lower positive end-expiratory pressures in patients with the acute respiratory distress syndrome. Clinical trial comparative study multicenter study randomized controlled trial research support, U.S. Gov't, P.H.S. N Engl J Med. 2004;351(4):327–36. https://doi.org/10.1056/NEJMoa032193.
96. Meade MO, Cook DJ, Guyatt GH, et al. Ventilation strategy using low tidal volumes, recruitment maneuvers, and high positive end-expiratory pressure for acute lung injury and acute respiratory distress syndrome: a randomized controlled trial. JAMA. 2008;299(6):637–45. https://doi.org/10.1001/jama.299.6.637.
97. Mercat A, Richard JC, Vielle B, et al. Positive end-expiratory pressure setting in adults with acute lung injury and acute respiratory distress syndrome: a randomized controlled trial. Comparative study multicenter study randomized controlled trial research support, non--U.S. Gov't. JAMA. 2008;299(6):646–55. https://doi.org/10.1001/jama.299.6.646.
98. Writing Group for the Alveolar Recruitment for Acute Respiratory Distress Syndrome Trial I, Cavalcanti AB, Suzumura EA, et al. Effect of lung recruitment and titrated positive end-expiratory pressure (PEEP) vs low PEEP on mortality in patients with acute respiratory distress syndrome: a randomized clinical trial. JAMA. 2017;318(14):1335–45. https://doi.org/10.1001/jama.2017.14171.
99. Hodgson CL, Cooper DJ, Arabi Y, et al. Maximal recruitment open lung ventilation in acute respiratory distress syndrome (PHARLAP): a phase II, multicenter, randomized, controlled trial. Am J Respir Crit Care Med. 2019;200:1363. https://doi.org/10.1164/rccm.201901-0109OC.
100. Nieman GF, Satalin J, Kollisch-Singule M, et al. Physiology in medicine: understanding dynamic alveolar physiology to minimize ventilator-induced lung injury. J Appl Physiol (1985). 2017;122(6):1516–22. https://doi.org/10.1152/japplphysiol.00123.2017.

Chapter 5
The Acutely Injured Lung Becomes Time/Press Dependent

Introduction

The time and pressure necessary to open or prevent re-collapse of viscoelastic lung tissue are not static but dependent upon the level of surfactant function and the degree of mechanical interdependence combined with parenchymal tethering on the walls of small airways. In the acutely injured lung, the loss of stabilizing factors discussed in Chap. 4 renders the lung *time-* and *pressure-dependent* (Fig. 5.1, green box). This means it will take more time for the alveoli to open and less time for them to collapse at any given airway pressure. It has been shown that repetitive alveolar collapse and expansion (RACE) can occur within the same time frame in adjacent airspace connected to the same terminal airway [1]. Excessive shear or "peeling" stress would impact endothelial cells without a protective ventilation strategy as the collapsed alveolar walls separate with each breath (Fig. 4.6). The collapsed or edema-filled tissue generates stress multipliers that will damage the normal surrounding tissue by excessive dynamic strain and overdistension (Figs. 2.6, 2.7, 4.3, 4.9, 4.10, and 4.11, Videos 4.4 and 4.5). Since acinar opening and collapse are time-dependent, adjusting ventilator inspiratory and expiratory time may be effective at opening and stabilizing the acutely injured lung.

Role of inspiratory and expiratory time and pressure on lung opening and stability. The distending force that inflates the lung is airway pressure. As discussed in Chap. 3, the lung changes volume in response to the distending force as a viscoelastic system. Using the spring and dashpot model to show the impact of an extended inspiratory time, we see a slow progressive movement of the dash in the pot without increasing the distending force, known as creep (Figs. 3.6 Viscoelastic Behavior–Lung Recruitment, Fig. 3.7, Video 3.6).

Supplementary Information The online version contains supplementary material available at https://doi.org/10.1007/978-3-031-66352-9_5.

© The Author(s), under exclusive license to Springer Nature Switzerland AG 2024

G. F. Nieman, N. M. Habashi, *Applied Physiology to Reduce Ventilator Induced Lung Injury*, https://doi.org/10.1007/978-3-031-66352-9_5

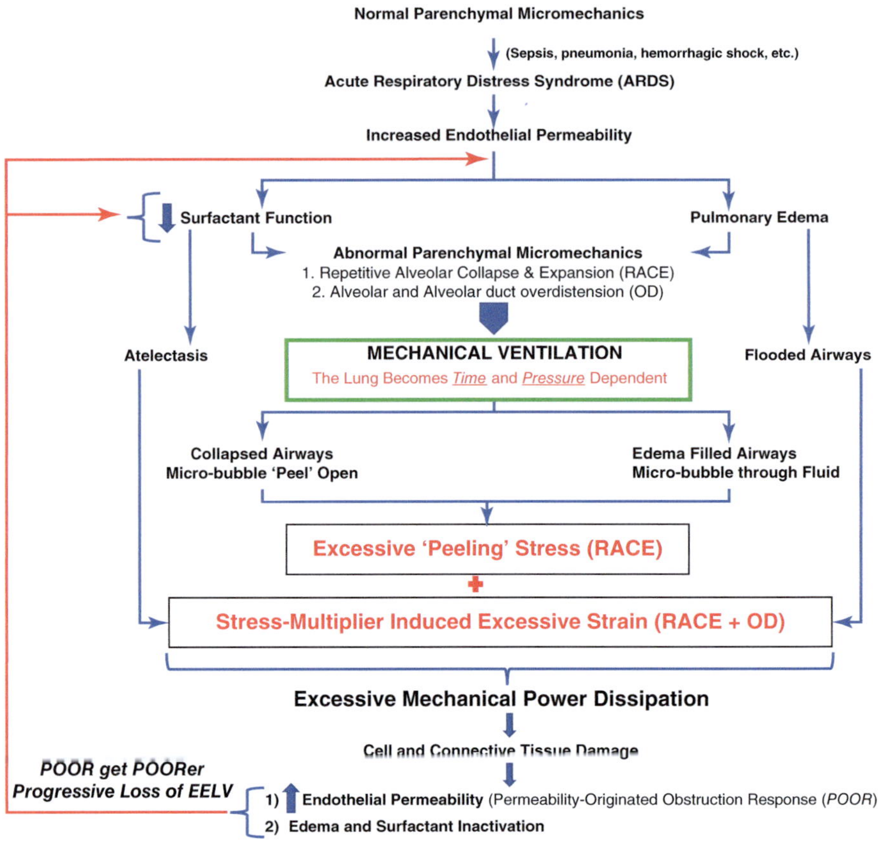

Fig. 5.1 The unifying hypothesis of how acute respiratory distress syndrome (ARDS) pathophysiology predisposes the lung to a secondary ventilator-induced lung injury (VILI). This chapter discusses how ARDS renders the lung *Time*- and *Pressure*-dependent (green box). This means it will take more time to open the collapsed lung and less time for it to re-collapse at any given airway pressure. Applied physiology suggests that an extended inspiratory and brief expiratory time would stabilize and then gradually reopen lung tissue that has become time and pressure-dependent

Boehme et al. utilized an ultrafast indwelling oxygen-sensing probe (UFIOP) in a piglet saline lavage acute respiratory distress syndrome (ARDS) model. They measured breath-to-breath changes in arterial partial pressure of oxygen (PaO_2), denoted as ΔPaO2, to evaluate dynamic repetitive alveolar collapse and expansion (RACE) [2]. Additionally, the researchers systematically altered airway pressure, observing dynamic changes in the partial pressure of oxygen (PO_2) to calculate recruitment and derecruitment time constants (TAU). They found that RACE does not occur in the normal lung but significantly increases following acute lung injury, especially with an Inspiratory:Expiratory (I:E) ratio of 1:4 that extends the expiratory time.

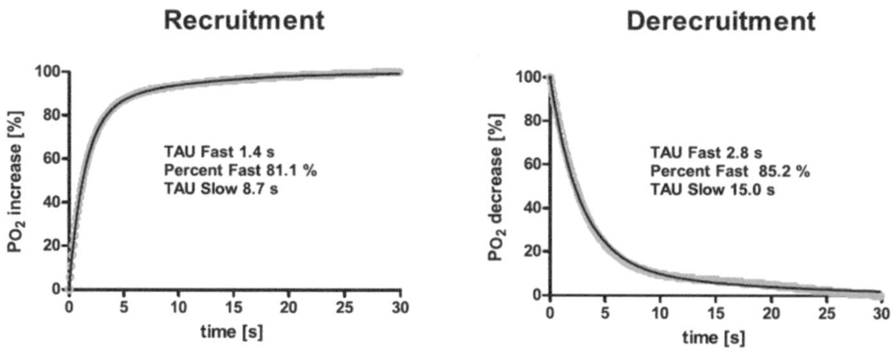

Fig. 5.2 Recruitment and derecruitment time constants (TAU) assessment using a PO_2/Time curve with the corresponding two-phase exponential model fit (dark line) in a porcine surfactant washout ARDS model. TAU for recruitment and derecruitment measured by multifrequency phase fluorimetry [2]

A two-phase (Fast and Slow) exponential model fit was best for analyzing TAU in the acutely injured lung (Fig. 5.2) [2]. They also found that recruitment TAU was much faster (fast 1.6 s, 78%; slow 9.2 s) than derecruitment (fast 3.1 s, 87%; slow 17.7 s) and that inverse ratio ventilation (IRV) of 4:1 (i.e., short expiratory time) significantly reduced RACE. Based on the time constants for dynamic cyclic recruitment and derecruitment (RACE), they concluded that a short expiratory time using IRV 4:1 can significantly reduce RACE, the primary mechanism of atelectrauma. Note the similarity between the inspiratory and expiratory TAU curves (Fig. 5.2) and the curve generated by a viscoelastic increase or decrease in volume (Fig. 3.6 Viscoelastic Behavior—Lung Recruitment—Lung Derecruitment).

Ma and Bates developed a computational model centered on symmetrical airway bifurcations to simulate alveolar collapse and re-opening dynamics. In this model, each branch possessed distinct critical pressures for collapse and re-opening [3]. Subsequently, they enhanced the model by incorporating alveolar interdependence, where adjacent alveoli's state (open or collapsed) influenced the critical opening and collapse pressures for each airway field [1]. This computational model was designed to replicate data obtained through synchrotron phase-contrast imaging, offering direct visualization of the time-dependent regional opening and re-collapse of acini and terminal airways [1]. Their study concluded that RACE over short time scales results from the intricate interactions between the time constants associated with alveolar opening and collapse, coupled with the mechanical interdependence among alveoli that share walls. This model provides valuable insights into the complex dynamics governing the behavior of alveoli and their impact on lung function.

In a rat model of acute respiratory distress syndrome (ARDS), varying airway pressures of 20, 30, or 40 cmH_2O were applied and maintained for 40 s, with measurements taken of both subpleural alveoli observed through in vivo microscopy and whole recruitment (Fig. 5.3) [4]. Utilizing in vivo microscopy allowed for the direct real-time measurement of alveolar opening following an increase in airway

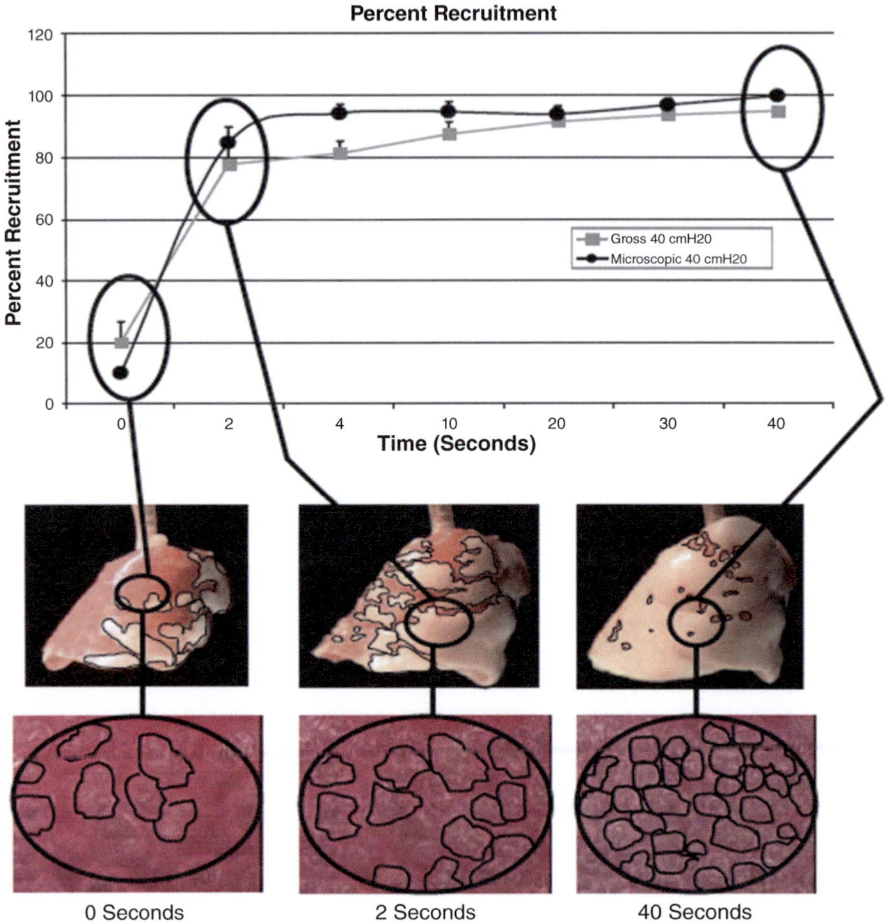

Fig. 5.3 The impact of inspiratory time on subpleural alveolar and whole lung recruitment. **The bottom panel** shows individual subpleural alveoli (black circles) and the entire lung before airway pressure is applied (0 Time–Seconds) and at 2 and 40 s after applying 40 cmH_2O pressure. The **top panel** is the graph depicting the percent of the microscopic field covered by inflated alveoli (black circles and line) or the percent of the lung surface with open lung tissue (gray square and line). Note that 40 cmH_2O was applied at T0 and held until T40; there was no increase in airway pressure over time. Rapid recruitment of lung tissue and alveoli occurred over the first 2 s of applied pressure and then gradual, continual recruitment over the entire 40 s without an increase in airway pressure [28]

pressure (Fig. 5.3). The study showed a two-second delay after applying airway pressure before alveoli or lung tissue initiated opening. This was followed by a rapid recruitment phase lasting 2 s, with continued gradual recruitment occurring over the subsequent 38 seconds (Fig. 5.3). A computational model supported the observation of continuous alveolar recruitment over an extended period without additional increases in airway pressure, a phenomenon known as creep (Fig. 3.7) [4].

The clinical significance of the two-second delay in alveolar opening is noteworthy, especially considering that the inspiratory time in conventional ventilator settings typically ranges from 0.5 to 1.0 s. This duration may not be sufficient for alveoli to fully recruit with each inspiration. Video 5.1 illustrates the impact of extending the inspiratory time from 1.0 s, typical of a conventional breath, to 5.0 s, representing the inspiratory time in Airway Pressure Release Ventilation (APRV) mode. Notably, continual recruitment is observed (depicted by dark red collapsed tissue turning pink when recruited) over the 5-s inspiratory hold without any increase in airway pressure (Fig. 3.7). Other studies have demonstrated a temporal lag in alveolar recruitment and collapse, supporting the above findings. Importantly, it's emphasized that not only is lung recruitment temporal but so is the chest wall, making the entire respiratory system time-dependent [5–7].

Dynamic alveolar inflation and deflation in the acutely injured lung involve a complex interplay of mechanical interactions between adjacent alveoli, surfactant function loss, and modifications in opening and collapse time constants. This results in the lung becoming time- and pressure-dependent [1, 8]. The closing pressure required for alveoli and small airways to collapse is influenced by the duration and intensity of these pressures, as indicated by fluid movement in the microenvironment [9].

In a rat ARDS model using conventional mechanical ventilation with V_T 6 cc/kg and PEEP 5 cmH_2O combined with a very short inspiratory and extended expiratory time, lung tissue and alveoli recruit during inspiration but re-collapse during expiration. Notably, the "baby lung" tissue on the outer edge of the acutely injured lung does not appear to be over-distending. Instead, the volume change is attributed to recruiting collapse (dark red) alveoli that re-collapse during expiration (Video 4.3) [10]. In contrast, the APRV mode with extended inspiratory and brief expiratory times results in homogenous ventilation without RACE (Video 5.3). These data support using inspiratory time to recruit and expiratory time to prevent re-collapse as an effective ventilatory method to maintain homogeneous ventilation and minimize RACE [10].

A rabbit ARDS model study investigated RACE prevention through expiratory time and pressure. Groups with high positive end-expiratory pressure (PEEP) and a prolonged expiratory time and those with low PEEP but a brief expiratory duration effectively stabilized alveoli. Despite having low PEEP and a short expiratory time, the latter group prevented cyclical recruitment and atelectasis as effectively as the high PEEP group without generating intrinsic PEEP (iPEEP). Moreover, decreasing expiratory duration improved cardiac output, systolic blood pressure, and mixed venous saturation compared to the high PEEP group. This suggests that a mechanism other than iPEEP, possibly an extremely short expiratory duration preventing alveolar collapse, plays a role in dynamic alveolar mechanics and atelectasis [11].

Neumann et al. demonstrated that an expiratory time <0.6 s would prevent RACE without extrinsic PEEP in three porcine ARDS models [12], supporting the Syring et al. study [11]. Lung opening was faster than collapse in all models, indicating that equal inspiratory and expiratory times (1:1) lead to progressive atelectasis with each breath. The oleic acid and endotoxin groups experienced a more rapid collapse, with

60%–70% occurring within 4 s, while the saline lavage group exhibited a 30% collapse. The differing rates of collapse suggest that factors beyond surfactant loss contribute to lung collapse, as seen in models with endothelial cell damage and high permeability pulmonary edema [6].

This group also demonstrated that achieving lung opening and stabilization in a porcine oleic acid ARDS model required specific combinations of parameters: (1) A plateau pressure (Pplat) >40 cmH_2O + PEEP >20 cmH_2O + an expiratory duration of 4.0 s or (2) Pplat >40 cmH_2O + PEEP <15 cmH_2O + an expiratory duration of less than 0.6 s was found to be necessary [5]. Longer inspiratory times with inverse ratio ventilation (IRV) did not significantly enhance lung recruitment. Atelectasis increased rapidly after a 0.6-s delay with PEEP levels of 10 and 15 cmH_2O, but stabilizing the lung during the 4 s of expiration was achieved with a PEEP of 20 cmH_2O.

However, the use of high PEEP was associated with increased volutrauma and hemodynamic impairment. The time constant for atelectasis remained consistent at 0.86 ± 0.67 s, regardless of the PEEP level, while the inspiratory time constant was 0.69 ± 0.54 s, with recruitment reaching 85% completion in 1.4 s. Unlike expiration, there was no delay period, highlighting the asymmetry between recruitment and re-collapse. Although the recruiting pressure was 15 cmH_2O above PEEP, atelectasis did not completely resolve even with a Pplat exceeding 40 cmH_2O [5]. These findings contrasted with a study by Albert et al., which observed a ~2-s delay in alveolar recruitment following an applied airway pressure, followed by a short burst of rapid recruitment and then continual gradual recruitment over the entire 40-s study period [4].

In a third study by the same group, IRV was compared with an inspiratory-to-expiratory (I:E) ratio of 3:1 without PEEP and conventional ventilation with an I:E ratio of 1:2 and 20 cmH_2O PEEP. The IRV group had inspiratory and expiratory times of 1.5 and 0.5 s, respectively. Interestingly, the conventional ventilation group exhibited a similar ability to stabilize the lung as the IRV group, with improved oxygenation and better-matched ventilation/perfusion (V/Q). Both groups utilized inspiratory pressure of 40 cmH_2O and tidal volumes of 12–15 mL/kg, values believed to be sufficiently high to cause volutrauma and atelectrauma. However, these parameters limit the clinical extrapolation of the study's findings, concluding that IRV did not offer advantages in lung stabilization compared to conventional ventilation [12]. Overall, the studies by Neumann presented mixed results regarding the effectiveness of time versus pressure in lung opening and stabilization [5].

Our group used a rat surfactant deactivation lung injury model with ventilation modes and settings identical to those in a previous study [13]. The objective was to assess the impact of inspiratory and expiratory airway time and pressure on subpleural alveolar opening and collapse, measured in real time using in vivo microscopy (Fig. 5.4) [14]. Two ventilation modes were compared: volume control ventilation (VCV) with a short inspiratory and long expiratory time, incorporating two levels of PEEP, and APRV with an extended time at inspiration and either very brief or extended expiratory time, generating two levels of time-controlled PEEP (TC-PEEP). Alveoli were color-coded yellow through computer image analysis,

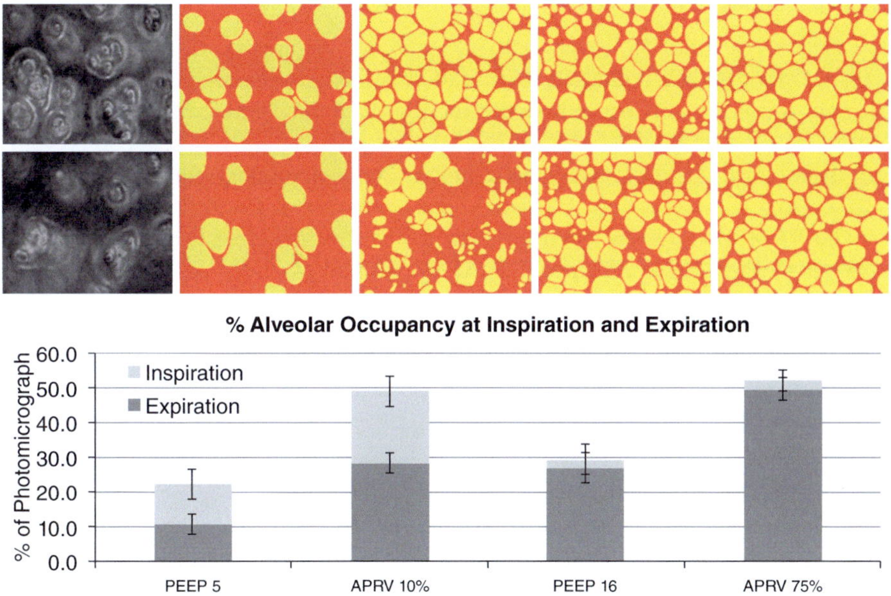

Fig. 5.4 Assessment of subpleural dynamic alveolar inflation and deflation using an in vivo microscope in a rat surfactant deactivation ARDS model using different combinations of end-expiratory pressure and inspiratory and expiratory. The inspiratory time was prolonged in both airway pressure release ventilation (APRV) groups. The expiratory time was adjusted to be brief (APRV 75%) or extended (APRV 10%). The termination of expiratory flow (T_{EF}), which determines the expiratory time, was identified by multiplying the peak expiratory flow (P_{EF}) by either 75% or 10% (P_{EF} L/min × 75% or P_{EF} × 10% = T_{EF} L/min) with the low pressure (P_{Low}) set to zero (see Chap. 8 for details) [17]. The volume-controlled (VCV) mode used either a positive end-expiratory pressure (PEEP) of 5 (PEEP 5) or 16 cmH_2O (PEEP 16). The inspiratory time was short, and a low tidal volume (6 cc/kg) was used. **TOP Panel**: Subpleural alveoli at Inspiration and Expiration in black and white as seen with the in vivo microscope. Alveoli were color-coded yellow by computer image analysis, with the red being areas of atelectasis. **BOTTOM Panel**: The bar graph shows the percent of the microscopic field covered by inflated alveoli (% of photomicrograph) at Inspiration (light gray) and Expiration (dark gray). The difference between the light and dark bar would be a measure of repetitive alveolar collapse and expansion (RACE). The extended inspiratory time recruited a similar number of alveoli in both APRV groups (~50% of photomicrograph). The VCV mode, even with PEEP 16, only recruited ~30% of the microscopic field. Only the APRV 75% group recruited many alveoli, preventing them from re-collapsing during expiration [14]

and the assessment focused on the percent surface area of the photomicrograph occupied by inflated alveoli (% of Photomicrograph). The amount of RACE was determined by the number of alveoli inflated at inspiration (light gray bar) and expiration (dark gray bar). (Fig. 5.4).

In the VCV mode, employing a standard inspiratory time and an extended expiratory time at a PEEP of 5 cmH_2O, there was no recruitment of alveoli at inspiration, and re-collapse at expiration occurred, resulting in a significant amount of RACE (difference between the light and dark gray bars) (Fig. 5.4). Increasing PEEP to 16 cmH_2O slightly improved recruitment and significantly reduced RACE.

Both APRV groups, with a long inspiratory time, recruited alveoli irrespective of the expiratory time. However, with an extended expiratory time (APRV 10%, ~1.0 s), many alveoli collapsed at expiration, leading to the highest RACE among all groups (i.e. the difference between the light and dark gray bars). Conversely, a very brief expiratory time (APRV 75%, ~0.15 s) proved highly effective in preventing alveolar collapse compared to a much longer expiratory time (APRV 10%, ~1.0 s) (Fig. 5.4).

The VCV mode, even when utilizing a PEEP of 16 cmH_2O, did not achieve alveolar recruitment as effectively as APRV with an extended inspiratory time, as illustrated in the bar graph of Fig. 5.4. Higher PEEP levels contributed to the stabilization of alveoli and a reduction in RACE, which was measured as the difference between light and dark gray bars. Notably, APRV 75% caused both alveolar stabilization and recruitment, as indicated in the bar graph of Fig. 5.4. Conversely, APRV 10% exhibited alveolar recruitment with the extended expiratory time, but this allowed the newly opened alveoli to re-collapse during expiration, resulting in a substantial amount of RACE.

In another study, the long inspiratory and very short expiratory duration was shown to maintain a homogeneous population of alveoli like that in a normal lung, whereas extending the expiratory duration resulted in a heterogeneous population of alveolar sizes and a significant collapse of alveoli with each breath [15]. These studies show by direct visualization that inspiratory time can be used to gradually 'ratchet' open collapsed lung tissue, and a very brief expiratory time, adjusted to changes in respiratory system compliance, will quickly stabilize alveoli.

Current experiments investigating the role of expiratory time and pressure on alveolar stabilization: Our group is actively investigating the impact of expiratory time and pressure on alveolar stabilization [16]. Using the APRV mode, if the expiratory time is sufficiently short, the lung does not have sufficient time to depressurize fully, maintaining a time-controlled PEEP (TC-PEEP). Our ongoing study is testing if the very brief expiratory time or the TC-PEEP it creates are the critical factors in stabilizing alveoli. The study involves a comparison between two groups of rats utilizing the APRV mode: (1) a TC-PEEP group that uses a very brief expiratory time (<0.5 seconds) and (2) a Set-PEEP group with PEEP adjusted to match the TC-PEEP level with a conventional expiratory time of 2.0 s. In this crossover study, he measured derecruitment of the same alveoli at the same level of PEEP but with a short and long expiratory time.

In this crossover study, we aim to measure derecruitment of the same alveoli at the same level of PEEP but with varying expiratory times. The experimental procedure involves anesthetizing rats ($n = 4$), surgically instrumenting them for vascular access, placing them on mechanical ventilation using the APRV mode, and opening the chest to expose the lung surface. Lung injury is induced by Tween-induced surfactant deactivation. An in vivo microscope is positioned on the lung surface, and dynamic subpleural mechanics is recorded in real time using a high-speed camera (Basler Aca1920 155fps). Images are exported every 0.007 s during expiration (Fig. 5.5).

To determine alveolar area at expiration, still images from all fields at end-expiration are exported from the video recordings. These images are then processed

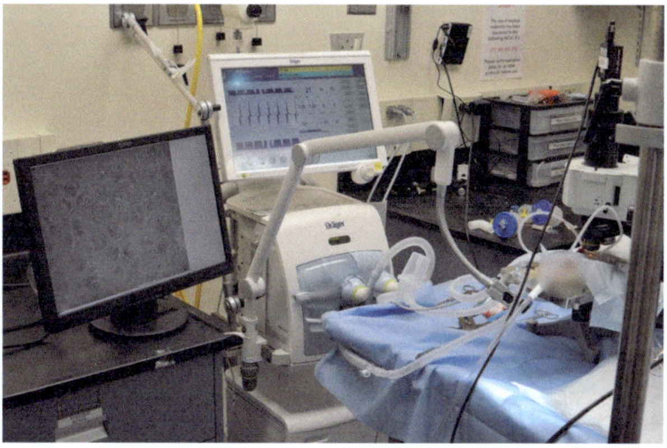

Fig. 5.5 Laboratory setup with a mechanical ventilator, a rat with the *in vivo* microscope on the lung surface, and the computer monitor capturing the chances in alveolar size during inspiration and expiration in real time

using Adobe Photoshop (CS6), where alveoli are delineated, and areas are filled in using computer image analysis. Different colors correspond to individual alveoli. Subsequently, these images are imported into ImagePro (MediaCybernetics) and configured to calculate the area per field based on the chosen color. This meticulous approach allows us to gather detailed insights into the dynamics of alveolar stabilization under varying expiratory times and pressures.

Images were captured from the end of inspiration to the end of expiration or until the alveolus completely collapsed. The alveolar area was then calculated based on the described method. The resolution for all recordings was standardized at 1920 × 1200 (2,304,000 pixels). The total alveolar surface area change within the microscopic field was quantified as a percentage (%) in alveolar area (pixels) from peak inspiration to end-expiration.

Two groups were studied: the TC-PEEP group, which used the Time-Controlled Adaptive Ventilation (TCAV) method to set the expiratory time. The termination of expiratory flow (T_{EF}) was determined by multiplying the peak expiratory flow (P_{EF}) by 75% (P_{EF} L/min × 75% = T_{EF} L/min) with the low pressure (P_{Low}) set to zero [17]. The very brief expiratory duration or T_{Low} (0.08 ± 0.03 s) using this method was insufficient for the lung to depressurize, generating a TC-PEEP. Alveolar collapse was always filmed in the TC-PEEP group first, and the PEEP level was recorded. **Set-PEEP group**: The P_{Low} was set to the TC-PEEP level measured during the first expiration, the T_{Low} increased to 2.0 s, and the collapse of the same alveolus was once again filmed. Thus, the same alveoli were filmed during exhalation with the same level of PEEP; the only difference was the expiratory time. See Chap. 8 for details on setting APRV using the TCAV method.

The same subpleural alveolus circled in both groups is seen in Frame-1 before the beginning of exhalation (Fig. 5.6). The alveolus was color-coded by computer image analysis. A frame-by-frame (150 frames/s) analysis of alveolar collapse was assessed for the entire expiratory phase. In the TC-PEEP group, there was only a slight decrease in alveolar size over the 9-frame exhalation phase during the brief Release Phase.

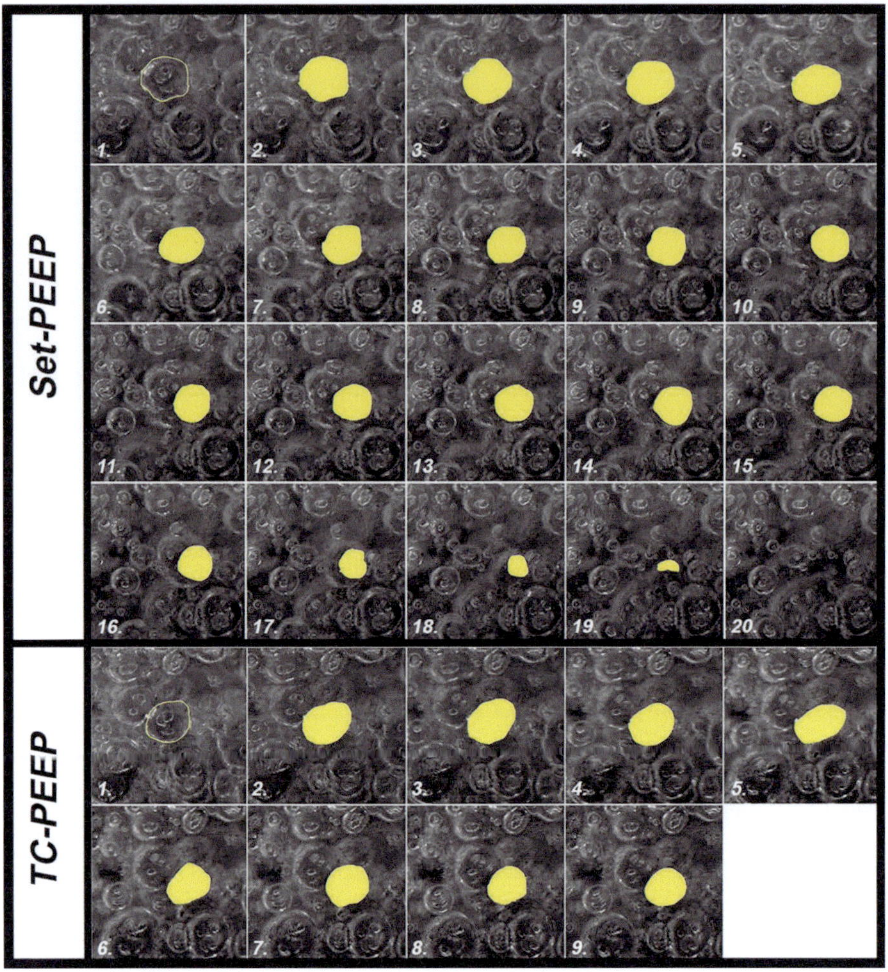

Fig. 5.6 (A) **TC-PEEP group:** The very brief expiratory duration (T_{Low}, 0.08 ± 0.03 s) was not sufficient time for the lung to depressurize, generating a Time-controlled PEEP (TC-PEEP). The amount of TC-PEEP was measured, the alveolar collapse was recorded, and the lung was reinflated. **Set-PEEP group**: The PEEP (P_{Low}) was set to match the TC-PEEP level, and the expiratory time (T_{Low}) increased to 2.0 s. The collapse of the same alveoli measured in the TC-PEEP group was filmed again. Thus, PEEP was identical in both groups, the only difference being expiratory time. A single subpleural alveolus is circled in frame 1 before the beginning of exhalation. Frame-by-frame analysis (150 frames/s) of the alveolar collapse was assessed for the entire expiratory phase. Only a slight decrease in alveolar size was seen in the 9-frames in the TC-PEEP group. In the Set-PEEP group, the alveolus has a significant volume loss at frame-16 followed by a rapid volume loss with complete collapse by frame-20

There was no significant difference in the initial expiratory alveolar collapse rate between groups with identical levels of Set- vs. TC-PEEP (Fig. 5.6 Frames 1–9). However, alveoli in the Set-PEEP group continued to collapse over the 2-s expiratory time (T_{Low}) (Fig. 5.6 Set-PEEP Frames 10–20, Video 5.2). In contrast, there was a significant loss of alveolar volume in frame-16 followed by a rapid derecruitment with a complete collapse by frame-20 in the Set-PEEP group with an extended expiratory duration. A higher-power photomicrograph shows the same alveoli color-coded yellow. Six of the seven alveoli did not collapse at end-expiration, but one alveolus (*) collapsed in the Set-PEEP group and did not collapse in the TC-PEEP group (Fig. 5.7b). The change in airway pressure and two individual alveolar areas over time during expiration with Set- versus TC-PEEP (Fig. 5.7a, b). In the Set-PEEP group, both alveoli continued to collapse over time (Figs. 3.6 Viscoelastic Behavior Expiration, 5.2 Derecruitment).

Figure 5.7 compares the decay in end-expiratory pressure and time with the collapse of a single alveolus (**a**) and a cluster of alveoli within the in vivo microscopic field (**b**) using Set- and TC-PEEP. The average loss of alveolar volume in all four rats during one expiration using Set- versus TC-PEEP is shown in Fig. 5.7c. The average percent change (%) in alveolar area (Pixels) at expiration was significantly higher in the TC-PEEP group vs. the Set-PEEP group (60.4% vs. 47.5%, $p < 0.05$), demonstrating reduced overall alveolar collapse (Fig. 5.7c). Figure 5.7d is a photomicrograph of the single alveolus (white outline and *) measured in Fig. 5.7a, and the cluster of alveoli (all yellow colorized alveoli) measured in Fig. 5.7b. This preliminary work suggests that a brief expiratory time is more effective at stabilizing alveoli and preventing collapse than an extended expiratory time at the same level of PEEP.

Combining an extended inspiratory time with a very brief expiratory time to stabilize and then recruit alveoli and alveolar ducts: Applied physiology suggests that stabilizing alveoli and minimizing RACE-induced atelectrauma is an essential initial step in a protective ventilation strategy. However, this is just the starting point, as a significant portion of the acutely injured lung with edema and surfactant abnormalities remains collapsed, contributing to stress multipliers that induce both atelectrauma and volutrauma (Figs. 2.6, 2.7, 4.3, 4.9, 4.10, and 4.11, Videos 4.4 and 4.5). Therefore, time and pressure are combined during inspiration and expiration to stabilize and reopen the lung.

Neither alveolar recruitment nor collapse can be determined using static measurements of airway pressure and lung volume during a breath-hold [18, 19]. These unseen *dynamic* time-related changes between peak and end-expiration with each breath cause mechanical damage to pulmonary tissue, resulting in VILI [2]. Dynamic computerized tomography (dCT), lung sounds, *in vivo* microscopy, and ultrafast indwelling oxygen-sensing probe (UFIOP) can all be used to measure and analyze dynamic RACE [20–23]. Both alveolar opening and collapse time constants need consideration to apply physiology to the timing of inspiration and expiration required to stabilize and reopen alveoli. Boehme et al. found that in the acutely injured lung, a two-phase (Fast and Slow) exponential model fit was optimal for analyzing TAU during both inspiration and expiration (Fig. 5.2) [2].

In a rat surfactant deactivation ARDS model, the impact of inspiratory and expiratory time and pressure on gas distribution within an acinus (alveoli vs. alveolar ducts) was tested using the APRV and volume-controlled (VCV) modes [13].

Figure 5.8a illustrates the microanatomical color code used on histologic samples, with alveoli coded in blue, alveolar ducts in green, and alveolar walls in red. Figure 5.8b provides an example of color coding in lung tissue. Results from the five study groups are presented in Fig. 5.8c. Control rats, not subjected to injury, were briefly ventilated before euthanasia and lung fixation. VCV groups, with V_T of 6 mL/kg, were ventilated with PEEP of either 5 or 16 cm H_2O. APRV groups were ventilated with an extended inspiratory phase (~2.0 s). The APRV 75% group had a very short expiratory time (T_{Low}) of 0.13 s, while the APRV 10% group had an extended expiratory time (0.40 s). See Chap. 8 for TLow setting methods. The inspiratory time (T_{High}) of ~2.0 s was 90% of each breath. Thus, VCV had a very short inspiratory and long expiratory time, whereas the APRV mode had an extended inspiratory and very brief expiratory time.

Fig. 5.7 Airway pressure/ alveolar area/time curve of a single alveolus (**a**) and a cluster of alveoli (**b**) that fill an in vivo microscopic field during a single expiration using Set- versus TC-PEEP at the same end-expiratory pressure but different expiratory times. The brief expiratory time in the TC-PEEP group reduced the size of alveolar collapse (blue solid line) compared to the Set-PEEP group with an extended expiratory time (red solid line) at the same pressure. Alveolar size is measured as the number of pixels on the photomicrograph. (**c**) Assessment of alveolar collapse was measured in all four rats and measured as a Percent Change in Alveolar Area (%) of all alveoli within a microscopic field. Reducing expiratory time (TC-PEEP) group significantly reduced alveolar collapse (blue bar) as compared to an extended expiratory time (red bar) (* = $P < 0.05$). The microscopic field used to generate the curves in **a** and **b** is shown in **d**. The single alveolus analyzed in **a** is outlined in white with an asterisk in the center (**d**). All colorized alveoli (yellow) in the microscopic field generated the curves in **b**. The percent alveolar occupancy was calculated as a percentage of alveolar air space in 1 microscopic field (1920 × 1280 pixels). Josh Satalin at Upstate Medical University generated the data

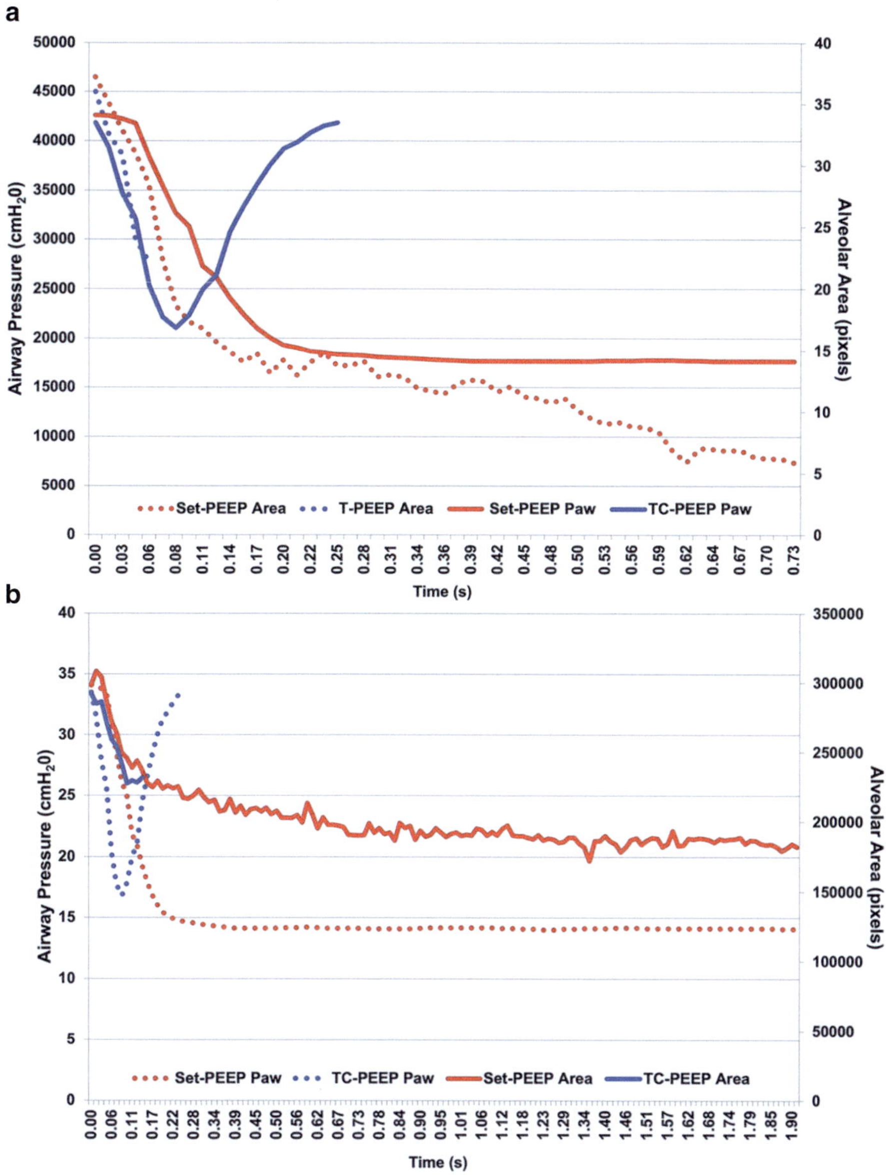
a
Airway Pressure (cmH$_2$0)
Alveolar Area (pixels)
Set-PEEP Area
T-PEEP Area
Set-PEEP Paw
TC-PEEP Paw
Time (s)
b
Airway Pressure (cmH$_2$0)
Alveolar Area (pixels)
Set-PEEP Paw
TC-PEEP Paw
Set-PEEP Area
TC-PEEP Area
Time (s)

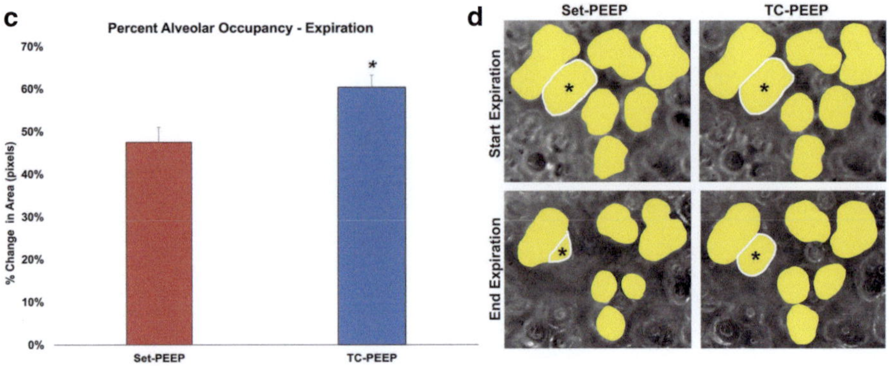

Fig. 5.7 (continued)

The primary finding of this study indicates that the VCV mode at both PEEP levels and APRV 10% group led to abnormal gas distribution in both the ducts and alveoli when compared with the normal control group (Fig. 5.8c). Most maldistribution was observed in the alveolar duct (overdistended) rather than the alveolus. The ducts in both VCV PEEP groups and the APRV 10% group were significantly enlarged, while alveoli in all three groups were smaller than those in normal control lung tissue [13]. However, compared to normal, this highly abnormal gas distribution (Fig. 5.8 Control), was nearly normalized by significantly increasing inspiratory time and shortening expiratory time (Fig. 5.8 APRV 75% group). Indeed, the APRV-75% group restored the alveolar/alveolar duct volume ratio to nearly that of the gas distribution in a normal uninjured lung [13]. This study highlights the importance of effectively managing inspiratory and expiratory time to protect the acutely injured lung. Similarly, pulmonary surfactant treatment has also been demonstrated to normalize gas distribution and the alveolar/alveolar duct strain relationship in the microenvironment of acutely injured lungs [24–26].

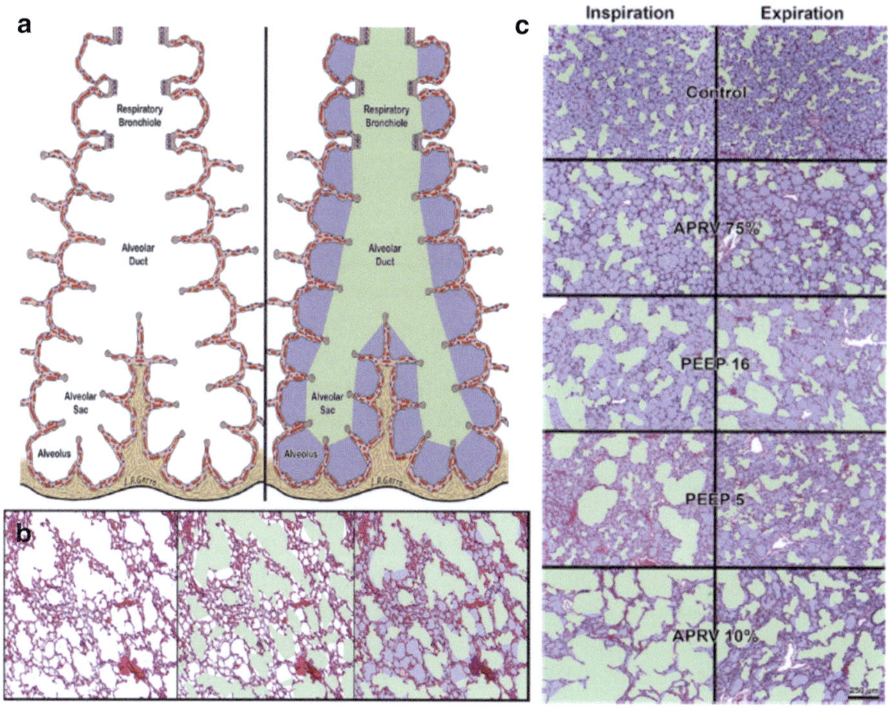

Fig. 5.8 Histologic assessment of gas distribution in alveoli and alveolar ducts in a rat surfactant deactivation ARDS model with four different combinations of airway pressures and times compared to a control uninjured group. In a surfactant deactivation plus high tidal volume (V_T) rat ARDS model, the airway pressure release ventilation (APRV) mode was used with the same extended inspiratory time. Two groups were studied **APRV 75%** group with a very brief expiratory time and the **APRV 10%** group with an extended expiratory time (see Fig. 5.4 for group descriptions). The volume-controlled mode (VCV) used a low V_T (6 cc/kg) with positive end-expiratory pressure (PEEP) of either 5 (**PEEP 5**) or 16cm$_2$O (**PEEP 16**) groups. In each animal, one lung was fixed at inspiration and the other lung at expiration. (**a**) Computer image analysis color coding for the amount of area occupied by each of the compartments of interest: Alveoli in blue, alveolar sacs, ducts, respiratory bronchioles in green, and alveolar walls and blood vessels in red. (**b**) Shows our color coding applied to the lung tissue histology. (**c**) Lung histology at Inspiration and Expiration from each of the four injured lung ventilation groups and a non-injured control group. In normal tissue (control group), alveoli (blue) occupy a little over half of the microscopic field, and the alveolar ducts (green) most of the remaining area. Gas distribution similar to that of the control group was seen in the APRV 75% group. The other three groups showed a maldistribution of gases with significant overdistention of the ducts (green) being most severe in the PEEP 5 and APRV 10% groups. This study demonstrates that in an injured lung, a mechanical breath with an extended time at inspiration and very brief expiratory time can effectively distribute gas within the alveoli and alveolar ducts similar to that seen in a normal lung [29]

Computational Models of Alveolar Stabilization Using Time and Pressure

A computational model of an acutely injured lung with surfactant dysfunction has shown that *in silico* "alveoli" can be stabilized to prevent atelectrauma using low V_T ventilation plus PEEP or APRV using a very brief expiratory duration. These data suggest that expiration timing may be as crucial as PEEP in eliminating RACE. Two two-time constants predict the time-dependent efficacy of APRV: lung emptying (τ_{rs}) and recruitment/derecruitment ($\tau_{R/D}$). The time constant τ_{rs} impacts the threshold of expiratory time over which RACE will develop. "Alveolar" instability *in silico* is exquisitely sensitive to slight changes in expiratory duration. For example, "alveoli" remain stable with an expiratory time ≤0.5 s, but the number of "alveoli" that collapse increases rapidly, with even slight increases (100th of a second) in expiratory duration. An atelectrauma index (I_{atelec}) calculation, defined as the total change in the fraction of open lung taking place per breath, identified the "alveolar" injury rate, assuming that "alveolar" instability will result in tissue damage. The atelectrauma index depends on $\tau_{R/D}$, and remains low if the expiratory duration is ≤0.5 s but rises rapidly if expiratory time is extended [27]. In our previous study, the biological results of time-dependent alveolar recruitment were accurately predicted by a mathematical model incorporating the effects of time and pressure [28].

This underscores the importance of computational models in understanding and predicting the dynamics of alveolar stabilization in acutely injured lungs, as well as identifying the threshold of expiratory time over which RACE will develop. The in silico "alveolar" instability is remarkably sensitive to slight changes in expiratory duration. For instance, "alveoli" remain stable with an expiratory time of ≤0.5 s, but a rapid increase in the number of collapsing "alveoli" occurs with even slight increases (100th of a second) in expiratory duration.

Summary

The acutely injured lung becomes *time*- and *pressure*-dependent. This means it will take more time for the lung to open and less time before it collapses at any airway pressure. Multiple studies have shown that an extended time at inspiration will progressively recruit alveoli, and a short expiratory time will prevent alveoli from re-collapsing. Thus, the time of the applied breath at both inspiration and expiration is critical in designing an MB_P that will stabilize and then reopen the acutely injured lung, which is necessary to minimize VILI. An extended inspiratory time can recruit alveoli (Fig. 5.3, Video 5.1), and a very brief expiratory time can prevent re-collapse (Figs. 5.6 and 5.7, Video 5.2) and, when combined, result in open and stable lung inflation (Video 5.3).

References

1. Broche L, Perchiazzi G, Porra L, Tannoia A, Pellegrini M, Derosa S, Sindaco A, Batista Borges J, Degrugilliers L, Larsson A, et al. Dynamic mechanical interactions between neighboring airspaces determine cyclic opening and closure in injured lung. Crit Care Med. 2017;45(4):687–94.
2. Boehme S, Bentley AH, Hartmann EK, Chang S, Erdoes G, Prinzing A, Hagmann M, Baumgardner JE, Ullrich R, Markstaller K, et al. Influence of inspiration to expiration ratio on cyclic recruitment and derecruitment of atelectasis in a saline lavage model of acute respiratory distress syndrome. Crit Care Med. 2015;43(3):e65–74.
3. Ma B, Bates JHT. Modeling the complex dynamics of derecruitment in the lung. Ann Biomed Eng. 2010;38(11):3466–77.
4. Albert SP, DiRocco J, Allen GB, Bates JH, Lafollette R, Kubiak BD, Fischer J, Maroney S, Nieman GF. The role of time and pressure on alveolar recruitment. J Appl Physiol. 2009;106(3):757–65.
5. Neumann P, Berglund JE, Mondejar EF, Magnusson A, Hedenstierna G. Effect of different pressure levels on the dynamics of lung collapse and recruitment in oleic-acid-induced lung injury. Am J Respir Crit Care Med. 1998;158(5 Pt 1):1636–43.
6. Neumann P, Berglund JE, Fernandez Mondejar E, Magnusson A, Hedenstierna G. Dynamics of lung collapse and recruitment during prolonged breathing in porcine lung injury. J Appl Physiol (1985). 1998;85(4):1533–43.
7. Stenqvist O, Gattinoni L, Hedenstierna G. What's new in respiratory physiology? The expanding chest wall revisited! Intensive Care Med. 2015;41:1110.
8. Schiller HJ, McCann UG 2nd, Carney DE, Gatto LA, Steinberg JM, Nieman GF. Altered alveolar mechanics in the acutely injured lung. Crit Care Med. 2001;29(5):1049–55.
9. Broche L, Pisa P, Porra L, Degrugilliers L, Bravin A, Pellegrini M, Borges JB, Perchiazzi G, Larsson A, Hedenstierna G, et al. Individual airway closure characterized in vivo by phase-contrast CT imaging in injured rabbit lung. Crit Care Med. 2019;47(9):e774–81.
10. Bates JHT, Smith BJ. Ventilator-induced lung injury and lung mechanics. Ann Transl Med. 2018;6(19):378.
11. Syring RS, Otto CM, Spivack RE, Markstaller K, Baumgardner JE. Maintenance of end-expiratory recruitment with increased respiratory rate after saline-lavage lung injury. J Appl Physiol (1985). 2007;102(1):331–9.
12. Neumann P, Berglund JE, Andersson LG, Maripu E, Magnusson A, Hedenstierna G. Effects of inverse ratio ventilation and positive end-expiratory pressure in oleic acid-induced lung injury. Am J Respir Crit Care Med. 2000;161(5):1537–45.
13. Kollisch-Singule M, Emr B, Smith B, Ruiz C, Roy S, Meng Q, Jain S, Satalin J, Snyder K, Ghosh A, et al. Airway pressure release ventilation reduces conducting airway micro-strain in lung injury. J Am Coll Surg. 2014;219(5):9.
14. Kollisch-Singule M, Emr B, Smith B, Roy S, Jain S, Satalin J, Snyder K, Andrews P, Habashi N, Bates J, et al. Mechanical breath profile of airway pressure release ventilation: the effect on alveolar recruitment and microstrain in acute lung injury. JAMA Surg. 2014;149(11):1138–45.
15. Kollisch-Singule M, Jain S, Andrews P, Smith BJ, Hamlington-Smith KL, Roy S, DiStefano D, Nuss E, Satalin J, Meng Q, et al. Effect of airway pressure release ventilation on dynamic alveolar heterogeneity. JAMA Surg. 2016;151(1):64–72.
16. Satalin J, Andrews P, Gatto LA, Habashi NM, Nieman GF. "Open the lung and keep it open": a homogeneously ventilated lung is a 'healthy lung'. Ann Transl Med. 2016;4(7):141.
17. Habashi NM. Other approaches to open-lung ventilation: airway pressure release ventilation. Crit Care Med. 2005;33(3 Suppl):S228–40.
18. Carvalho AR, Bergamini BC, Carvalho NS, Cagido VR, Neto AC, Jandre FC, Zin WA, Giannella-Neto A. Volume-independent elastance: a useful parameter for open-lung positive end-expiratory pressure adjustment. Anesth Analg. 2013;116(3):627–33.

19. Caironi P, Cressoni M, Chiumello D, Ranieri M, Quintel M, Russo SG, Cornejo R, Bugedo G, Carlesso E, Russo R, et al. Lung opening and closing during ventilation of acute respiratory distress syndrome. Am J Respir Crit Care Med. 2010;181(6):578–86.
20. David M, Karmrodt J, Bletz C, David S, Herweling A, Kauczor HU, Markstaller K. Analysis of atelectasis, ventilated, and hyperinflated lung during mechanical ventilation by dynamic CT. Chest. 2005;128(5):3757–70.
21. Vena A, Rylander C, Perchiazzi G, Giuliani R, Hedenstierna G. Lung sound analysis correlates to injury and recruitment as identified by computed tomography: an experimental study. Intensive Care Med. 2011;37(8):1378–83.
22. Baumgardner JE, Markstaller K, Pfeiffer B, Doebrich M, Otto CM. Effects of respiratory rate, plateau pressure, and positive end-expiratory pressure on PaO2 oscillations after saline lavage. Am J Respir Crit Care Med. 2002;166(12 Pt 1):1556–62.
23. Hartmann EK, Boehme S, Bentley A, Duenges B, Klein KU, Elsaesser A, Baumgardner JE, David M, Markstaller K. Influence of respiratory rate and end-expiratory pressure variation on cyclic alveolar recruitment in an experimental lung injury model. Crit Care. 2012;16(1):R8.
24. Knudsen L, Lopez-Rodriguez E, Berndt L, Steffen L, Ruppert C, Bates JHT, Ochs M, Smith BJ. Alveolar micromechanics in bleomycin-induced lung injury. Am J Respir Cell Mol Biol. 2018;59(6):757–69.
25. Wilson TA, Bachofen H. A model for mechanical structure of the alveolar duct. J Appl Physiol Respir Environ Exerc Physiol. 1982;52(4):1064–70.
26. Haefeli-Bleuer B, Weibel ER. Morphometry of the human pulmonary acinus. Anat Rec. 1988;220:401–14.
27. Bates JHT, Gaver DP, Habashi NM, Nieman GF. Atelectrauma versus volutrauma: a tale of two time-constants. Crit Care Explor. 2020;2(12):e0299.
28. Albert SP, DiRocco J, Allen GB, Bates JH, Lafollette R, Kubiak BD, Fischer J, Maroney S, Nieman GF. The role of time and pressure on alveolar recruitment. J Appl Physiol (1985). 2009;106(3):757–65.
29. Kollisch-Singule M, Emr B, Smith B, Ruiz C, Roy S, Meng Q, Jain S, Satalin J, Snyder K, Ghosh A, et al. Airway pressure release ventilation reduces conducting airway micro-strain in lung injury. J Am Coll Surg. 2014;219(5):968–76.

Chapter 6
Applied Physiologic Analysis of Clinically Tested Protective Ventilation Strategies

Introduction

Given the absence of pharmacologic treatments for the acutely injured lung in clinical practice [1–3], the current management of Acute Respiratory Distress Syndrome (ARDS) relies on supportive measures, with the mechanical ventilator playing a pivotal role. The dual nature of mechanical ventilation, both therapeutic and potentially harmful depending on its application, underscores the need for an optimal strategy in ventilating the injured lung.

ARDS induces an increase in lung microvascular permeability, leading to altered alveolar mechanics characterized by repetitive alveolar collapse and expansion (RACE) and overdistension (OD) of alveolar and alveolar ducts (Fig. 6.1, top green box). It is now recognized that RACE and OD contribute to excessive "peeling" stress during inflation, causing separation of alveolar walls and generating regional stress multipliers, resulting in excessive strain (Fig. 6.1, lower green box).

Efforts in evidence-based medicine to identify an optimal ventilation strategy for ARDS have yielded limited specific recommendations. The current standard of care for ARDS involves the use of a low tidal volume (V_T—6 mL/kg ideal body weight) and plateau pressure (Pplat) along with empirical suggestions regarding positive end-expiratory pressure (PEEP) levels [4] and the recent addition of prone positioning [5]. Despite the comprehensive understanding of ventilator-induced lung injury (VILI) mechanisms, as discussed in Chaps. 2, 4, and 5, it seems somewhat curious that with the much-improved understanding of ARDS pathophysiology (Chaps. 4 and 5), the current standard of care would use more components of the MB_P to protect the lung from VILI.

Supplementary Information The online version contains supplementary material available at https://doi.org/10.1007/978-3-031-66352-9_6.

© The Author(s), under exclusive license to Springer Nature Switzerland AG 2024

G. F. Nieman, N. M. Habashi, *Applied Physiology to Reduce Ventilator Induced Lung Injury*, https://doi.org/10.1007/978-3-031-66352-9_6

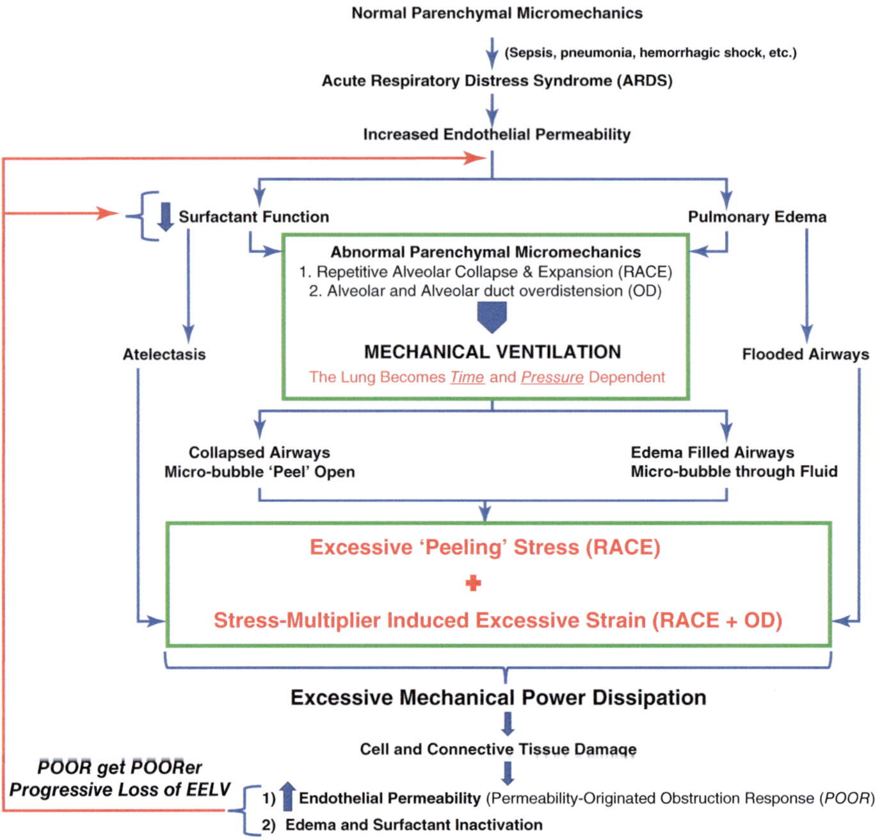

Fig. 6.1 The unifying hypothesis of the pathophysiologic mechanisms associated with acute respiratory distress syndrome (ARDS) that predisposes the lung to a secondary ventilator-induced lung injury (VILI). This chapter discusses the physiologic correctness of the current ventilator strategies on RACE and OD (green box) that have been tested in randomized controlled trials (RCTs) on ARDS patients in relation to minimizing the mechanisms that cause lung tissue damage (lower green box) in order to improve outcome

ARDSnet ARMA method: Clinical trials, such as the seminal ARDSnet ARMA trial, often compare two straightforward choices to determine what is best for the average patient population. However, this approach presents two key challenges: (1) further refinement of the prescription becomes challenging due to statistical power limitations, making it difficult to determine, for instance, whether a tidal volume of 5 or 7 is superior to 6 mL/kg, and (2) in a highly heterogeneous disease like ARDS, the average optimal choice may not be the best for an individual patient. Addressing both of these challenges could be achieved through clinical trials exploring personalized management approaches. For instance, tailoring the choice of tidal volume in ARDS based on each patient's specific characteristics, rather than adopting a one-size-fits-all approach, should yield improved outcomes for individual patients. This personalized approach could enhance the effectiveness of clinical trials and reduce the number of patients needed to demonstrate significant benefits.

It's important to note that a low V_T alone does not prevent repetitive alveolar collapse and expansion (RACE) in the ARDS lung (Video 4.3). In the presence of inadequate PEEP leading to a low end-expiratory lung volume (EELV), low V_T may result in the inflation of alveoli during inspiration, followed by re-collapse during expiration (i.e., RACE). An illustrative example involves an excised rat lung model with surfactant deactivation-induced ARDS ventilated with a V_T of 6 cc/kg and a PEEP of 5cmH_2O using conventional mechanical ventilation (CMV) in volume-controlled mode (Video 4.3 and 6.1 CMV). Lung tissue recruits during inspiration (transitioning from red atelectasis to pink open tissue) but re-collapses during expiration. In contrast, when employing the Time-Controlled Adaptive Ventilation (TCAV) method to set and adjust the airway pressure release ventilation (APRV) mode, the V_T is not fixed but rather a product of inspiratory time, pressure, and expiratory time (Chap. 8).

In the same rat ARDS model, the TCAV method successfully recruited the entire lung, normalizing EELV. Despite a V_T of 11 cc/kg, there was no tissue collapse during expiration because the EELV was maintained at a normal level (Video 6.1 TCAV). This highlights the potential benefits of personalized ventilation strategies by preventing detrimental effects in the ARDS lung. The challenge in testing personalized approaches lies in the complexity of patient-specific prescriptions, as there are often considerably more intricate options than simple one-size-fits-all strategies. Focusing on personalized prescriptions grounded in an understanding of underlying pathophysiology is crucial. However, this presents a significant challenge given biology's virtually limitless multi-scale complexity. Even with detailed knowledge of pathologic mechanisms, there is no guarantee that it will be sufficient to guide effective therapy, as seen in the case of permissive hypercapnia. Only when proven clinically acceptable did allowing arterial PCO_2 to rise above normal levels was conventionally advocated by pulmonary physiologists. Nevertheless, the current understanding of VILI pathophysiology supports the rationalized design of personalized ventilation strategies for the injured lung, potentially improving current clinical practice.

As detailed in previous Chaps. 2, 4, and 5, most mechanisms of VILI pathophysiology manifest at the microscale (Figs. 2.6 and 2.7, Videos 4.4 and 4.5), while the parameters defining traditional modes and methods of protective mechanical ventilation (primarily low V_T and Pplat and PEEP adjusted to oxygenation) are chosen from a macroscale perspective. The impact of these parameters on the microenvironment is neither linear nor intuitive. For instance, despite the intuitive assumption that over-inflating the lung should be a primary mechanism of injury (Fig. 2.3), recent studies suggest that this is not the case [6–8]. Supporting this concept, the prone position mitigated experimental lung injury during ventilation with a relatively large V_T, suggesting that the protective mechanism was reduced RACE rather than decreased OD [9].

Recognition is growing that ventilating the injured lung based solely on OD of the "baby lung" concept (Fig. 2.3) does not ensure lung protection across all patient populations [10–12]. Therefore, the search for alternative strategies is ongoing. One concept under scrutiny is that the mechanical power delivered to the lungs during a breath is detrimental since power is presumably required to damage lung tissue. However, this is complicated by the fact that most of the energy delivered during inspiration is elastic in nature and is returned during expiration. The exercise literature reveals that the mechanical power in the normal lung during exercise can be as much as 19 times greater than the average power associated with lung injury in ARDS patients [13–17]. This suggests that lung tissue is not primarily injured by the energy *delivered* during inspiration but rather by the energy that is *not returned* at expiration and is instead dissipated within the tissue [18]. Recent findings by Mellenthin et al. indicate that this dissipated energy can be a useful predictor of ventilator-induced lung injury (VILI) in mice [19].

Moreover, insights from the exercise literature indicate that the normal homogeneous lung is considerably more resistant to damage at high mechanical power than the heterogeneously injured lung [20–24]. This emphasizes the importance of understanding the dynamic relationship between mechanical energy and lung resilience, shedding light on potential factors influencing lung injury in various contexts, including exercise and ARDS.

Current protective ventilation would appear to be beset by two conundrums, but fortunately, they are not intractable problems:

1. The ARMA Low V_T method has not further reduced ARDS-related mortality, suggesting OD of the "baby lung" is not the primary mechanism driving VILI [11, 12, 25]. Recent evidence points to regional alveolar instability and collapse as the main mechanisms causing both atelectrauma and volutrauma (Figs. 2.6, 2.7, 4.3, 4.9, 4.10, and 4.11, Videos 4.4 and 4.5) [26–28].
2. If heterogeneous regional lung instability and collapse are the mechanical damage mechanisms, the OLA should eliminate localized excessive lung strain and minimize VILI, but randomized controlled trials (RCTs) suggest otherwise [29–33]. Analysis of the current OLA strategies demonstrates that they were ineffective at reopening the lung, based on the low C_{RS} and PaO_2/FiO_2 ratios that were not significantly different than the Control low V_T group [33–35]. The current OLA methods did not take into account dynamic alveolar opening and collapse time constants and thus did not eliminate regional lung instability and collapse, the mechanisms of VILI in the microenvironment (Figs. 5.3, 5.4, and 5.8, Videos 5.1, 5.2, and 5.3) [36–38].

Using our understanding that alveoli open and collapse as a time-dependent system suggests that increasing the duration of inspiration will progressively recruit alveoli (Fig. 5.3, Videos 5.1, 8.1, and 8.4). In contrast, a very short expiratory duration will curtail collapse (Fig. 5.6, Videos 5.2, 8.4, 8.6, and 8.7) [39–44]. The concept of alveolar opening and collapse time constants has been around for several decades [43–47]. Still, it has yet to receive widespread acceptance from the medical community, and thus, the use of time-controlled protective ventilation is relegated to patients with refractory hypoxemia as a rescue mode [48, 49].

The low V_T ARMA method has been taught to physicians and staff who manage ARDS patients for over two decades and is thus far and away the most understood method of protective mechanical ventilation. This is critical since the same ventilation protocol must be used over all three shifts in an ICU with changes in faculty and staff treating the ARDS patient (Table 6.1). Most critical care ventilators can deliver the ARMA method, and there has been a positive RCT. There are two main problems with the ARMA method: (i) OD of the remaining normal lung tissue (i.e., the "baby lung") might not be the primary mechanism driving progressive VILI (Chap. 4), and (ii) the low V_T and Pplat may allow for progressive lung collapse and loss of EELV pushing the lung into the "VILI Vortex" (Fig. 2.4) [50].

It is possible that some of the components of the ARMA method are not physiologically correct since the goal is to prevent OD of normal tissue, which current data suggests is not a primary mechanism of VILI (Chap. 4). Recent meta and statistical analyses have shown that ARDS-related mortality has not been further reduced since the ARMA study was published in 2000, supporting the physiologic evidence that without modification and personalization, the ARMA method is ineffective at reducing ARDS-related mortality (Table 6.1) [11, 12, 25].

Table 6.1 ARDSnet LV_T ARMA method

	Yes	Maybe	No
Ease of use:	√		
Physician knowledge:	√		
Physician acceptance:	√		
Available in most ICUs:	√		
Positive RCT:	√		
Positive meta-analyses:			√
Physiologic correctness:			√
Were physiologic goals met:	√		

- Physiologic goal: To minimize overdistension of the remaining normal lung
  - Normal lung tissue was likely not overdistended
  - Recent evidence suggests that the normal lung is very resistant to damage caused by overdistension and thus is not the primary mechanism driving VILI
  - Regional alveolar instability and collapse causing overdistension and dynamic strain-induced damage to alveoli and alveolar ducts in the normal tissue surrounding these lesions is believed to be the mechanism driving VILI
- Constrained to ventilating a heterogeneous lung
  - This method does not attempt to eliminate stress multipliers
  - Progressive loss of end expiratory lung volume (EELV) with low ventilation volumes and pressures force the lung into the "VILI Vortex"
  - Large volume of atelectatic lung can cause secondary lung pathologies
- One size fit all settings not based on lung pathophysiology
  - New concept: base settings on driving pressure to personalize treatment
- PEEP set based on oxygenation
  - May not be sufficient to prevent progressive loss of EELV
  - May not be sufficient to prevent repetitive alveolar collapse and expansion (RACE)
- The lung is not stable or open and thus VILI can occur

Open Lung Approach (OLA)

The OLA correctly targets the physiologic mechanisms of VILI, specifically regional alveolar instability and collapse in the microenvironment. It aims to eliminate both by increasing PEEP with or without recruitment maneuvers (RM) (Table 6.2). While the ventilation strategy of OLA is identical to the ARMA method, the addition of higher PEEP with or without RMs needs to be better understood and accepted, given the variations in the RM protocols [51]. Although the physiologic targets align to reduce VILI in OLA randomized controlled trials (RCTs), there is no clear evidence that the objective of achieving an open and stable lung was met. Analysis of recent large failed OLA RCTs showed no conclusive evidence of durable lung recruitment. On day 7 of the study, the respiratory system static compliance was 34.5 (32.5–36.5) mL/cmH_2O, and the PaO_2/FiO_2 ratio was 267.7 (250.0–275.4), indicating that the lungs of these patients were not fully open and contained a significant amount of unstable or collapsed tissue. This suggests that the physiologic goals of the OLA strategy were not achieved (refer to Table 6.2). If the lung is not stable and open, VILI mechanisms remain in play (Figs. 2.6, 2.7, 2.8, 4.3, 4.6, 4.7, and 4.9, Videos 2.1, 4.4, and 4.5). Even maximal lung recruitment with a titrated

Table 6.2 Open lung approach (OLA)

	Yes	Maybe	No
Ease of use:		√	
Physician knowledge:		√	
Physician acceptance:		√	
Available in most ICUs:	√		
Positive RCT:			√
Positive meta-analyses:			√
Physiologic correctness:	√		
Were physiologic goals met:			√

- Physiologic goal: Inflate the entire lung converting to homogeneous ventilation
  - If homogeneous ventilation is accomplished, it would eliminate regional alveolar instability and collapse the mechanisms driving VILI
  - However, the current OLA method did not effectively open the lung
    No clear X-rays data
    Normal blood gases were not achieved
    Normal respiratory system compliance (C_{RS}) was not achieved
- Opening the majority of collapsed tissue rapidly is problematic
  - If a large amount of lung tissue with dysfunctional surfactant is rapidly opened (over seconds or minutes) it would be very unstable
  - The only ventilator 'tool' to keep this unstable tissue open using conventional ventilation is airway pressure in the form of PEEP
  - If PEEP is set too high, there will be hemodynamic compromise
  - If PEEP is set too low, repetitive alveolar collapse and expansion (RACE) will occur causing atelectrauma
- The lung is not stable or open and thus VILI can occur

PEEP and very low V_T strategy neither fully opens the lung (evidenced by a PaO_2/FiO_2 ratio of 267.7) nor reduces ventilator-free days or mortality [31].

Another issue with current OLA methods is the rapid recruitment strategy that attempts to open the lung over a few seconds or minutes. Patients requiring RMs often have severe ARDS with a large volume of the lung without functioning surfactant. Rapidly opening a large volume of surfactant-depleted lung would require very high PEEP to keep it open. However, this poses challenges, as insufficient PEEP can lead to alveoli re-collapsing or developing RACE. The physician faces the difficult decision of keeping the lung open with high PEEP at the risk of heart failure or allowing the lung to re-collapse and destabilize, risking VILI (Table 6.2).

The physician has an alternative "tool" to PEEP, which is using expiratory time to stabilize the lung (Chap. 5). Direct visualization has shown that a very brief expiratory time can prevent alveolar collapse compared to a longer time at the same level of PEEP (Figs. 5.6 and 5.7, Videos 5.2). This introduces a potential avenue for managing lung stability without the negative impact on hemodynamics associated with high PEEP.

High-Frequency Oscillation Ventilation (HFOV)

HFOV targets the physiologic mechanisms of VILI, specifically regional alveolar instability and collapse (Table 6.3). It aims to eliminate both by using very low V_T to prevent RACE and maintain a high constant Pplat with CO_2 and O_2, moved along a pressure gradient generated by quasi-sinusoidal flow oscillations, to recruit atelectatic tissue (Table 6.3). Unlike the OLA, which uses the ARMA method with the addition of higher PEEP and RMs, HFOV is a distinct mode of mechanical ventilation. However, its limited understanding, acceptance, and availability in the Intensive Care Unit (ICU) might have contributed to the failure of this mode in Randomized Controlled Trials (RCTs). Although minimal data on lung function was published in the OSCAR and OSCILLATE RCTs studies, the PaO_2 and FiO_2 were published so that the PaO_2/FiO_2 ratio could be calculated. The PaO_2/FiO_2 on day 7 was 169 in the OSCILLATE trial [34], and on day 3 was 217 in the OSCAR trial, [35] suggesting that the physiologic goal of an open lung was not attained in either study (Table 6.3). Thus, the mechanisms driving VILI in the microenvironment would not have been eliminated. Dreyfuss et al. reviewed the possible reasons for the negative results in clinical studies using the HFOV mode [52].

Kaczka's group has shown that HFOV results in a maldistribution of oscillatory flow when ventilating a heterogeneously injured lung, predisposing these regions to high parenchymal strain and injury [53]. They also demonstrated that multi-frequency oscillatory ventilation (MFOV) may improve lung protection by reducing strain magnitude and spatial gradients compared with conventional mechanical ventilation or HFOV [54].

Table 6.3 High frequency oscillatory ventilation (HFOV)

	Yes	Maybe	No
Ease of use:			√
Physician knowledge:			√
Physician acceptance:		√	
Available in most ICUs:			√
Positive RCT:			√
Positive meta-analyses:			√
Physiologic correctness:	√		
Were physiologic goals met:		√	

- Physiologic goal: Inflate the entire lung converting to homogeneous ventilation
  - If homogeneous ventilation is accomplished it would eliminate regional alveolar instability and collapse the mechanisms driving VILI
  - However, no evidence that HFOV effectively open the lung
    No clear X-rays
    No normal blood gases
    No normal respiratory system compliance (C_{RS})
    Low PaO_2/FiO_2 ratio
- The optimal method to set and adjust the HFOV mode may not have been used
  - Robust studies to identify the optimal method to set and adjust the HFOV mode have not been conducted
  - It is possible that the lack of experience using HFOV by some of the physicians in the RCT negatively impacted outcomes pressure in the form of PEEP
- The lung is not stable or open and thus VILI can occur

Microvascular permeability does not vary linearly with increased airway pressure, but rather, a threshold must be crossed, followed by an exponential increase in high permeability edema [55, 56]. The extended time at higher airway pressure with HFOV could have reached this threshold much sooner, exacerbating pulmonary edema formation. Lastly, long-term atelectasis is associated with numerous additional lung pathologies (Chap. 2, *Problems caused by long-term atelectasis*) [57, 58].

The OSCILLATE and OSCAR studies suggest that minimizing the V_T while failing to open the lung is not lung protective. The very small V_Ts associated with HFOV should have minimized RACE. Does this mean that alveolar instability and atelectrauma are not primary VILI mechanisms? This is highly unlikely since much evidence exists demonstrating the role of RACE in VILI-induced tissue injury and inflammation [59–61]. If RACE does not occur on HFOV, why wasn't mortality reduced? The lungs of these patients appeared to have a significant degree of atelectasis, evidenced by the low PaO_2/FiO_2 ratio, exposing an extensive amount of tissue would be subjected to stress multipliers even if they were static and not dynamic (Figs. 2.7, 4.9, 4.10, and 4.11, Videos 2.1 and 4.5). It has been shown that even static overdistension, similar to that delivered by HFOV, can cause severe damage, leading to increased alveolar epithelial permeability [62]. The airway pressure differential between the collapsed or edema-filled tissue and the surrounding open alveoli would concentrate the stress lines even if this pressure differential was relatedly constant (Fig. 1.1 Edema green arrow, Figs. 2.7, 4.9, 4.10, and 4.11, Videos 2.1 and 4.5).

Ramcharran et al., using a heterogeneous lung injury model and the airway pressure release ventilation (APRV) mode, made ventilator adjustments to vary the amount of lung tissue overdistension (OD) and recruitment/derecruitment (RD). Four combinations of more (OD↑) or less (OD↓), lung overdistension (OD), and more (RD↑) or less (RD↓) were studied (Fig. 6.2). Combining more OD and RD (OD↑RD↑) caused the most lung injury, and minimizing both (OD↓RD↓) caused the least. However, both OD and RD alone (OD↑RD↓ and OD↓RD↑) were able to generate some degree of lung damage. Also, the normal tissue (baby lung) suffered minimal injury even when ventilated with OD↑RD↑, suggesting that OD of the baby lung is not the primary mechanism driving VILI.

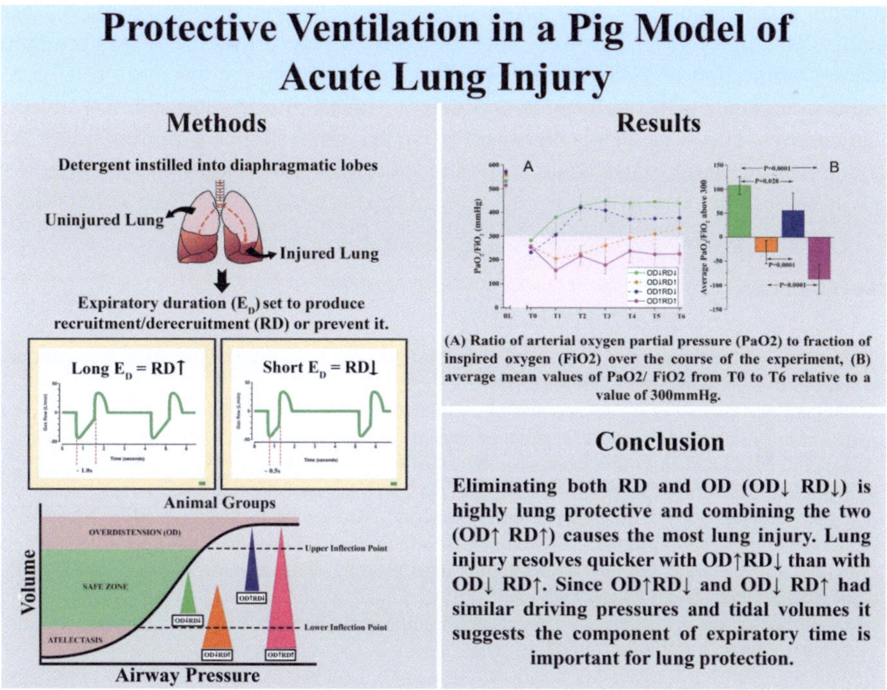

Fig. 6.2 The ventilator-induced lung injury (VILI) mechanisms of lung overdistension (OD) or volutrauma and recruitment/derecruitment (RD) atelectrauma on lung function and injury were tested using a porcine heterogeneous lung injury model. Ventilator adjustments were made to cause more (OD↑) or less (OD↓) lung overdistension and more (RD↑) or less (RD↓) lung recruitment/derecruitment [63]. The study showed that OD plus RD (OD↑RD↑) caused the most lung injury, and minimizing both (OD↓RD↓) caused the least. Both OD and RD alone (OD↑RD↓ and OD↓RD↑) generated some lung damage. The normal lung tissue suffered little injury even when ventilated with OD↑RD↑

Summary

VILI is a frequent and often fatal consequence of supportive care for ARDS patients. Current lung-protective ventilation strategies focus on reducing OD of the remaining normal lung tissue by targeting low V_T, assuming this is the primary mechanism for lung protection. The supposed rationale is on the macroscale and assumes that the small volume of open lung tissue will be subjected to gross volutrauma if V_T and Pplat are not significantly reduced (Fig. 2.3). However, recent animal studies suggest that atelectrauma (i.e., RACE) is the principal instigator and disseminator of VILI that, once started, becomes susceptible to further injury from OD in a permeability-originated obstructive response (*POOR*)-get-POORer vicious cycle (Fig. 4.11). The implication is that mechanical ventilation should prioritize avoiding cyclic RACE with each breath. How to achieve this in a patient-specific manner remains an open question. Still, promising results have been obtained using a time-controlled adaptive ventilation (TCAV) method to set and adjust the airway pressure release ventilation (APRV) mode. This strategy leverages the disparate time constants associated with recruitment and derecruitment to open and stabilize alveoli and airways. This approach is highly effective in animal studies at minimizing VILI and preventing progressive acute lung injury. Chapter 8 will focus on this topic.

References

1. Boyle AJ, Mac Sweeney R, McAuley DF. Pharmacological treatments in ARDS; a state-of-the-art update. BMC Med. 2013;11:166.
2. Duggal A, Ganapathy A, Ratnapalan M, Adhikari NK. Pharmacological treatments for acute respiratory distress syndrome: systematic review. Minerva Anestesiol. 2015;81(5):567–88.
3. Spieth PM, Zhang H. Pharmacological therapies for acute respiratory distress syndrome. Curr Opin Crit Care. 2014;20(1):113–21.
4. Acute Respiratory Distress Syndrome Network, Brower RG, Matthay MA, Morris A, Schoenfeld D, Thompson BT, Wheeler A. Ventilation with lower tidal volumes as compared with traditional tidal volumes for acute lung injury and the acute respiratory distress syndrome. N Engl J Med. 2000;342(18):1301–8.
5. Guerin C, Reignier J, Richard JC. Prone positioning in the acute respiratory distress syndrome. N Engl J Med. 2013;369(10):980–1.
6. Jain SV, Kollisch-Singule M, Satalin J, Searles Q, Dombert L, Abdel-Razek O, Yepuri N, Leonard A, Gruessner A, Andrews P, et al. The role of high airway pressure and dynamic strain on ventilator-induced lung injury in a heterogeneous acute lung injury model. Intensive Care Med Exp. 2017;5(1):25.
7. Seah AS, Grant KA, Aliyeva M, Allen GB, Bates JHT. Quantifying the roles of tidal volume and PEEP in the pathogenesis of ventilator-induced lung injury. Ann Biomed Eng. 2011;39(5):1505–16.
8. Protti A, Andreis DT, Monti M, Santini A, Sparacino CC, Langer T, Votta E, Gatti S, Lombardi L, Leopardi O, et al. Lung stress and strain during mechanical ventilation: any difference between statics and dynamics? Crit Care Med. 2013;41(4):1046–55.

9. Xin Y, Cereda M, Hamedani H, Pourfathi M, Siddiqui S, Meeder N, Kadlecek S, Duncan I, Profka H, Rajaei J, et al. Unstable inflation causing injury. Insight from prone position and paired computed tomography scans. Am J Respir Crit Care Med. 2018;198(2):197–207.
10. Maca J, Jor O, Holub M, Sklienka P, Bursa F, Burda M, Janout V, Sevcik P. Past and present ARDS mortality rates: a systematic review. Respir Care. 2017;62(1):113–22.
11. Bellani G, Laffey JG, Pham T, Fan E, Brochard L, Esteban A, Gattinoni L, van Haren F, Larsson A, McAuley DF, et al. Epidemiology, patterns of care, and mortality for patients with acute respiratory distress syndrome in intensive care units in 50 countries. JAMA. 2016;315(8):788–800.
12. Fan E, Brodie D, Slutsky AS. Acute respiratory distress syndrome: advances in diagnosis and treatment. JAMA. 2018;319(7):698–710.
13. Kallet RH, Branson RD. Respiratory controversies in the critical care setting. Do the NIH ARDS Clinical Trials Network PEEP/FIO2 tables provide the best evidence-based guide to balancing PEEP and FIO2 settings in adults? Respir Care. 2007;52(4):461–75; discussion 475–467.
14. Kallet RH, Daniel BM, Garcia O, Matthay MA. Accuracy of physiologic dead space measurements in patients with acute respiratory distress syndrome using volumetric capnography: comparison with the metabolic monitor method. Respir Care. 2005;50(4):462–7.
15. Chiumello D, Pelosi P, Croci M, Bigatello LM, Gattinoni L. The effects of pressurization rate on breathing pattern, work of breathing, gas exchange and patient comfort in pressure support ventilation. Eur Respir J. 2001;18(1):107–14.
16. L'Her E, Deye N, Lellouche F, Taille S, Demoule A, Fraticelli A, Mancebo J, Brochard L. Physiologic effects of noninvasive ventilation during acute lung injury. Am J Respir Crit Care Med. 2005;172(9):1112–8.
17. Gattinoni L, Tonetti T, Cressoni M, Cadringher P, Herrmann P, Moerer O, Protti A, Gotti M, Chiurazzi C, Carlesso E, et al. Ventilator-related causes of lung injury: the mechanical power. Intensive Care Med. 2016;42(10):1567–75.
18. Marini JJ. How I optimize power to avoid VILI. Crit Care. 2019;23(1):326.
19. Mellenthin MM, Seong SA, Roy GS, Bartolak-Suki E, Hamlington KL, Bates JHT, Smith BJ. Using injury cost functions from a predictive single-compartment model to assess the severity of mechanical ventilator-induced lung injuries. J Appl Physiol (1985). 2019;127(1):58–70.
20. Guenette JA, Querido JS, Eves ND, Chua R, Sheel AW. Sex differences in the resistive and elastic work of breathing during exercise in endurance-trained athletes. Am J Physiol Regul Integr Comp Physiol. 2009;297(1):R166–75.
21. Guenette JA, Witt JD, McKenzie DC, Road JD, Sheel AW. Respiratory mechanics during exercise in endurance-trained men and women. J Physiol. 2007;581(Pt 3):1309–22.
22. Harms CA, Wetter TJ, McClaran SR, Pegelow DF, Nickele GA, Nelson WB, Hanson P, Dempsey JA. Effects of respiratory muscle work on cardiac output and its distribution during maximal exercise. J Appl Physiol (1985). 1998;85(2):609–18.
23. Dominelli PB, Molgat-Seon Y, Bingham D, Swartz PM, Road JD, Foster GE, Sheel AW. Dysanapsis and the resistive work of breathing during exercise in healthy men and women. J Appl Physiol (1985). 2015;119(10):1105–13.
24. Cross TJ, Sabapathy S, Beck KC, Morris NR, Johnson BD. The resistive and elastic work of breathing during exercise in patients with chronic heart failure. Eur Respir J. 2012;39(6):1449–57.
25. Pham T, Serpa Neto A, Pelosi P, Laffey JG, De Haro C, Lorente JA, Bellani G, Fan E, Brochard LJ, Pesenti A, et al. Outcomes of patients presenting with mild acute respiratory distress Syndrome: insights from the LUNG SAFE study. Anesthesiology. 2019;130(2):263–83.
26. Cressoni M, Chiurazzi C, Gotti M, Amini M, Brioni M, Algieri I, Cammaroto A, Rovati C, Massari D, di Castiglione CB, et al. Lung inhomogeneities and time course of ventilator-induced mechanical injuries. Anesthesiology. 2015;123(3):618–27.
27. Cereda M, Xin Y, Hamedani H, Bellani G, Kadlecek S, Clapp J, Guerra L, Meeder N, Rajaei J, Tustison NJ, et al. Tidal changes on CT and progression of ARDS. Thorax. 2017;72(11):981–9.

28. Cereda M, Xin Y, Meeder N, Zeng J, Jiang Y, Hamedani H, Profka H, Kadlecek S, Clapp J, Deshpande CG, et al. Visualizing the propagation of acute lung injury. Anesthesiology. 2016;124(1):121–31.
29. Brower RG, Lanken PN, MacIntyre N, Matthay MA, Morris A, Ancukiewicz M, Schoenfeld D, Thompson BT. Higher versus lower positive end-expiratory pressures in patients with the acute respiratory distress syndrome. N Engl J Med. 2004;351(4):327–36.
30. Meade MO, Cook DJ, Guyatt GH, Slutsky AS, Arabi YM, Cooper DJ, Davies AR, Hand LE, Zhou Q, Thabane L, et al. Ventilation strategy using low tidal volumes, recruitment maneuvers, and high positive end-expiratory pressure for acute lung injury and acute respiratory distress syndrome: a randomized controlled trial. JAMA. 2008;299(6):637–45.
31. Hodgson CL, Cooper DJ, Arabi Y, King V, Bersten A, Bihari S, Brickell K, Davies A, Fahey C, Fraser J, et al. Maximal recruitment open lung ventilation in acute respiratory distress syndrome (PHARLAP): a phase II, multicenter, randomized, controlled trial. Am J Respir Crit Care Med. 2019;200:1363–72.
32. Mercat A, Richard JC, Vielle B, Jaber S, Osman D, Diehl JL, Lefrant JY, Prat G, Richecoeur J, Nieszkowska A, et al. Positive end-expiratory pressure setting in adults with acute lung injury and acute respiratory distress syndrome: a randomized controlled trial. JAMA. 2008;299(6):646–55.
33. Writing Group for the Alveolar Recruitment for Acute Respiratory Distress Syndrome Trial I, Cavalcanti AB, Suzumura EA, Laranjeira LN, Paisani DM, Damiani LP, Guimaraes HP, Romano ER, Regenga MM, Taniguchi LNT, et al. Effect of lung recruitment and titrated positive end-expiratory pressure (PEEP) vs low PEEP on mortality in patients with acute respiratory distress syndrome: a randomized clinical trial. JAMA. 2017;318(14):1335–45.
34. Ferguson ND, Cook DJ, Guyatt GH, Mehta S, Hand L, Austin P, Zhou Q, Matte A, Walter SD, Lamontagne F, et al. High-frequency oscillation in early acute respiratory distress syndrome. N Engl J Med. 2013;368(9):795–805.
35. Young D, Lamb SE, Shah S, MacKenzie I, Tunnicliffe W, Lall R, Rowan K, Cuthbertson BH, Group OS. High-frequency oscillation for acute respiratory distress syndrome. N Engl J Med. 2013;368(9):806–13.
36. Carvalho AR, Zin WA. Respiratory system dynamical mechanical properties: modeling in time and frequency domain. Biophys Rev. 2011;3(2):71.
37. Suki B, Bates JH. Lung tissue mechanics as an emergent phenomenon. J Appl Physiol (1985). 2011;110(4):1111–8.
38. Nieman GF, Satalin J, Kollisch-Singule M, Andrews P, Aiash H, Habashi NM, Gatto LA. Physiology in medicine: understanding dynamic alveolar physiology to minimize ventilator-induced lung injury. J Appl Physiol (1985). 2017;122(6):1516–22.
39. Takahashi A, Bartolak-Suki E, Majumdar A, Suki B. Changes in respiratory elastance after deep inspirations reflect surface film functionality in mice with acute lung injury. J Appl Physiol (1985). 2015;119(3):258–65.
40. Neumann P, Berglund JE, Mondejar EF, Magnusson A, Hedenstierna G. Effect of different pressure levels on the dynamics of lung collapse and recruitment in oleic-acid-induced lung injury. Am J Respir Crit Care Med. 1998;158(5 Pt 1):1636–43.
41. Gattinoni L, Vagginelli F, Chiumello D, Taccone P, Carlesso E. Physiologic rationale for ventilator setting in acute lung injury/acute respiratory distress syndrome patients. Crit Care Med. 2003;31(4 Suppl):S300–4.
42. Kollisch-Singule M, Emr B, Smith B, Roy S, Jain S, Satalin J, Snyder K, Andrews P, Habashi N, Bates J, et al. Mechanical breath profile of airway pressure release ventilation: the effect on alveolar recruitment and microstrain in acute lung injury. JAMA Surg. 2014;149(11):1138–45.
43. Boehme S, Bentley AH, Hartmann EK, Chang S, Erdoes G, Prinzing A, Hagmann M, Baumgardner JE, Ullrich R, Markstaller K, et al. Influence of inspiration to expiration ratio on cyclic recruitment and derecruitment of atelectasis in a saline lavage model of acute respiratory distress syndrome. Crit Care Med. 2015;43(3):e65–74.

44. Albert SP, DiRocco J, Allen GB, Bates JH, Lafollette R, Kubiak BD, Fischer J, Maroney S, Nieman GF. The role of time and pressure on alveolar recruitment. J Appl Physiol (1985). 2009;106(3):757–65.
45. Lachmann B. Open up the lung and keep the lung open. Intensive Care Med. 1992;18(6):319–21.
46. Neumann P, Berglund JE, Fernandez Mondejar E, Magnusson A, Hedenstierna G. Dynamics of lung collapse and recruitment during prolonged breathing in porcine lung injury. J Appl Physiol (1985). 1998;85(4):1533–43.
47. Markstaller K, Eberle B, Kauczor HU, Scholz A, Bink A, Thelen M, Heinrichs W, Weiler N. Temporal dynamics of lung aeration determined by dynamic CT in a porcine model of ARDS. Br J Anaesth. 2001;87(3):459–68.
48. Facchin F, Fan E. Airway pressure release ventilation and high-frequency oscillatory ventilation: potential strategies to treat severe hypoxemia and prevent ventilator-induced lung injury. Respir Care. 2015;60(10):1509–21.
49. Mireles-Cabodevila E, Kacmarek RM. Should airway pressure release ventilation be the primary mode in ARDS? Respir Care. 2016;61(6):761–73.
50. Marini JJ, Gattinoni L. Time course of evolving ventilator-induced lung injury: the "shrinking baby lung". Crit Care Med. 2020;48(8):1203–9.
51. Dianti J, Tisminetzky M, Ferreyro BL, Englesakis M, Del Sorbo L, Sud S, Talmor D, Ball L, Meade M, Hodgson C, et al. Association of positive end-expiratory pressure and lung recruitment selection strategies with mortality in acute respiratory distress syndrome: a systematic review and network meta-analysis. Am J Respir Crit Care Med. 2022;205(11):1300–10.
52. Dreyfuss D, Ricard JD, Gaudry S. Did studies on HFOV fail to improve ARDS survival because they did not decrease VILI? On the potential validity of a physiological concept enounced several decades ago. Intensive Care Med. 2015;41(12):2076–86.
53. Kaczka DW. Oscillatory ventilation redux: alternative perspectives on ventilator-induced lung injury in the acute respiratory distress syndrome. Curr Opin Physio. 2021;21:36–43.
54. Herrmann J, Gerard SE, Shao W, Hawley ML, Reinhardt JM, Christensen GE, Hoffman EA, Kaczka DW. Quantifying regional lung deformation using four-dimensional computed tomography: a comparison of conventional and oscillatory ventilation. Front Physiol. 2020;11:14.
55. de Prost N, Dreyfuss D, Saumon G. Evaluation of two-way protein fluxes across the alveolo-capillary membrane by scintigraphy in rats: effect of lung inflation. J Appl Physiol (1985). 2007;102(2):794–802.
56. Parker JC, Townsley MI, Rippe B, Taylor AE, Thigpen J. Increased microvascular permeability in dog lungs due to high peak airway pressures. J Appl Physiol Respir Environ Exerc Physiol. 1984;57(6):1809–16.
57. Zeng C, Lagier D, Lee JW, Vidal Melo MF. Perioperative pulmonary atelectasis: part I. Biology and mechanisms. Anesthesiology. 2022;136(1):181–205.
58. Lagier D, Zeng C, Fernandez-Bustamante A, Vidal Melo MF. Perioperative pulmonary atelectasis: part II. Clinical implications. Anesthesiology. 2022;136(1):206–36.
59. Nieman GF, Gatto LA, Habashi NM. Impact of mechanical ventilation on the pathophysiology of progressive acute lung injury. J Appl Physiol (1985). 2015;119(11):1245–61.
60. Slutsky AS, Ranieri VM. Ventilator-induced lung injury. N Engl J Med. 2013;369(22):2126–36.
61. Uhlig U, Uhlig S. Ventilation-induced lung injury. Compr Physiol. 2011;1(2):635–61.
62. Egan EA, Nelson RM, Olver RE. Lung inflation and alveolar permeability to non-electrolytes in the adult sheep in vivo. J Physiol. 1976;260(2):409–24.
63. Ramcharran H, Bates JHT, Satalin J, Blair S, Andrews PL, Gaver DP, Gatto LA, Wang G, Ghosh AJ, Robedee B, et al. Protective ventilation in a pig model of acute lung injury: timing is as important as pressure. J Appl Physiol (1985). 2022;133(5):1093–105.
64. Hess DR. Recruitment maneuvers and PEEP titration. Respir Care. 2015;60(11):1688–704.
65. Halter JM, Steinberg JM, Schiller HJ, DaSilva M, Gatto LA, Landas S, Nieman GF. Positive end-expiratory pressure after a recruitment maneuver prevents both alveolar collapse and recruitment/derecruitment. Am J Respir Crit Care Med. 2003;167(12):1620–6.

Chapter 7
It's Not the Wand; It's the Wizard: It's Not Just the Mode but the Method Used to Set and Adjust the Mode that Is Lung Protective

Introduction

The significance of acute respiratory distress syndrome (ARDS) [1] has been underscored by the recent Severe Acute Respiratory Syndrome Coronavirus 2 (SARS-CoV-2) pandemic, commonly known as COVID-19. The global health crisis arising from SARS-CoV-2 frequently results in a distinct form of lung injury termed COVID-induced Acute Respiratory Distress Syndrome (CARDS) [2]. CARDS specifically impacts the pulmonary vascular endothelium, disrupting the lungs' ability to autoregulate blood flow. This disruption culminates in acute respiratory failure, characterized by a high mortality rate. While mechanical ventilation is a crucial tool for managing ARDS or CARDS, setting and adjusting a ventilator mode are as vital as the mode itself.

In the seminal Acute Respiratory Management Approach (ARMA) randomized controlled trial (RCT) on ARDS patients, two methods for setting and adjusting volume assist-control ventilation (VCV) were tested. The first group used low tidal volume (LV_T - V_T < 6 mL/kg of predicted body weight (PBW)] combined with low plateau pressure (Pplat <30 cm/H_2O], while the second group used higher V_T [HV_T - 12 mL/kg of PBW] and allowed a higher Pplat [>30 and <50 cm/H_2O] [3]. Notably, exceptions to the protocol permitted the V_T in the low V_T group to be increased up to 8 mL/kg if severe dyspnea occurred, as long as Pplat remained <30 cm/H_2O, resulting in a mean tidal volume of 6.5 ± 1.4 mL/kg on day 7, indicating some patients received nearly 8 mL/kg. Additionally, Pplat was allowed to exceed the group limits (30 and 50 cmH_2O, respectively) if the pH was <7.15. The physiologic goals of the ARMA method were to (i) "protect" the normal lung "baby lung" tissue from overdistension (OD—volutrauma) using low V_T and Pplat (Fig. 2.3), (ii) "rest" collapsed, edema-filled, or atelectatic lung tissue by excluding it from the ventilatory cycle, and (iii) minimize repetitive alveolar collapse and

© The Author(s), under exclusive license to Springer Nature Switzerland AG 2024

G. F. Nieman, N. M. Habashi, *Applied Physiology to Reduce Ventilator Induced Lung Injury*, https://doi.org/10.1007/978-3-031-66352-9_7

expansion (RACE)-induced atelectrauma and progressive loss of end-expiratory lung volume (EELV) by adjusting positive end-expiratory pressure (PEEP) based on oxygenation. Results of the ARMA trial showed a statistically significant reduction in mortality of 8.8% using the *same mode* with only a *slight change in the method* of setting the mode (6 vs 12 cc/kg V_T) [3]. Subsequently, the ARMA method became the current standard-of-care method for patients with ARDS, and the protocol for this method is listed in Fig. 7.1.

A key takeaway from the ARMA study was that the method of setting and adjusting the mode, rather than the mode itself, is critical to improve patient outcomes. Despite this, the importance of the method is often overlooked when assessing treatment efficacy, particularly in modes like airway pressure release ventilation (APRV).

Ventilator settings must be directed by lung pathophysiology. It is well known that the VCV mode per se is neither lung protective nor injurious. Instead, the specific combination of settings and adjustments made to the mode has been shown to affect outcomes. The conclusion of the 2000 ARMA study was not that VCV was or was not lung protective but that the LV_T method was more lung protective than the HV_T method.

However, further analysis by Deans et al. of the ARMA data from 2587 eligible patients who were excluded for technical reasons from participating in the original ARMA study suggests that low V_T did not necessarily reduce ARDS-related mortality but rather than high V_T increased mortality [4]. In fact, the V_T in the excluded patients was approximately 10 mL/kg PBW, yet their mortality was comparable to the low V_T group (31.7% versus 31.0%). The study also found a significant association between group allocation of high or low V_T and respiratory system compliance (C_{RS}) regarding mortality. Increasing V_T in patients with lower C_{RS} increased mortality (42% vs. 29%), whereas increasing tidal volume decreased mortality in patients with higher C_{RS} (21% vs. 37%; $P = 0.003$) (Fig. 7.2). This suggests that ventilator settings should be guided by the patient's lung mechanics and pathophysiology (i.e., C_{RS}), and that personalized ventilator settings may be more critical to patient outcomes than the ventilator mode itself.

Another example of a protocol that fails to consider patient physiology is the REST trial, which further reduced tidal volume from the "standard" 6 mL/kg to 4 mL/kg when the Pplat exceeded 30 cm/H_2O. Veno-venous extracorporeal carbon dioxide removal (VV-ECCO2R) was used to manage uncontrolled $PaCO_2$ elevation with such low V_Ts. However, mortality was higher (41.5%) in the study group with V_Ts of 3–4 mL/kg versus the control group (39.5%) with V_Ts of 6 mL/kg, despite achieving lower Pplat and driving pressure (ΔP). Additionally, the 3–4 mL/kg group experienced worsened oxygenation (likely due to lung derecruitment), increases in mechanical ventilation power (secondary to elevated respiratory rate), PEEP, and inspiratory gas flow (due to brief inspiratory times), and nearly double the use of neuromuscular blocking medications (42.1% versus 21.5%) [5].

These observations have been confirmed in a secondary analysis of 1096 patients enrolled in five RCTs of lower vs. higher tidal volume ventilatory strategies in ARDS [6]. This analysis shows that the mortality benefit of ventilation with lower V_T is more significant in patients with higher elastance (i.e., lower C_{RS}) [4]. Using

ARDSnet

NIH NHLBI ARDS Clinical Network
Mechanical Ventilation Protocol Summary

INCLUSION CRITERIA: Acute onset of

1. $PaO_2/FiO_2 \leq 300$ (corrected for altitude)
2. Bilateral (patchy, diffuse, or homogeneous) infiltrates consistent with pulmonary edema
3. No clinical evidence of left atrial hypertension

PART I: VENTILATOR SETUP AND ADJUSTMENT

1. Calculate predicted body weight (PBW)
   Males = 50 + 2.3 [height (inches) - 60]
   Females = 45.5 + 2.3 [height (inches) -60]
2. Select any ventilator mode
3. Set ventilator settings to achieve initial V_T = 8 ml/kg PBW
4. Reduce V_T by 1 ml/kg at intervals ≤ 2 hours until V_T = 6ml/kg PBW.
5. Set initial rate to approximate baseline minute ventilation (not > 35 bpm).
6. Adjust V_T and RR to achieve pH and plat eau pressure goals below.

OXYGENATION GOAL: PaO_2 55-80 mmHg or SpO_2 88-95%
Use a minimum PEEP of 5 cm H_2O. Consider use of incremental FiO_2/PEEP combinations such as shown below (not required) to achieve goal.

Lower PEEP/higher FiO2

FiO_2	0.3	0.4	0.4	0.5	0.5	0.6	0.7	0.7
PEEP	5	5	8	8	10	10	10	12

FiO_2	0.7	0.8	0.9	0.9	0.9	1.0
PEEP	14	14	14	16	18	18-24

Higher PEEP/lower FiO2

FiO_2	0.3	0.3	0.3	0.3	0.3	0.4	0.4	0.5
PEEP	5	8	10	12	14	14	16	16

FiO_2	0.5	0.5-0.8	0.8	0.9	1.0	1.0
PEEP	18	20	22	22	22	24

PLATEAU PRESSURE GOAL: ≤ 30 cm H_2O
Check Pplat (0.5 second inspiratory pause), at least q 4h and after each change in PEEP or V_T.
If Pplat > 30 cm H_2O: decrease V_T by 1ml/kg steps (minimum = 4 ml/kg).
If Pplat < 25 cm H_2O and V_T < 6 ml/kg , increase V_T by 1 ml/kg until Pplat > 25 cm H_2O or V_T = 6 ml/kg.
If Pplat < 30 and breath stacking or dys-synchrony occurs: may increase V_T in 1ml/kg increments to 7 or 8 ml/kg if Pplat remains ≤ 30 cm H_2O.

Fig. 7.1 The ARDSnet protocol for using the ARMA method to set and adjust conventional ventilator modes using a low tidal volume, low plateau pressure protective ventilation strategy

pH GOAL: 7.30-7.45
Acidosis Management: (pH < 7.30)
If pH 7.15-7.30: Increase RR until pH > 7.30 or $PaCO_2 < 25$ (Maximum set RR = 35).

If pH < 7.15: Increase RR to 35.
If pH remains < 7.15, V_T may be increased in 1 ml/kg steps until pH > 7.15 (Pplat target of 30 may be exceeded).
May give $NaHCO_3$
Alkalosis Management: (pH > 7.45) Decrease vent rate if possible.

I: E RATIO GOAL: Recommend that duration of inspiration be ≤ duration of expiration.

PART II: WEANING

A. Conduct a SPONTANEOUS BREATHING TRIAL daily when:
1. $FiO_2 \leq 0.40$ and PEEP ≤ 8 OR $FiO_2 \leq 0.50$ and PEEP ≤ 5.
2. PEEP and FiO_2 ≤ values of previous day.
3. Patient has acceptable spontaneous breathing efforts. (May decrease vent rate by 50% for 5 minutes to detect effort.)
4. Systolic BP ≥ 90 mmHg without vasopressor support.
5. No neuromuscular blocking agents or blockade.

B. SPONTANEOUS BREATHING TRIAL (SBT):
If all above criteria are met and subject has been in the study for at least 12 hours, initiate a trial of UP TO 120 minutes of spontaneous breathing with FiO2 ≤ 0.5 and PEEP ≤ 5:
1. Place on T-piece, trach collar, or CPAP ≤ 5 cm H_2O with PS ≤ 5
2. Assess for tolerance as below for up to two hours.
   a. $SpO_2 \geq 90$: and/or $PaO_2 \geq 60$ mmHg
   b. Spontaneous $V_T \geq 4$ ml/kg PBW
   c. RR ≤ 35/min
   d. pH ≥ 7.3
   e. No respiratory distress (distress= 2 or more)
      - ➢ HR > 120% of baseline
      - ➢ Marked accessory muscle use
      - ➢ Abdominal paradox
      - ➢ Diaphoresis
      - ➢ Marked dyspnea
3. If tolerated for at least 30 minutes, consider extubation.
4. If not tolerated resume pre-weaning settings.

Definition of UNASSISTED BREATHING
(Different from the spontaneous breathing criteria as PS is not allowed)

1. Extubated with face mask, nasal prong oxygen, or room air, OR
2. T-tube breathing, OR
3. Tracheostomy mask breathing, OR
4. CPAP less than or equal to 5 cm H_20 **without pressure support or IMV assistance.**

Fig. 7.1 (continued)

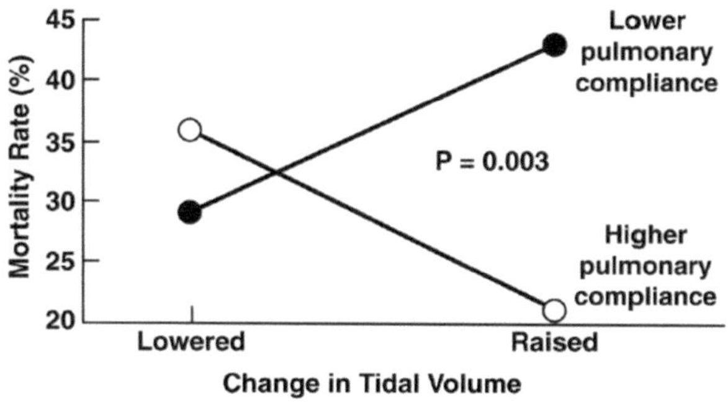

Fig. 7.2 Interaction between tidal volume (V_T) size and respiratory system compliance (C_{RS}) on mortality. Using the same volume assist-control [20] mode, a ***Lower*** V_T reduced mortality in patients with low C_{RS} but increased mortality in patients with high lung C_{RS}. A ***Higher*** V_T had the opposite impact on mortality, increasing mortality in patients with low C_{RS}, and decreasing mortality in patients with high lung C_{RS} [4]

parallel logic, we suggest that ventilator mode settings should be adjusted according to individual lung pathophysiology, regardless of the ventilator mode used. Just as the volume of intravenous fluid needed for optimal resuscitation is not the same for everyone and must consider factors such as cardiac status, vascular endothelial tone, current intravascular volume, and dynamic response to a volume challenge, ventilator settings must be personalized to the patient's pathophysiology.

The Airway Pressure Release Ventilation (APRV) mode: The APRV mode was developed in 1987 and has been the subject of extensive study with varied methods for setting and adjusting, leading to diverse outcomes. Unlike conventional modes, such as Volume Control Ventilation (VCV), there is no consensus on the optimal method to set and adjust APRV [7]. The multitude of approaches in clinical trials has contributed to significant outcome variations [8–12]. Acknowledging that outcomes depend heavily on the method used to set the mode, it becomes essential to recognize that APRV, as a mode, cannot be definitively categorized as lung protective or harmful; instead, one method of setting and adjusting APRV may prove superior to another (Fig. 7.3). Indeed, a review showed that the wide variety of methods used to set and adjust APRV undoubtedly significantly impact patient outcomes (Fig. 7.4) [13–15]. Many myths and misconceptions attributed to the APRV mode have recently been debunked [16].

Multiple RCTs have been designed to test different methods to set and adjust the same conventional ventilator mode, with changes most often involving modification of the size of the V_T and magnitude of the PEEP [1, 3, 17–22]. Other RCTs compare modes, usually using the VCV mode and the ARMA method as the control group, with modes such as high-frequency oscillatory ventilation (HFOV) or APRV [10, 23–25]. Some of these RCTs showed improved outcomes compared to standard of care, [25, 26] and others worsened outcomes (Table 2.1) [10, 23, 25, 27]. What was overlooked in all of these RCTs was the method used to set and adjust the HFOV and APRV modes, and as shown in the above studies, slight variation in the method can significantly impact outcomes.

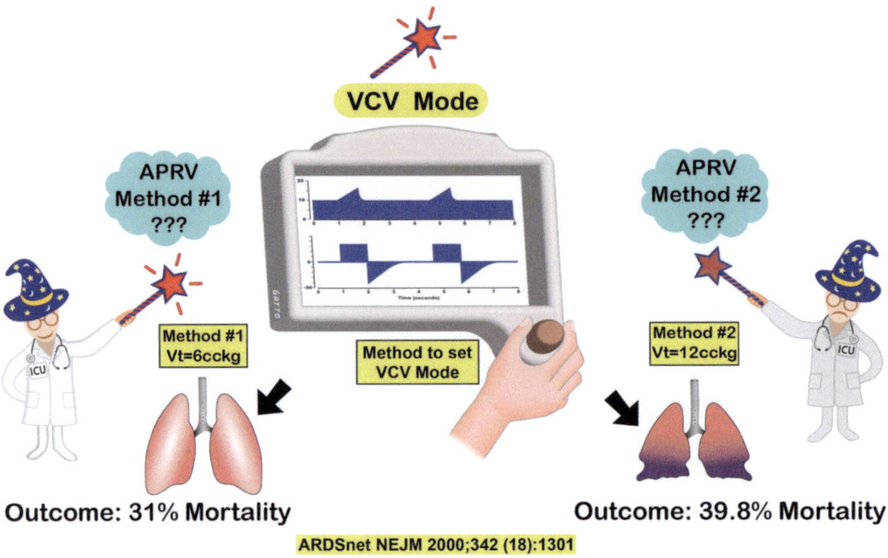

Fig. 7.3 *It's not the Wand it's the Wizard.* The same volume assist-controlled (VCV) mode (Wand) set using two different methods (Wizards) results in different outcomes. In this example, the ARMA study patients received either a low or high tidal volume (V_T) (6 vs 12 mL/kg predicted body weight (PBW) delivered using the same mode [VCV]). The low V_T method had significantly lower mortality (31%) than the high V_T method (39.8%) [3]. This illustrates that the mode selected is less important than the method used to set and adjust the mode to determine treatment efficacy: *It's not the Wand; it's the Wizard.* If the method to set the VCV mode plays a role in patient outcome, it is logical to postulate that the same is true about the method used to set and adjust the airway pressure release ventilation (APRV) mode

Fig. 7.4 Pressure/time waveforms from four published studies using the Airway Pressure Release Ventilation (APRV) mode illustrate the tremendous variability in the methods used to set APRV. These highly variable settings may impact outcomes in basic science studies or randomized controlled trials using the APRV mode (Fig. 7.3) [13]. (**a**) Stock 1987 used an expiratory duration of 1.27 s and 60% continuous positive airway pressure (CPAP) with a respiratory rate (RR) of 20 breaths/min [7]. (**b**) Davis decreased the respiratory rate (RR) by prolonging the inspiratory and expiratory durations and used a continuous positive airway pressure (CPAP) time (60%) similar to that of Stock [39]. (**c**) Gama de Abreau simulated conventional ventilation with a prolonged expiratory time and a brief time at inspiration [40]. Finally, (**d**) Roy used the Time-Controlled Adaptive Ventilation (TCAV) method with a brief adaptive expiratory duration based on lung compliance and an extended inspiratory time occupying ~90% of each breath [41]

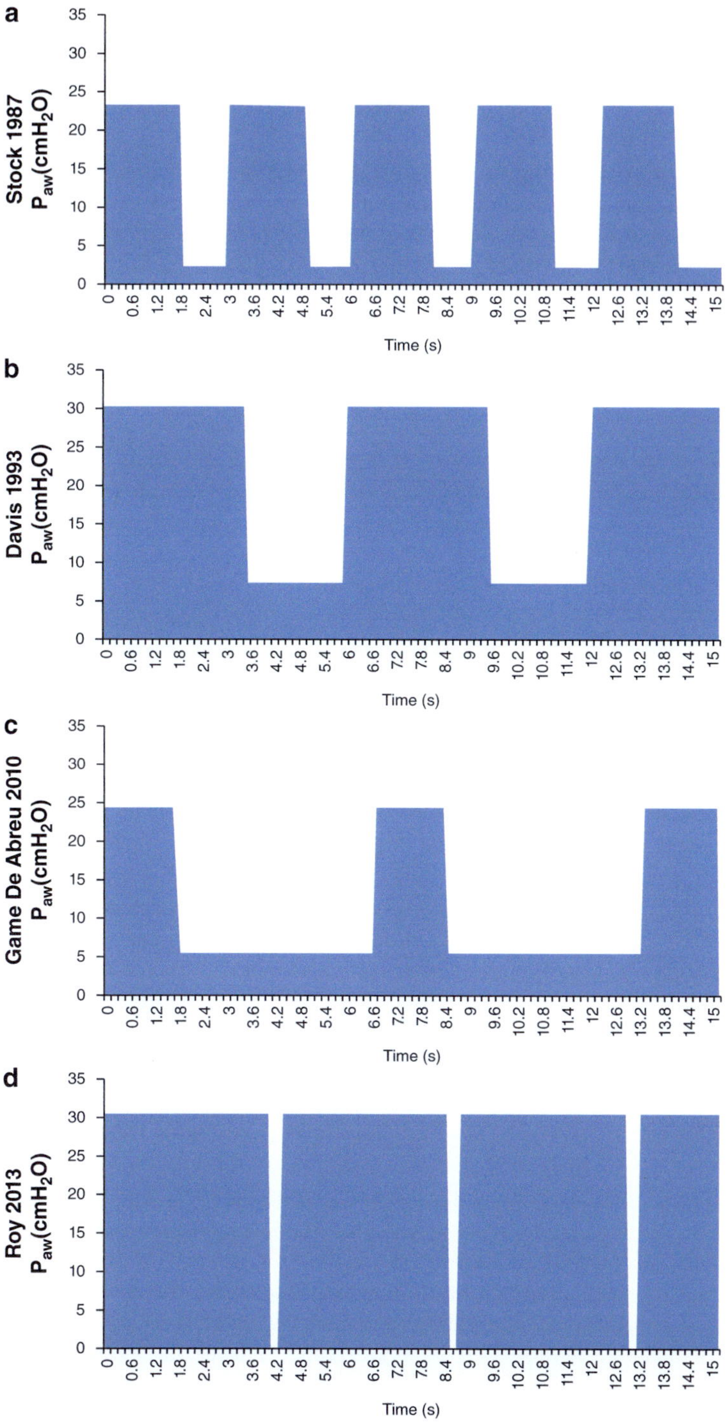
a
Stock 1987
Paw(cmH2O)
35
30
25
20
15
10
5
0
0 0.6 1.2 1.8 2.4 3 3.6 4.2 4.8 5.4 6 6.6 7.2 7.8 8.4 9 9.6 10.2 10.8 11.4 12 12.6 13.2 13.8 14.4 15
Time (s)
b
Davis 1993
Paw(cmH2O)
35
30
25
20
15
10
5
0
0 0.6 1.2 1.8 2.4 3 3.6 4.2 4.8 5.4 6 6.6 7.2 7.8 8.4 9 9.6 10.2 10.8 11.4 12 12.6 13.2 13.8 14.4 15
Time (s)
c
Game De Abreu 2010
Paw(cmH2O)
35
30
25
20
15
10
5
0
0 0.6 1.2 1.8 2.4 3 3.6 4.2 4.8 5.4 6 6.6 7.2 7.8 8.4 9 9.6 10.2 10.8 11.4 12 12.6 13.2 13.8 14.4 15
Time (s)
d
Roy 2013
Paw(cmH2O)
35
30
25
20
15
10
5
0
0 0.6 1.2 1.8 2.4 3 3.6 4.2 4.8 5.4 6 6.6 7.2 7.8 8.4 9 9.6 10.2 10.8 11.4 12 12.6 13.2 13.8 14.4 15
Time (s)

The significance of the method over the mode is exemplified by the ARMA study, revealing that even slight changes in the method of applying VCV mode can have a substantial impact on patient outcomes (Fig. 7.3). Instead of analyzing studies based solely on the mode used (HFOV or APRV), a more informative approach would involve stratifying studies by ventilator settings for subgroup analysis [15]. It would be akin to averaging mortality outcomes from both V_Ts in the ARMA study (6 and 12 mL/kg) and concluding that VCV is not lung protective [3]. One reason for this oversight is that there is little or no data to identify the optimal methods to set and adjust HFOV, and only recent optimal settings and methods have been investigated for APRV.

The Time-Controlled Adaptive Ventilation (TCAV) Method to set and adjust the APRV mode: To design an effective protective ventilation strategy, the entire MB_P must be considered [28]. We and others have extensively studied and reviewed the TCAV method to set and adjust the APRV mode and have demonstrated that slight deviations from the TCAV method will significantly reduce lung-protective efficacy (Video 8.5) [29–33]. The TCAV method is based on our understanding that ARDS pathophysiology renders the lung time- and pressure-dependent. This means that the lung will take more time to open and less time to re-collapse at any given airway pressure. Thus, reducing the expiratory duration will prevent alveolar collapse (Video 6.1—TCAV), and extending the inspiratory time will gradually recruit collapsed tissue (Video 5.1). When an extended inspiratory time is combined with a short expiratory time to prevent the newly open tissue from re-collapsing, the acutely injured lung can be ventilated in an open and stable condition, minimizing VILI (Videos 8.2 TCAV-P_{EF} 75%, 8.4 TCAV Method, 8.6-P_{EF}×75%).

Thus, the TCAV method uses the MB_P component of inspiratory and expiratory *time* first to stabilize alveoli, preventing RACE-induced atelectrauma, and then gradually "ratchets" open collapsed tissue over an extended period (hours or even days) (Fig. 8.8). This treatment sequence of rapidly stabilizing the lung and then gradually recruiting is critical since atelectrauma is a key mechanism driving VILI (Fig. 8.1). This sequence is in direct contrast to the current open lung approach [34], which attempts to rapidly (seconds or minutes) recruit most of the lung first with high airway pressure and then attempt to stabilize the newly recruited tissue using titrated PEEP.

When using the TCAV method, lung stability is attained with an adequately set expiratory duration during the Release Phase (T_{Low}) (Fig. 8.3 TCAV Method, Release Phase), which is directed by changes in C_{RS} using the expiratory flow curve that pairs V_T to C_{RS} (i.e., low C_{RS} = LV_T and vice versa) (Figs. 8.4, 8.5, 8.6, 8.7, 8.9, and 8.10) [31, 33]. Physiologically incorrect adjusting of T_{Low} to achieve a specific V_T, increase minute ventilation, or reduce $PaCO_2$, as seen in recent studies, may dramatically increase alveolar instability and RACE-induced atelectrauma. [10, 12] In addition, if the T_{Low} is not correctly set (Peak expiratory flow × 75% vs. 10%) and paired with an extended inspiratory duration (T_{High}) at high pressure (P_{High}), the number of unstable alveoli will be exacerbated because the extended inspiratory time will recruit alveoli, but they will re-collapse during each Release Phase (Figs. 5.4 and 5.8).

In a recent RCT testing APRV efficacy on COVID-19 patients, although oxygenation and C_{RS} were augmented, mortality was not improved. We postulate these results reflect extending $T_{High,}$ providing alveolar recruitment and improved gas exchange, but incorrectly set and extended expiratory duration (T_{Low}), allowing RACE-induced atelectrauma. [12] Dynamic alveolar collapse can be immediately neutralized with an appropriately set T_{Low} (Peak expiratory flow × 75%) (Figs. 8.7 and 8.8, Videos 8.2, 8.3, 8.4, and 8.5) [32]. Still, reaeration of densely collapsed lung regions may require several hours to days, depending on ARDS severity (Fig. 8.1 Gradual Lung Recruitment). We postulate that the TCAV method uses an *Inflate and Brake* method to "ratchet" method to open a small volume of lung tissue with each breath, [32] similar to the way a full-term newborn opens their collapsed and fluid-filled lung at birth (Fig. 8.8) [35].

Once collapsed lung regions are re-aerated, they must be stented open with appropriate airway *pressure* and *time* (Fig. 8.2) until a functional surfactant system is re-established. This is critical since this newly recruited lung tissue is still time- and pressure-dependent, and without properly set APRV re-collapse and RACE will not be prevented, even though the chest X-ray and blood gases suggest the lung has "healed" (Fig. 8.9b). Thus, using APRV with incorrectly set times and pressures is equivalent to not setting PEEP sufficiently high to prevent re-collapse and RACE following a recruitment maneuver [10] [14, 36]. Alveolar recruitment with inadequate PEEP-induced alveolar stabilization or preventing progressive loss of EELV is a possible pathophysiologic explanation for why using RMs in recent RCTs did not influence ARDS-related mortality [34, 37, 38].

Summary

The ARMA study demonstrated the importance of the method used to set the VCV mode on patient outcomes (Fig. 7.3). Thus, when analyzing studies using the APRV mode, they must be stratified by the methods used to set and adjust the mode [15]. A negative outcome using APRV cannot be solely attributed to the mode alone since it is possible the protocol used to set APRV was not based on sound physiologic evidence of efficacy, significantly reducing the lung-protective capability of the mode. The TCAV method is the most extensively studied protocol for setting APRV and uses a dual treatment strategy of both inspiratory and expiratory time and pressure to first stabilize and then gradually reopen the lung [31–33]. There is a continuing and critical need to identify optimal methods to set and adjust any ventilator mode for ARDS patients, with the goal of personalizing the settings by an individual patient's lung mechanics. In the next chapter, we will discuss the applied physiology of the TCAV method to set and adjust the APRV mode.

References

1. Brower RG, Lanken PN, MacIntyre N, Matthay MA, Morris A, Ancukiewicz M, Schoenfeld D, Thompson BT, National Heart L, Blood Institute ACTN. Higher versus lower positive end-expiratory pressures in patients with the acute respiratory distress syndrome. N Engl J Med. 2004;351(4):327–36.
2. Habashi NM, Camporota L, Gatto LA, Nieman G. Functional pathophysiology of SARS-CoV-2-induced acute lung injury and clinical implications. J Appl Physiol (1985). 2021;130(3):877–91.
3. Acute Respiratory Distress Syndrome N, Brower RG, Matthay MA, Morris A, Schoenfeld D, Thompson BT, Wheeler A. Ventilation with lower tidal volumes as compared with traditional tidal volumes for acute lung injury and the acute respiratory distress syndrome. N Engl J Med. 2000;342(18):1301–8.
4. Deans KJ, Minneci PC, Cui X, Banks SM, Natanson C, Eichacker PQ. Mechanical ventilation in ARDS: one size does not fit all. Crit Care Med. 2005;33(5):1141–3.
5. McNamee JJ, Gillies MA, Barrett NA, Perkins GD, Tunnicliffe W, Young D, Bentley A, Harrison DA, Brodie D, Boyle AJ, et al. Effect of lower tidal volume ventilation facilitated by extracorporeal carbon dioxide removal vs standard care ventilation on 90-day mortality in patients with acute hypoxemic respiratory failure: the REST randomized clinical trial. JAMA. 2021;326(11):1013–23.
6. Goligher EC, Costa ELV, Yarnell CJ, Brochard LJ, Stewart TE, Tomlinson G, Brower RG, Slutsky AS, Amato MPB. Effect of lowering Vt on mortality in acute respiratory distress syndrome varies with respiratory system elastance. Am J Respir Crit Care Med. 2021;203(11):1378–85.
7. Stock MC, Downs JB, Frolicher DA. Airway pressure release ventilation. Crit Care Med. 1987;15(5):462–6.
8. Andrews PL, Shiber JR, Jaruga-Killeen E, Roy S, Sadowitz B, O'Toole RV, Gatto LA, Nieman GF, Scalea T, Habashi NM. Early application of airway pressure release ventilation may reduce mortality in high-risk trauma patients: a systematic review of observational trauma ARDS literature. J Trauma Acute Care Surg. 2013;75(4):635–41.
9. Janssen M, Meeder JHJ, Seghers L, den Uil CA. Time controlled adaptive ventilation as conservative treatment of destroyed lung: an alternative to lung transplantation. BMC Pulm Med. 2021;21(1):176.
10. Hirshberg EL, Lanspa MJ, Peterson J, Carpenter L, Wilson EL, Brown SM, Dean NC, Orme J, Grissom CK. Randomized feasibility trial of a low tidal volume-airway pressure release ventilation protocol compared with traditional airway pressure release ventilation and volume control ventilation protocols. Crit Care Med. 2018;46(12):1943–52.
11. Ganesan SL, Jayashree M. Reply to Daxon and to Kyo et al. Am J Respir Crit Care Med. 2018;198(11):1460–2.
12. Ibarra-Estrada MA, Garcia-Salas Y, Mireles-Cabodevila E, Lopez-Pulgarin JA, Chavez-Pena Q, Garcia-Salcido R, Mijangos-Mendez JC, Aguirre-Avalos G. Use of airway pressure release ventilation in patients with acute respiratory failure due to COVID-19: results of a single-center randomized controlled trial. Crit Care Med. 2022;50(4):586–94.
13. Jain SV, Kollisch-Singule M, Sadowitz B, Dombert L, Satalin J, Andrews P, Gatto LA, Nieman GF, Habashi NM. The 30-year evolution of airway pressure release ventilation (APRV). Intensive Care Med Exp. 2016;4(1):11.
14. Habashi N, Andrews P, Roy S, Sadowitz B, Nieman G, Gatto LA. Up in smoke: airway pressure release ventilation must be applied correctly to protect the lung. Crit Care Med. 2012;40(3):1040–1; author reply 1041–1042. https://doi.org/10.3390/jcm13092690
15. https://doi.org/10.3390/jcm13092690.
16. Andrews P, Shiber J, Madden M, Nieman GF, Camporota L, Habashi NM. Myths and misconceptions of airway pressure release ventilation: getting past the noise and on to the signal. Front Physiol. 2022;13:928562.

17. Amato MB, Barbas CS, Medeiros DM, Magaldi RB, Schettino GP, Lorenzi-Filho G, Kairalla RA, Deheinzelin D, Munoz C, Oliveira R, et al. Effect of a protective-ventilation strategy on mortality in the acute respiratory distress syndrome. N Engl J Med. 1998;338(6):347–54.
18. Brower RG, Shanholtz CB, Fessler HE, Shade DM, White P Jr, Wiener CM, Teeter JG, Dodd-o JM, Almog Y, Piantadosi S. Prospective, randomized, controlled clinical trial comparing traditional versus reduced tidal volume ventilation in acute respiratory distress syndrome patients. Crit Care Med. 1999;27(8):1492–8.
19. Brochard L, Roudot-Thoraval F, Roupie E, Delclaux C, Chastre J, Fernandez-Mondejar E, Clementi E, Mancebo J, Factor P, Matamis D, et al. Tidal volume reduction for prevention of ventilator-induced lung injury in acute respiratory distress syndrome. The Multicenter Trail Group on Tidal Volume Reduction in ARDS. Am J Respir Crit Care Med. 1998;158(6):1831–8.
20. Talmor D, Sarge T, Malhotra A, O'Donnell CR, Ritz R, Lisbon A, Novack V, Loring SH. Mechanical ventilation guided by esophageal pressure in acute lung injury. N Engl J Med. 2008;359(20):2095–104.
21. Meade MO, Cook DJ, Guyatt GH, Slutsky AS, Arabi YM, Cooper DJ, Davies AR, Hand LE, Zhou Q, Thabane L, et al. Ventilation strategy using low tidal volumes, recruitment maneuvers, and high positive end-expiratory pressure for acute lung injury and acute respiratory distress syndrome: a randomized controlled trial. JAMA. 2008;299(6):637–45.
22. Mercat A, Richard JC, Vielle B, Jaber S, Osman D, Diehl JL, Lefrant JY, Prat G, Richecoeur J, Nieszkowska A, et al. Positive end-expiratory pressure setting in adults with acute lung injury and acute respiratory distress syndrome: a randomized controlled trial. JAMA. 2008;299(6):646–55.
23. Young D, Lamb SE, Shah S, MacKenzie I, Tunnicliffe W, Lall R, Rowan K, Cuthbertson BH, Group OS. High-frequency oscillation for acute respiratory distress syndrome. N Engl J Med. 2013;368(9):806–13.
24. Ferguson ND, Slutsky AS, Meade MO. High-frequency oscillation for ARDS. N Engl J Med. 2013;368(23):2233–4.
25. Zhou Y, Jin X, Lv Y, Wang P, Yang Y, Liang G, Wang B, Kang Y. Early application of airway pressure release ventilation may reduce the duration of mechanical ventilation in acute respiratory distress syndrome. Intensive Care Med. 2017;43(11):1648–59.
26. Joseph DAK, Baltazar GA, Jacquez RA, Islam S, Stright A, Divers J, Brathwaite CEM, Petrone P. A pilot study of patients with COVID–19-related respiratory failure utilizing airway pressure release ventilation (APRV). Innov Surg Interv Med. 2020;1(1):3–8.
27. Ferguson ND, Cook DJ, Guyatt GH, Mehta S, Hand L, Austin P, Zhou Q, Matte A, Walter SD, Lamontagne F, et al. High-frequency oscillation in early acute respiratory distress syndrome. N Engl J Med. 2013;368(9):795–805.
28. Kollisch-Singule M, Emr B, Smith B, Roy S, Jain S, Satalin J, Snyder K, Andrews P, Habashi N, Bates J, et al. Mechanical breath profile of airway pressure release ventilation: the effect on alveolar recruitment and microstrain in acute lung injury. JAMA Surg. 2014;149(11):1138–45.
29. Habashi NM. Other approaches to open-lung ventilation: airway pressure release ventilation. Crit Care Med. 2005;33(3 Suppl):S228–40.
30. Nieman GF, Satalin J, Andrews P, Aiash H, Habashi NM, Gatto LA. Personalizing mechanical ventilation according to physiologic parameters to stabilize alveoli and minimize ventilator induced lung injury (VILI). Intensive Care Med Exp. 2017;5(1):8.
31. Nieman GF, Al-Khalisy H, Kollisch-Singule M, Satalin J, Blair S, Trikha G, Andrews P, Madden M, Gatto LA, Habashi NM. A physiologically informed strategy to effectively open, stabilize, and protect the acutely injured lung. Front Physiol. 2020;11:227.
32. Nieman G, Kollisch-Singule M, Ramcharran H, Satalin J, Blair S, Gatto LA, Andrews P, Ghosh A, Kaczka DW, Gaver D, et al. Unshrinking the baby lung to calm the VILI vortex. Crit Care. 2022;26(1):242.
33. Nieman GF, Gatto LA, Andrews P, Satalin J, Camporota L, Daxon B, Blair SJ, Al-Khalisy H, Madden M, Kollisch-Singule M, et al. Prevention and treatment of acute lung injury with

time-controlled adaptive ventilation: physiologically informed modification of airway pressure release ventilation. Ann Intensive Care. 2020;10(1):3.
34. Writing Group for the Alveolar Recruitment for Acute Respiratory Distress Syndrome Trial I, Cavalcanti AB, Suzumura EA, Laranjeira LN, Paisani DM, Damiani LP, Guimaraes HP, Romano ER, Regenga MM, Taniguchi LNT, et al. Effect of lung recruitment and titrated positive end-expiratory pressure (PEEP) vs low PEEP on mortality in patients with acute respiratory distress syndrome: a randomized clinical trial. JAMA. 2017;318(14):1335–45.
35. Tingay DG, Farrell O, Thomson J, Perkins EJ, Pereira-Fantini PM, Waldmann AD, Ruegger C, Adler A, Davis PG, Frerichs I. Imaging the respiratory transition at birth: unraveling the complexities of the first breaths of life. Am J Respir Crit Care Med. 2021;204(1):82–91.
36. Batchinsky AI, Burkett SE, Zanders TB, Chung KK, Regn DD, Jordan BS, Necsoiu C, Nguyen R, Hanson MA, Morris MJ, et al. Comparison of airway pressure release ventilation to conventional mechanical ventilation in the early management of smoke inhalation injury in swine. Crit Care Med. 2011;39(10):2314–21.
37. Cui Y, Cao R, Wang Y, Li G. Lung recruitment maneuvers for ARDS patients: a systematic review and meta-analysis. Respiration. 2020;99(3):264–76.
38. Pensier J, de Jong A, Hajjej Z, Molinari N, Carr J, Belafia F, Chanques G, Futier E, Azoulay E, Jaber S. Effect of lung recruitment maneuver on oxygenation, physiological parameters and mortality in acute respiratory distress syndrome patients: a systematic review and meta-analysis. Intensive Care Med. 2019;45(12):1691–702.
39. Davis K Jr, Johnson DJ, Branson RD, Campbell RS, Johannigman JA, Porembka D. Airway pressure release ventilation. Arch Surg. 1993;128(12):1348–52.
40. Gama de Abreu M, Cuevas M, Spieth PM, Carvalho AR, Hietschold V, Stroszczynski C, Wiedemann B, Koch T, Pelosi P, Koch E. Regional lung aeration and ventilation during pressure support and biphasic positive airway pressure ventilation in experimental lung injury. Crit Care. 2010;14(2):R34.
41. Roy S, Habashi N, Sadowitz B, Andrews P, Ge L, Wang G, Roy P, Ghosh A, Kuhn M, Satalin J, et al. Early airway pressure release ventilation prevents ARDS-a novel preventive approach to lung injury. Shock. 2013;39(1):28–38.

Chapter 8
Novel Time-Controlled Adaptive Ventilation Method to Minimize VILI

A Paradigm Shift in Lung-Protective Mechanical Ventilation

The current Acute Respiratory Management Approach (ARMA) low tidal volume (V_T) and low airway pressure protective ventilation strategy for patients with acute respiratory distress syndrome (ARDS) can be viewed as a Protect the Lung Approach (PLA). The primary goal of PLA is to prevent overdistension-induced tissue damage in the remaining normal tissue, referred to as the "baby lung," caused by high ventilation volumes and pressures (Fig. 2.3). Additionally, the strategy aims to allow the collapsed atelectatic tissue to "rest" by keeping it out of the ventilatory cycle [1].

A variation of this method, known as the Open Lung Approach (OLA), also utilizes low V_T and airway pressures. However, it emphasizes forcibly recruiting collapsed tissue over a very brief period using various recruitment maneuver (RM) protocols [2]. If respiratory failure worsens with either the PLA or OLA, a standard rescue option is to use extracorporeal membrane oxygenation (ECMO) to exchange oxygen and carbon dioxide. This generally involves utilizing very low V_T to achieve "Lung Rest" defined as not ventilating collapsed lung tissue [3]. While the concept of lung rest is intuitively understood, it needs to be more well-defined physiologically, and its implementation varies significantly among published studies [4, 5]. This can lead to continued deterioration of the small portion of the functioning "baby lung," which descends further into the VILI vortex [6] often described as "ECMO lung" or "lung white out" post-ECMO, [7–10]. Significant loss of end expiratory lung volume (EELV) makes the lung highly susceptible to VILI. Despite these strategies, as reviewed in Chap. 2, recent large randomized controlled trials (RCTs) have shown increased mortality with OLA, and multiple statistical and meta-analyses have indicated no reduction in ARDS-related mortality using the ARMA PLA (Table 2.1).

Supplementary Information The online version contains supplementary material available at https://doi.org/10.1007/978-3-031-66352-9_8.

© The Author(s), under exclusive license to Springer Nature Switzerland AG 2024

G. F. Nieman, N. M. Habashi, *Applied Physiology to Reduce Ventilator Induced Lung Injury*, https://doi.org/10.1007/978-3-031-66352-9_8

A shift toward utilizing applied physiology in designing protective mechanical breaths is crucial to improving outcomes for ARDS patients. It is essential to analyze the entire Mechanical Breath Profile (MB_P), including all airway volumes, pressures, flows, rates, and the time they are applied during inspiration and expiration. Understanding the alteration in dynamic alveolar mechanics caused by ARDS is critical in designing a logical lung-protective MB_P, as discussed in Chaps. 2–4. These chapters reviewed the following: (i) the presumed lung pathophysiology (i.e., overdistension of the baby lung) on which current ARMA LV_T strategies are based (Fig. 2.3), (ii) the current evidence that the actual pathophysiology that drives ventilator-induced lung injury (VILI) is regional alveolar instability and stress multipliers (Figs. 2.6 and 2.7), (iii) normal alveolar and alveolar duct (acinar) dynamic mechanics during tidal ventilation (Figs. 3.3, 3.4, and 3.5), and (iv) how ARDS-induced pathophysiology changes acinar mechanics in a way that predisposes the lung to a secondary VILI (Figs. 2.6, 2.7, 4.3, 4.6, 4.7, and 4.9, Videos 4.4 and 4.5). The altered acinar mechanics driven by regional alveolar instability and stress multipliers are identified as the mechanisms causing VILI. If altered acinar mechanics are the mechanism driving VILI, then the applied physiologic solution is to normalize mechanics using a mechanical breath. Repetitive alveolar collapse and expansion (RACE). The solution seems obvious: stabilize and reopen the lung, eliminating the mechanisms driving progressive tissue damage that push the lung into the VILI vortex (Fig. 8.1) [6]. However, this solution has been much more challenging than anticipated, and the current OLA methods designed to fulfill these goals have failed to reduce ARDS-related mortality (Table 2.1), as reviewed in Chap. 6 [11].

The proposed solution first stabilizes and then gradually reopens the lung, eliminating the mechanisms driving progressive tissue damage. The Time-Controlled Adaptive Ventilation (TCAV) method to set and adjust the Airway Pressure Release Ventilation (APRV) mode has effectively achieved this goal. TCAV represents a Stabilize Lung Approach (SLA) designed to rapidly stabilize lung tissue and gradually reopen atelectatic tissue over hours or days, pulling the lung out of the VILI vortex (Fig. 8.1).

In simple terms, we need to use the mechanical breath as a "cast" to stabilize the "*broken*" ARDS lung from the inside until it heals, for the same reason we put a cast on a broken arm until the bone heals (Fig. 8.2) [12]. What are the components of the MB_P can we use to accomplish this goal? Applying our knowledge of physiology, we know that the lung becomes *time*- and *pressure*-dependent (Chap. 5). This means it will take more *time* for the alveoli to open and less *time* to re-collapse at any airway pressure. The obvious solution is to use the MB_P component of time at inspiration and expiration to accomplish our goal of an open and stable lung. The TCAV method to set and adjust the APRV mode is the most studied method to set APRV and has been shown to effectively cast open the ARDS lung until it heals (Fig. 8.2), [13–40] pulling the lung from the VILI vortex (Fig. 8.1), and is a paradigm shift from the PLA and OLA strategies.

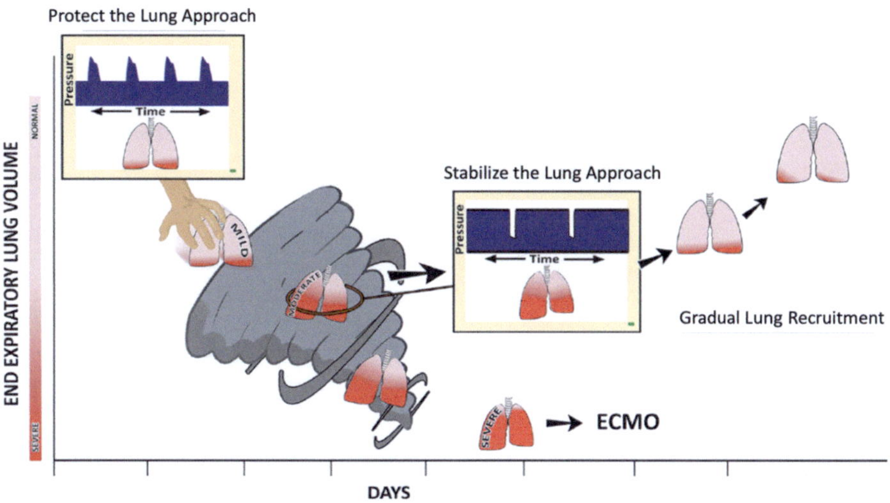

Fig. 8.1 Diagram of ARDS pathogenesis with a progressively collapsing "baby lung" resulting in a "VILI Vortex." Using the *Protect the Lung Approach* (PLA), low tidal volume and plateau airway pressure can push the lung into the VILI vortex with continual collapse over time, advancing lung disease from mild to moderate to severe ARDS. Without intervention, acute respiratory failure will occur, necessitating the use of extra-corporal membrane oxygenation (ECMO) as a rescue measure. The mechanical breath must rapidly stabilize lung tissue to pull the lung from the VILI vortex, preventing repetitive alveolar collapse and expansion (RACE). The time-controlled adaptive ventilation (TCAV) method is used to set and adjust the airway pressure release ventilation (APRV) mode to effectively accomplish the goals of the *Stabilize the Lung Approach* (SLA). Progressive lung tissue collapse and RACE are prevented using a combination of a time-controlled positive end-expiratory pressure (TC-PEEP) and a very brief Release Phase, not giving sufficient time for alveoli to collapse (Fig. 8.3, Release Phase, TC-PEEP, 5.6 and 5.7, Videos 5.3 and 8.2). Using a combination of an extended inspiratory time (Fig. 8.3 CPAP Phase, Videos 5.1 and 8.1) to recruit alveoli with long opening time constants and an inflate and brake "ratcheting" open of small volumes of lung tissue with each breath (Fig. 8.8), atelectatic lung will be gradually reopened over hours or days

The TCAV method strategically utilizes an extended time at inspiration (T_{High}), creating a continuous positive airway pressure (CPAP) phase and a very brief expiratory time (T_{Low}), creating a Release Phase (Fig. 8.3). This approach takes advantage of the lungs' viscoelastic behavior, employing the brief Release Phase to prevent the re-collapse of alveoli with very short time constants (Fig. 5.4 Expiration APRV 75%, Figs. 5.6, 5.7, and 5.8 Expiration APRV 75%, Videos 3.7, 5.2, and 8.2). Rapid stabilization of the lung sets the stage for the extended inspiratory time, allowing for the gradual reopening of lung tissue with long opening time constants (Figs. 5.3 and 5.4 Inspiration APRV 10% & 75%, Videos 3.6, 5.1, and 8.1). The brief Release Phase acts as a "brake" to stabilize alveoli, minimizing RACE-induced atelectrauma and preventing progressive loss of EELV (Fig. 5.4 Expiration APRV 75%, Figs. 5.6, 5.7, and 5.8 Expiration APRV 75%, Video 3.7, 5.2, and 5.3).

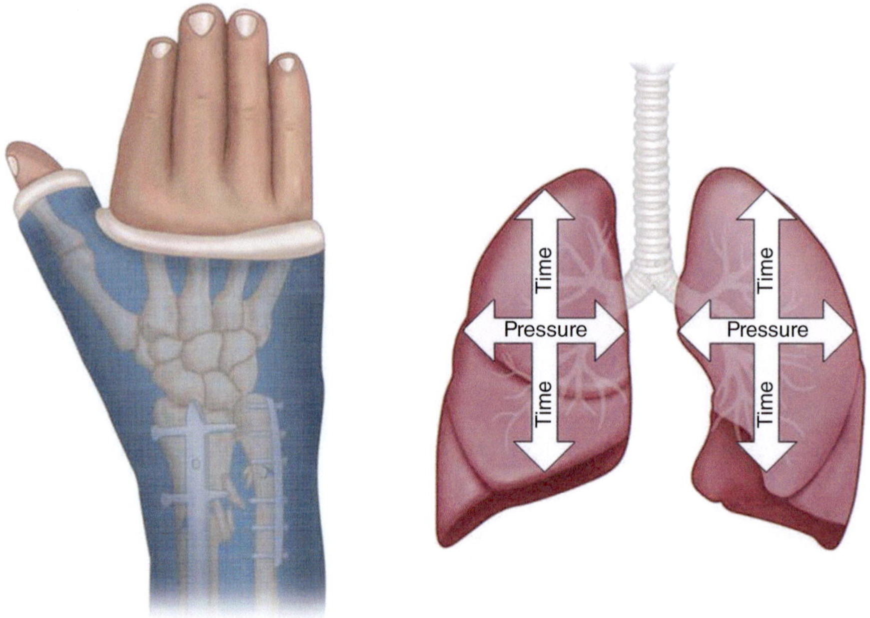

Fig. 8.2 The pathophysiology associated with ARDS renders the lung unstable, much like the instability resulting from a broken arm. An external cast is placed on the arm to stabilize the fractured bone until it heals. The unstable ARDS lung also needs a cast until it heals to prevent further mechanical injury (VILI) caused by regional alveolar instability and collapse. The ARDS lung is cast from the inside using the Time-controlled Adaptive Ventilation (TCAV) method to set and adjust the airway pressure release ventilation (APRV) mode (Figs. 5.4 APRV 75%, 5.8, APRV 75%, 8.14a; Videos 5.2 and 8.6). The "cast" combines an appropriately brief expiratory duration and a time-controlled PEEP (TC-PEEP), preventing alveolar collapse during expiration by two mechanisms - *Time* and *Pressure* (Fig. 5.4 Expiration APRV 75%, Videos 5.3, 8.2, and 8.6)

The critical aspect of the TCAV method lies in its adaptability and is characterized by its personalized features. The duration of the Release Phase is precisely set based on changes in respiratory system elastance (E_{RS}), which is measured as the slope of the expiratory flow curve ($Slope_{EF}$) (Fig. 8.3, Slope of expiratory flow). Adjustment is analyzed by observing the graphic of the flow time course during the passive exhalation of the Release Phase, emphasizing TCAV's ability to meet evolving individual patient needs. Personalized and dynamic adjustment using the TCAV method ensures adaptation to evolving respiratory mechanics throughout the patient's illness. By tuning the ventilator settings to individual patient needs, the TCAV method aims to achieve adequate lung protection. It gradually stabilizes and reopens distal air spaces, addressing the dynamic nature of respiratory mechanics in conditions like ARDS.

Figure 8.4a shows the correlation between decreasing respiratory system compliance (C_{RS}) with V_T and expiratory time using the $Slope_{EF}$ to set expiratory duration (T_{Low}). Female Yorkshire pigs ($n = 4$) were anesthetized, surgically prepared, and

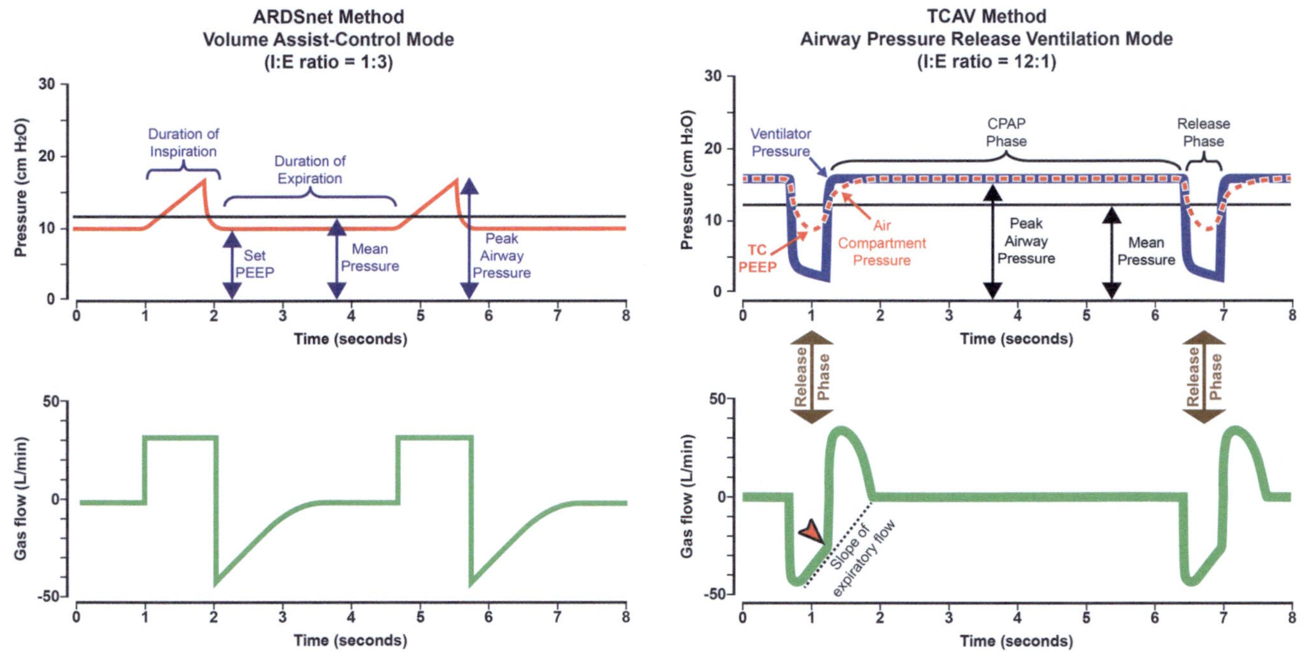

Fig. 8.3 Pressure/flow and volume/flow curves using the conventional volume assist-control mode and the low tidal volume ARDSnet method, and the Airway Pressure Release Ventilation (APRV) mode set and adjusted by the time-controlled adaptive ventilation (TCAV) method. The main difference in the mechanical breath profile (i.e., all airway pressures, volumes, flows, rates, and the *time* they are applied during inspiration and expiration) of the TCAV method as compared with the ARDSnet method is the extended inspiratory duration (Continuous Positive Airway Pressure—CPAP Phase) and very brief expiratory duration (Release Phase). The slope of the expiratory flow curve is a breath-by-breath measure of respiratory system compliance (C_{RS}) (Figs. 8.5, 8.6, and 8.7). It is used to set the length of the Release Phase by determining the termination of the expiratory flow (red arrowhead) point when the lung is reinflated to the CPAP Phase. The Release Phase is sufficiently brief that the lung does not have time to depressurize fully, maintaining a time-controlled positive end-expiratory pressure (TC-PEEP, red dashed line). Thus, the TCAV method rapidly stabilizes alveoli by two mechanisms: *time* and *pressure*

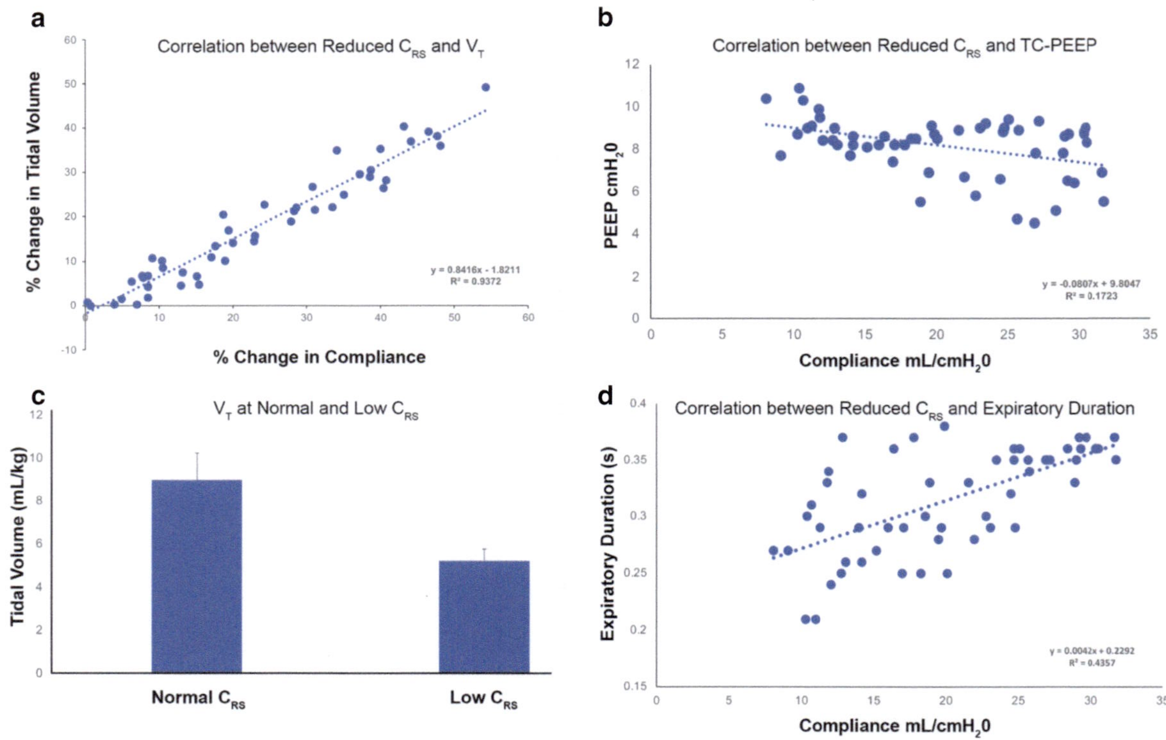

Fig. 8.4 Key to the Time-controlled Adaptive Ventilation (TCAV) method efficacy is that the changes in tidal volume (V_T), Time-controlled PEEP (TC-PEEP), and the Release Phase duration (T_{Low}) are *coupled* with changes in respiratory system compliance (C_{RS}). Note the tight correlation between a decrease in C_{RS} and a reduction in both V_T (**a**, **c**) and T_{Low} (**d**), as well as an increase in TC-PEEP (**b**). Thus, V_T, $T_{Low,}$ and TC-PEEP are all coupled with changes in C_{RS}. The average V_T with the lowest C_{RS} was less than 6 cc/kg (**c**). Because C_{RS} and V_T are coupled, the TCAV method will never deliver a high V_T into collapsed edema-filled lungs with low C_{RS}. Scott Cooper and Gregory Wetmore at Upstate Medical University generated these data

ventilated with the TCAV method to set and adjust the APRV mode. Chest wall compliance (C_{CW}) was progressively decreased in the normal animal and following acute lung injury by Tween instillation. Briefly, via bronchoscopy, a 3% Tween solution (0.75 mL/kg) was instilled into the left and right diaphragmatic lobes. Chest wall compliance was increased by progressively tightening a T-Pod pelvic orthotic around the animal's chest.

At each stage of reduced C_{CW}, both in the normal and then in the acutely injured lung, we measured changes in time-controlled PEEP (TC-PEEP) (Fig. 8.4b), in V_T (Fig. 8.4c) and in expiratory duration (T_{Low}) (Fig. 8.4a, d), with each progressive decrease in C_{CW}. These data clearly show the tight correlation between reduced V_T and T_{Low} with lower C_{RS} (Fig. 8.4a), personalizing the size of the V_T to lung physiology as measured by C_{RS}. Thus, the TCAV method will deliver a small V_T to a collapsed stiff lung, keeping driving pressure (ΔP) safe. As C_{RS} goes down, expiratory time gets shorter (Fig. 8.4d), decreasing the time for the lung to depressurize and increasing TC-PEEP (Fig. 8.4b). Then, as the lung gradually recruits (Fig. 8.1 Gradual Lung Recruitment) and C_{RS} increases, V_T will likewise increase, and driving pressure (ΔP) will fall into the normal range because $\Delta P = V_T/C_{RS}$ (Fig. 8.5). Scott Cooper and Gregory Wetmore generated these data at Upstate Medical University. These data have been confirmed in a recently published study [41].

It's Not the Wand; It's the Wizard

The physiologic importance of how the APRV mode is set and adjusted has been discussed previously (Chap. 7), but it must once again be stressed. This is true of any mode and was clearly shown in the ARMA study establishing a V_T of 6 cc/kg and plateau pressure (Pplat) at or below 30 cm/H_2O significantly reduce mortality as compared with a V_T of 12 cc/kg and Pplat greater than 30 cm/H_2O both using the volume-assist control (VCV) mode (Fig. 7.3). There are many ways to set and adjust the APRV mode (Fig. 7.4), and some methods are not personalized, adaptive, or based on the physiologic principles of dynamic alveolar opening and collapse, as discussed in Chaps. 3–5. The TCAV method is the most studied method to set and adjust the APRV mode. It is personalized to the patient's C_{RS} and thus adaptive as the lung gets better or worse (Fig. 8.5) [13–40]. A recent systematic review showed that there are currently no clinical studies that have precisely used the TCAV method and that modifications to the TCAV protocol that have been used are not always physiologically sound. Indeed, 68% of the published studies set the expiratory time arbitrarily without scientific rigor [42].

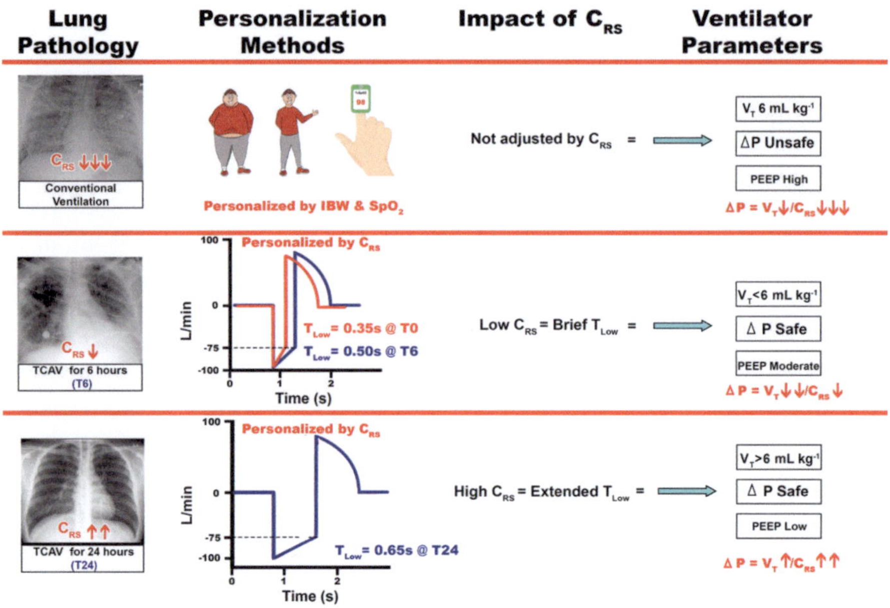

Fig. 8.5 A graphic abstract highlighting how the Time-controlled Adaptive Ventilation (TCAV) method *Personalizes* the duration of the Release Phase (T_{Low}) based on changes in the slope of the expiratory flow curve ($Slope_{EF}$) (Fig. 8.3 TCAV, Release Phase), which is a breath-by-breath measurement of respiratory system compliance (C_{RS}). Conventional lung-protective methods personalize ventilator adjustments (tidal volume V_T, PEEP, and FiO_2) based on ideal body weight (IBW) and oxygen saturation. TCAV is an excellent recruiting tool that has shown progressive improvements in X-rays over time (TCAV T6 → T24h). The lower the C_{RS}, the steeper the $Slope_{EF}$ and the shorter the time at expiration (T0 = 0.35 s; T6 = 0.50 s; and T24 = 0.65 s), reducing V_T size and increasing the time-controlled PEEP (TC-PEEP) (Fig. 8.4). The steeper $Slope_{EF}$ is caused by increased lung recoil with low C_{RS}, resulting in a rapid expiratory gas flow (Fig. 8.6b, large blue arrow). As the lung reopens (TCAV T6—T24), there is a progressive increase in C_{RS}, reducing lung recoil and slowing expiratory gas flow (Fig. 8.6a, small blue arrow). Since V_T and T_{Low} duration are *coupled* with changes in C_{RS} as acute lung injury improves, T_{Low} gets longer and V_T size increases (TCAV T24, T_{Low} 0.65 s, V_T > 6 cc/kg). If the lung worsens, the opposite would occur: T_{Low} would get shorter and V_T smaller (TCAV for 6 h, T_{Low} ~ 0.5 s, V_T < 6 cc/kg). Keeping the V_T low with low C_{RS} will help to keep the driving pressure (ΔP) in the safe range when combined with progressive lung recruitment (improvement in X-rays) since $\Delta P = V_T/C_{RS}$.

Understanding the Physiology of TCAV

There are many myths concerning TCAV efficacy that have mostly been debunked, [18] and multiple publications have discussed the applied physiology of TCAV and the mechanisms of action for the brief expiratory time, the extended inspiratory time, [12, 15–17, 43–45], and the inflate and brake ratchet that will be reviewed in the following sections [46]. The TCAV method delivers a small V_T to a collapsed and stiff lung, thereby maintaining a safe driving pressure (ΔP) (Figs. 8.5 and 8.6). As the lung gradually reopens, the C_{RS} improves, the V_T increases, and the ΔP falls within the normal range (Fig. 8.6). Despite the potential benefits of TCAV, there is a recognized need for a comprehensive large-scale RCT comparing the TCAV

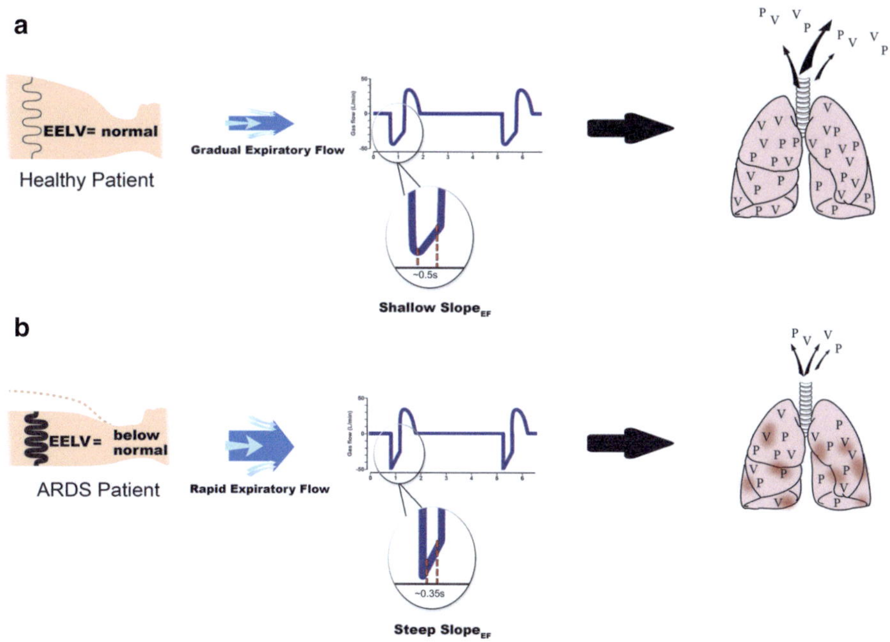

Fig. 8.6 The mechanism by which lung and chest wall recoil (thin or thick springs) modifies expiratory time using the Time-controlled Adaptive Ventilation (TCAV) method. (**a**) A healthy patient has a low lung and chest wall recoil (thin Spring) due to a functioning surfactant system, and End-Expiratory Lung Volume (EELV) is normal. The low recoil will result in a gradual expiratory flow (small blue arrow), resulting in a shallow slope of the expiratory flow curve ($Slope_{EF}$), resulting in an expiratory time of ~0.5 s. This relatively long expiratory duration will allow more volume (V) and pressure (P) to escape the lung, generating a tidal volume (V_T) >6 cc/kg and a low time-contolled positive end expiratory pressure (TC-PEEP). (**b**) An ARDS patient with significantly increased lung and chest wall C_{RS} (thick spring) with a low EELV with dysfunctional surfactant and pulmonary edema. The high recoil causes a rapid expiratory flow (large blue arrow), resulting in a steep $Slope_{EF,}$ significantly reducing the expiratory time (0.35 s). The very brief expiratory time will allow little volume (V) or pressure (P) to exit the lung during exhalation, resulting in a very low V_T and higher TC-PEEP (Fig. 8.4)

method with the ARMA method. Such a trial would be essential in determining the widespread adoption of TCAV in clinical practice.

The primary mechanism of action in the TCAV method revolves around establishing a brief expiratory time (T_{Low}) to rapidly stabilize the lung, thereby preventing atelectrauma and impeding progressive collapse. This is essential for preventing the lung from entering the progressive VILI vortex (Fig. 8.1). The TCAV method accomplishes this by employing "time control" to fine-tune the T_{Low} based on the lung and chest wall recoil forces measured by changes in C_{RS}. This adjustment limits its collapse and maintains the EELV regardless of ARDS severity. As ARDS severity increases, C_{RS} decreases, which is caused by loss of pulmonary surfactant function and airway edema, which increases chest wall recoil (Fig. 8.6b) [47–49].

Why is this critical? Increasing lung recoil makes the lung *time*- and *pressure*-dependent (Chap. 5), significantly decreasing alveolar collapse time constants and increasing opening time constants. Thus, the lower the $C_{RS,}$ the greater the lung recoil and shorter the expiratory time (Release Phase) necessary to prevent alveolar collapse. This personalizes the Release Phase as the patient's lung improves or worsens (C_{RS}↑↑ or C_{RS}↓↓↓) (Fig. 8.5). The TCAV method of setting the Release Phase couples the C_{RS}, V_T, ΔP, and TC-PEEP such that a low C_{RS} will result in a very brief Release Phase that will increase TC-PEEP (less time for the lung to depressurize), reduce V_T (less time to exhale gas volume) which in turn will keep ΔP in the safe range ($\Delta P = V_T/C_{RS}$) (Fig. 8.5).

Unlike PEEP, which sets a pressure to regulate a volume (i.e., EELV) indirectly, the TCAV method focuses on time control, directly manipulating integrals of volume (flow and time) during the Release Phase. By implementing a brief expiratory time, TCAV ensures that lung volume loss is minimized, thus preserving EELV. This dynamic approach is instrumental in preventing the lung from the progressive VILI vortex, offering a noninvasive, real-time, targeted, and effective strategy for lung protection (Figs. 8.1 and 8.5).

In TCAV, the Release Phase is calibrated to minimize EELV loss during the depressurization of the Release Phase by controlling the termination of expiratory flow (T_{EF}) (Fig. 8.7c). The expiratory time for the Release Phase is deliberately set,

Fig. 8.7 The applied physiology of setting the expiratory time (T_{Low}) necessary to minimize alveolar collapse during expiration based on changes in respiratory system compliance (C_{RS}) measured as the slope of the expiratory flow curve ($Slope_{EF}$) (Fig. 8.3, Release Phase). (**a**) A patient with a NORMAL lung recoil (thin spring) during passive exhalation. The flow/time curve during the Release Phase (T_{Low}) at the beginning of expiration (green dot) and at end-expiration (red star) (Fig. 8.3, Release Phase). The C_{RS} of the normal lung is high with low lung recoil (thin black spring). The lung can empty to atmospheric pressure (Flow 0 L/min) while maintaining normal end-expiratory lung volume (EELV), roughly 2–3 L of gas volume. The $Slope_{EF}$ is shallow (NORMAL SLOPE), taking ~2 s for the lung to entirely empty. A functioning pulmonary surfactant system prevents lung collapse at atmospheric pressure, and EELV remains normal. The flow/time curve seen on the ventilator monitor is blue. (**b**) A patient with acute respiratory distress syndrome during passive exhalation. Loss of surfactant function and pulmonary edema decrease C_{RS}, causing high lung recoil (thick black spring). This results in a steep $Slope_{EF}$ (ARDS, solid black line) compared with a normal slope (NORMAL, dashed blue line). As a result, the lung empties rapidly (~1 s), resulting in a marked reduction in End-Expiratory Lung Volume (EELV green star) (Fig. 8.6b, Large blue arrow). The flow/time curve is seen on the ventilator monitor in blue. (**c**) A patient with ARDS was ventilated during passive exhalation using the TCAV method (yellow line). The TCAV method uses a percentage of the peak expiratory flow (P_{EF}) rate to set the Release Phase (T_{Low}) (Fig. 8.3, Release Phase). The physician sets the T_{Low} at the termination of the expiratory flow (T_{EF}) point (red star), which is calculated by the equation: P_{EF} (L/min) × 75% = T_{EF} (L/min). The lung is reinflated to the CPAP Phase at the T_{EF} point (red star) (Fig. 8.3, CPAP Phase). This will result in a sufficiently brief T_{Low} to prevent depressurization, maintaining a time-controlled PEEP (Fig. 8.3, Release Phase, TC-PEEP), or sufficient time for the alveoli to collapse. Stabilizing alveoli and preventing progressive lung collapse maintain a near-normal EELV, pulling the lung from the VILI vortex (Fig. 8.1). The TCAV method is personalized based on each patient's lung mechanics, measured by the change in the $Slope_{EF,}$ which assesses C_{RS}. A low C_{RS} generates rapid expiratory flow, and a steep $Slope_{EF}$ reduces expiratory time (T_{Low}) (Fig. 8.6b). In our example using our equation P_{EF} 100 L/min × 75% = T_{EF} 75 L/min, the T_{Low} is set to terminate exhalation at 75 L/min (red star), resulting in a T_{Low} for ARDS ≤0.5 s (Video 8.3). To summarize, in the ARDS lung, the $Slope_{EF}$ (yellow line) is steep, and the T_{EF} is reached rapidly (≤0.5 s) (red star), at which point the lung is reinflated (red line) to the CPAP Phase (P_{High})

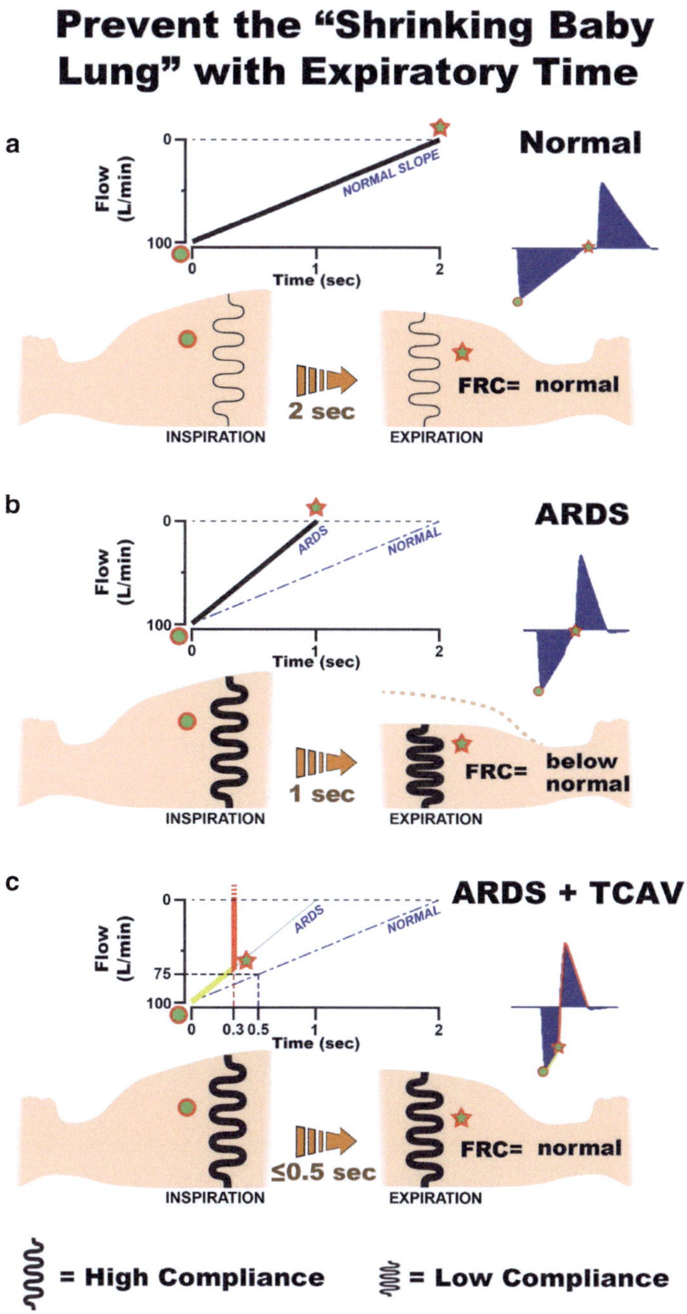
Prevent the "Shrinking Baby Lung" with Expiratory Time
a
Normal
Flow (L/min)
0
100
Time (sec)
0
1
2
NORMAL SLOPE
INSPIRATION
2 sec
EXPIRATION
FRC= normal
b
ARDS
ARDS
NORMAL
1 sec
FRC= below normal
c
ARDS + TCAV
75
0.3
0.5
≤0.5 sec
FRC= normal
= High Compliance
= Low Compliance

scrutinized, and adjusted based on C_{RS}. The significance of this lies in the patients' dynamic evolution, as they may experience improvement or deterioration in respiratory mechanics during the course of respiratory failure.

It is common to encounter worsening lung or chest wall E_{RS} as the severity of ARDS increases. Loss of pulmonary surfactant function, airspace edema, and a stiffening chest wall contribute to these challenges. By closely monitoring and adapting the expiratory time in response to changes in E_{RS}, the ventilator settings can be optimized to accommodate the evolving respiratory mechanics of the patient. This adaptability is crucial for providing personalized and effective care and reestablishing lung protection targets, particularly when the patient's respiratory status may vary over time (Fig. 8.5). If the evolving lung mechanics are ignored, previous "lung protection targets" become invalidated.

Such alterations in respiratory mechanics are evident in the changing elastic recoil forces and can be non-invasively observed in real-time spirometry at the bedside. This manifestation is discernible through changes in the $Slope_{EF}$ curve. Monitoring these real-time changes allows for dynamic adjustments in the Release Phase, ensuring that the ventilator settings remain aligned with the patient's evolving respiratory mechanics. This personalized and adaptive approach is crucial for effective lung protection and preventing complications associated with ARDS (Fig. 8.5).

TCAV Mechanisms of Action—A Brief Expiratory Time

Increasing lung recoil results in the lung increasing both times- and pressure-dependency, significantly reducing alveolar collapse time constants and increasing opening time constants. Therefore, the lower the C_{RS}, the greater the lung recoil, and the briefer the expiratory time (Release Phase) needed to prevent alveolar collapse. This dynamic approach personalizes the Release Phase according to the evolving patient's lung condition, reflected as C_{RS} changes (Figs. 8.6 and 8.7).

The method of setting the Release Phase is intricately designed to interconnect C_{RS}, V_T, ΔP, and EELV. For example, in the case of low C_{RS} E_{RS}, a very brief Release Phase is required, decreasing T_{Low} (expiratory time), simultaneously reducing V_T, and increasing EELV (less time to exhale gas volume) (Fig. 8.6). This orchestration aims to maintain ΔP within the safe range by linking V_T with C_{RS} (low C_{RS} = low V_T), calculated as $\Delta P = V_T/C_{RS}$ (Fig. 8.6).

To visualize the impact of this approach, consider comparing a healthy patient with normal C_{RS} (Fig. 8.7a) and an ARDS patient with low C_{RS} (Fig. 8.7b). The adjustments in the Release Phase are tailored to each patient's specific respiratory mechanics, showcasing the method's adaptability in optimizing expiratory gas flow and preserving lung function. This dynamic coupling provides real-time alignment of C_{RS}, V_T, ΔP, and EELV to evolve with the individual needs and conditions of the patient, ensuring a personalized and effective ventilation strategy.

Passive exhalation to atmospheric pressure in a healthy patient results in a gradual expiratory flow and a relatively large V_T (Fig. 8.6a). Conversely, in an ARDS patient with high elastic recoil force, there is a reduction in the total inspired gas volume and an increase in expiratory flow. This leads to rapid loss of EELV and is particularly noticeable as the severity of ARDS increases. As ARDS becomes more severe, the expiratory time during the Release Phase and the V_T decrease (Fig. 8.6b).

These adjustments are guided by changes in lung physiology measured through C_{RS} and are better understood in the context of passive exhalation. The altered dynamics in the ARDS patient reflect the challenges posed by increased lung recoil, emphasizing the need for precise adjustments in ventilator settings. The TCAV method's adaptability ensures that expiratory parameters are finely tuned (sub-second) to the evolving respiratory mechanics of the patient, providing tailored respiratory support in response to the specific conditions associated with ARDS.

The TCAV method of setting the Release Phase promotes alveolar stability, preventing complications associated with increases in dynamic lung tissue strain. By considering the patient's condition with real-time spirometry (i.e. $Slope_{EF}$) and adjusting expiratory time that changes the size of the V_T, and TC-PEEP the ventilator can effectively respond to the patient's specific needs, contributing to improved respiratory support and overall care. The TCAV method distinguishes itself by utilizing both time and pressure to stabilize alveoli, providing a unique advantage over conventional methods that focus solely on pressure. In comparison, it has been demonstrated that using a brief T_{Low} is more effective at stabilizing alveoli compared to a longer expiratory time at the same or higher levels of PEEP (Figs. 5.6 and 5.7, Video 5.2) [50, 51].

Studies have shown that the TCAV method's brief expiratory time prevents rapid alveolar collapse and expansion (RACE) and recruits more alveoli than the extended expiratory time currently used in the ARMA method [22, 29, 52]. The distribution of gas within the alveoli and alveolar ducts is normalized using a long inspiratory and very brief expiratory duration in TCAV, whereas high PEEP with a standard expiratory time in conventional methods does not achieve the same effect (Figs. 5.4, 5.6, 5.7, and 5.8) [28].

To address changes in C_{RS}, the expiratory time (Release Phase) is reassessed and adjusted to prevent RACE and loss of EELV, reflecting changes in lung and chest wall pathophysiology, as seen in the spirometry of the $Slope_{EF}$. As C_{RS} decreases, in conditions like ARDS, the increased lung recoil results in rapid lung emptying and decreased EELV, resulting in a steeper $Slope_{EF}$. Unless the Release Phase is adjusted accordingly (Fig. 8.6), the EELV will begin to fall. This dynamic adaptation based on changes in E_{RS} is crucial for preventing complications and optimizing ventilator settings for individualized patient care at a given time in the course of their illness.

The TCAV method uses time and pressure to stabilize alveoli, a distinct advantage over conventional methods that only use pressure. Of the two we have shown that using a brief expiratory time is more effective at stabilizing alveoli compared with a longer expiratory time at the same PEEP (Figs. 5.6 and 5.7, Video 5.2). A brief expiratory time was shown to prevent RACE and recruit more alveoli more effectively (Fig. 5.4—Inspiration & Expiration APRV 75%) than 16 cmH_2O of PEEP with an extended expiratory time currently used in the ARMA method (Fig. 5.4—PEEP 16). Distribution of gas within the alveoli and alveolar ducts was normalized using a long inspiratory and very short expiratory duration (Fig. 5.8—APRV 75%) but not with high PEEP using a standard expiratory time Fig. 5.8—PEEP 16). The efficacy of the TCAV method to stabilize and open the lung can be seen in excised rat lungs using a surfactant deactivation ARDS model (Video 5.3) in contrast with using conventional inspiratory and expiratory times with a V_T of 6 cc/kg and a PEEP of 5 cmH_2O (Video 4.3) using the same ARDS rat model [Unpublished observations]. Others have confirmed the impact of brief expiratory time on alveolar collapse [50, 51].

The above data suggests that TCAV gradually recruits the lung using an *Inflate & Brake* "Ratchet" mechanism. This mechanism gradually recruits the lung over an extended period, ranging from hours to days, depending on the severity of ARDS when TCAV is initially applied (Fig. 8.8). A "Ratchet" is illustrated by the analogy of a bucket being moved up a well, where the ratchet arm prevents the bucket from moving back into the well (Fig. 8.8). The TCAV method involves rapid lung inspiration combined with an extended breath-hold (CPAP Phase) to recruit alveoli with each breath. A very brief expiration acts as a *Brake* to prevent the re-collapse of the newly opened tissue (Fig. 8.8). Videos and illustrations provide insight into how the brief Release Phase prevents alveolar collapse during expiration (Videos 5.1, 5.2, 8.1, and 8.2, Fig. 5.4 Expiration APRV 75%, Figs. 5.6, and 5.7). This dynamic and adaptive approach highlights the potential of the TCAV method for gradual and sustained recruitment of the lung tissue in patients with ARDS.

Expiratory Time Is Personalized and Adaptive

To stabilize alveoli and prevent the progressive loss of EELV using the TCAV method, the expiratory duration is set and adjusted based on changes in C_{RS}. As C_{RS} falls, expiratory time shortens, and the V_T is reduced. As C_{RS} increases, expiratory time lengthens, and V_T is increased. The method of setting the Release Phase is as follows: The Peak Expiratory Flow (P_{EF}) L/min is multiplied by 75%, and this will identify the Termination of Expiratory Flow (T_{EF}) L/min point (P_{EF} 100 L/min × 75% = T_{EF} 75 L/min) at which point (expiratory flow hits 75 L/min) the physician sets the T_{Low} to stop exhalation and reinflate to the CPAP Phase (Fig. 8.7c Inspiration red line and green star).

In this example, the clinician adjusts the Release Phase time so that the T_{EF} occurs at 75 L/min, at which point the lung is reinflated to the CPAP Phase (Fig. 8.7c EELV green star). T_{EF} is reached at ~0.5 s and sufficiently brief that EELV remains at the normal volume in the ARDS patient (Fig. 8.7c EELV green star). The flow/time curve on the ventilator in blue shows that the lung is reinflated long before atmospheric pressure is reached, maintaining a EELV using both time and pressure (Fig. 8.7c blue flow/time curve green star). As the change of the $Slope_{EF}$ steepens,

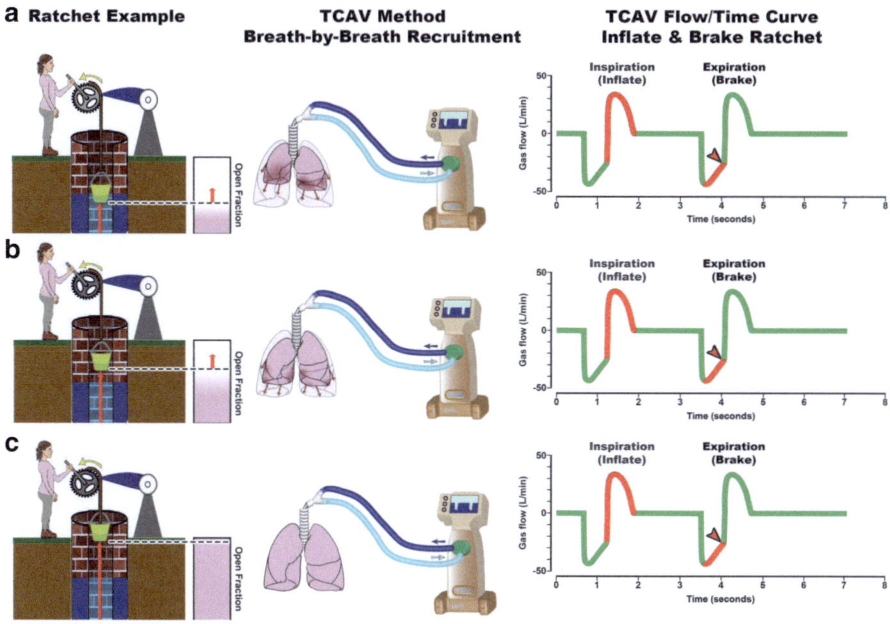

Fig. 8.8 Unlike the current rapid recruitment maneuver methods that attempt to open the entire lung in seconds or minutes, the Time-controlled Adaptive Ventilation (TCAV) method "ratchets" open the acutely injured lung one breath at a time over hours or days. (**a**) *Ratchet Example*: A ratchet is a device that progressively moves an object in one direction while preventing it from moving in the opposite direction. In the example, the woman pulls on the ratchet arm, slowly moving the pail of water up the well. When the woman releases the ratchet arm, the pawl hooks into a cog on the ratchet wheel, preventing the bucket from moving back down the well. (**b**) *TCAV Method Breath-by-Breath Recruitment*: Similar to the bucket progressively moving up the well, the TCAV method slowly ratchets open small amounts of lung tissue with each breath and prevents the re-collapse of this tissue. (**c**) *TCAV Flow/Time Curve Inflate & Brake Ratchet*: The mechanism by which TCAV ratchets open the lung can be seen in the flow/time curve. The inflation (inflate) portion of the ratchet is accomplished with rapid lung reinflation (red flow line) from the termination of the expiratory flow (T_{EF}) point. The expiration (brake) portion of the ratchet is accomplished with a very brief expiratory time (red flow line, red arrowhead). Thus, a small portion of lung tissue is recruited with each breath (inflate, red line), and re-collapse is prevented during expiration (Brake, red line, and arrowhead)
The inflate and brake Ratchet method of gradual lung recruitment is taken from "Nature's Playbook." The full-term healthy newborn has the same problem as the clinician treating a patient with ARDS—how to reinflate the collapsed fluid-filled lung. The newborn takes a large rapid inspiration to begin a "cry," moving fluid out of the airway into the interstitial space, recruiting a portion of lung tissue. During expiration, as the newborn cries, the lung begins to depressurize, and fluid moves back into the airway, reducing lung volume. The newborn applies a brake to lung reflooding and collapse by stopping active expiration and partially closing the glottis. At each end-expiration, there is a slight increase in functional residual capacity (FRC), progressively ratcheting open the fluid-filled lung

adjustment of the expiratory time (Release Phase) is required. (Videos 8.2 TCAV P_{EF} 75% and 8.3).

To calculate the T_{Low}, the P_{EF} is multiplied by 75% to determine the T_{EF} point. Video 8.3 shows how using the same equation and the same P_{EF} will change the expiratory time with a change in the $Slope_{EF}$. In our example, the P_{EF} is −60 L/min and using our equation: P_{EF} 60 L/min × 75% = T_{EF} 45 L/min. Thus, the physician would adjust the T_{Low} to terminate expiratory flow (T_{EF}) at 45 L/min. Normal lung C_{RS} and recoil result in a gradual expiratory flow with a shallow $Slope_{EF,}$ and the expiratory time is 0.6 s (Video 8.3). Using the same equation and P_{EF} in the ARDS lung, the low C_{RS} and high recoil result in a rapid expiratory flow (Fig. 8.6b Blue arrow) and a steep $Slope_{EF}$, and the expiratory time has significantly decreased to 0.3 s (Video 8.3). The longer expiratory time (0.6 s) in a normal lung will allow more gas to exit so that V_T will be larger (>8–12 cc/kg) (Fig. 8.6a), but driving pressure (ΔP) would be low since the normal lung would have a high C_{RS} ($\Delta P = V_T/C_{RS}$). The brief expiratory time (0.3 s) in the ARDS lung allows the minimal escape of gas (Fig. 8.6b), and subsequently, the V_T is often much smaller (≤6 cc/kg). This is critical since if V_T is not reduced, the lower C_{RS} in the ARDS lung would push the ΔP into the danger range (Fig. 8.5 Conventional Ventilation).

The typical progression of lung improvement when converted from conventional to TCAV ventilation in a patient with severe ARDS is seen in Fig. 8.9a–d. **Day 0**—Conventional ventilation in a patient with severe ARDS (white out X-ray) using the PLA method low V_T of 6 mL/kg, a PEEP of 18 cmH_2O, and low C_{RS} resulting in a dangerously high driving pressure (ΔP). **Day 1**—Conversion to TCAV with a very short Release Phase (0.35 s), resulting in a very small V_T (5.0 mL/kg). The ΔP has been lowered by a combination of the low V_T and improved C_{RS} (X-ray improvement). **Day 2**—Change in the $Slope_{EF}$ with improved C_{RS} (further improvement in the X-ray) increased the Release Phase (0.5 s) and V_T (8.2 mL/kg). The number of Release Phases has decreased, with much of the minute ventilation (MVe) being performed by spontaneous ventilation (gold waves). The ΔP has fallen into the safe zone (9.7 cmH_20) because of the vastly improved C_{RS}. **Day 3**—The lung has been fully recruited (Black X-ray), and all of the MVe is by spontaneous ventilation (gold waves). The brain now controls the V_T (spontaneous ventilation with a V_T 6.8 mL/kg), the ΔP is in the normal range (5.4 cmH_2O), and the patient is ready to wean off the ventilator.

Using the TCAV method, the expiratory time is personalized and adaptive (Figs. 8.5, 8.6, and 8.7, Video 8.3) and functions as a closed-loop feedback system to achieve a stable lung that permits and promotes a wave of gradual air space reopening (Fig. 8.10). The *Input* or desired effect of the TCAV closed-loop system is an Open & Stable lung. The *Controller* used to maintain the Input requirements sets the expiratory time using the P_{EF} and our equation (P_{EF} × 75% = T_{EF}). The *Effector* of our closed-loop system is the expiratory duration or T_{Low} (Release Phase), which is the time it takes the expiratory flow to hit the T_{EF} point (Video 8.3). The *Output* of the closed-loop system is the changes in C_{RS} and chest wall recoil (Figs. 8.6 and 8.7), thereby modifying the $Slope_{EF}$ (Figs. 8.6 and 8.7, Video 8.3).

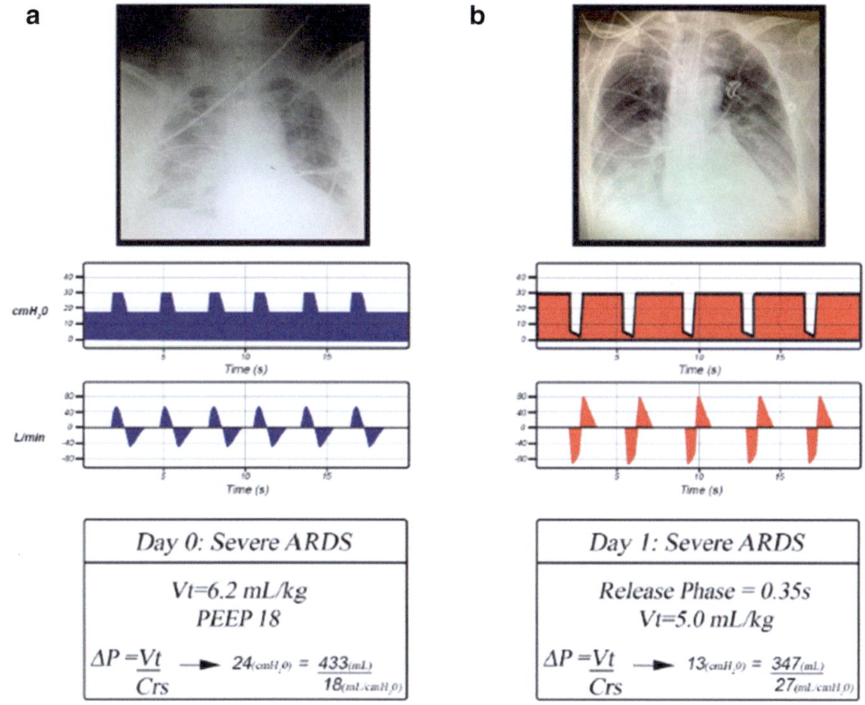

Fig. 8.9 A representation of the typical progressive improvement in lung inflation as seen following the application of the Time-controlled Adaptive Ventilation (TCAV) method on a patient with severe ARDS. (**a**) A patient with severe ARDS on Day 0 with a white-out X-ray using the ARDSnet low tidal volume (V_T) protective ventilation method and the volume-controlled mode. Plateau pressure is maxed out (30 cmH_2O), PEEP 18 cmH_2O, and V_T 6.2 mL/kg. The driving pressure (ΔP) is high (24 cmH_2O) because of the very low respiratory system compliance (C_{RS}—18 mL/cmH_2O). (**b**) On Day 1 of TCAV, the lung is still in severe ARDS, with a slight improvement in X-ray and a concomitant increase in C_{RS} (27 mL/cmH_2O). The Continuous Positive Airway Pressure (CPAP) Phase, known as $T_{High,}$ is still elevated at 30 cmH_2O with extended time at high pressure (T_{High}). The acutely injured lung still has high recoil (Figs. 8.6 and 8.7), so the Release Phase, also known as $T_{Low,}$ is very brief (0.35 s), resulting in a very low V_T (5.0 mL/kg). The lung remains open even with a loss of surfactant function because the TCAV method has applied an internal *time* and *pressure* cast that prevents lung collapse (Fig. 8.2). The small V_T combined with improving C_{RS} has reduced the ΔP to 13 cmH_2O. (**c**) Day 2 on TCAV shows a marked improvement in the chest X-ray, with most of the lung now open. The patient is spontaneously breathing (gold waves) and contributing significantly to their minute ventilation (MVe), so the number of Release Phases can be significantly reduced. The CPAP Phase pressure has been greatly reduced, and the Release Phase duration increased (0.5 s), which increases the V_T to 8.2 mL/kg. Although the V_T has increased, the C_{RS} has also increased (59 mL/cmH_2O), causing the ΔP to fall into the normal range (9.7 cmH_2O). (**d**) Day 3, and the patient is ready to wean. The lung is fully opened, and the patient is providing all of their MVe, so there is no need for a Release Phase. CPAP can now be gradually lowered as long as it doesn't result in lung collapse. The spontaneous breath has a V_T of 6.8 mL/kg, and the C_{RS} is normal, as is the ΔP

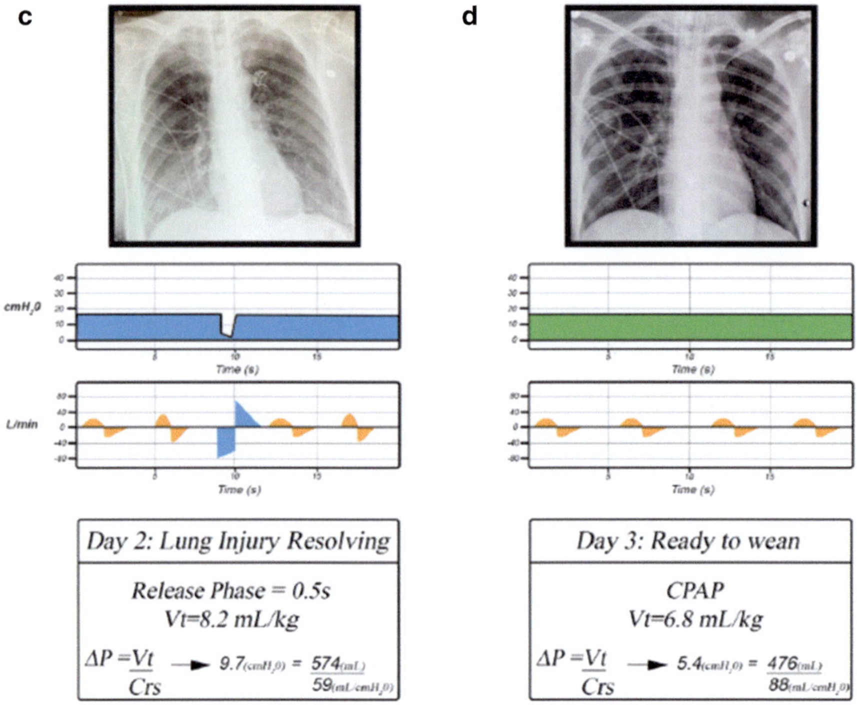

Fig. 8.9 (continued)

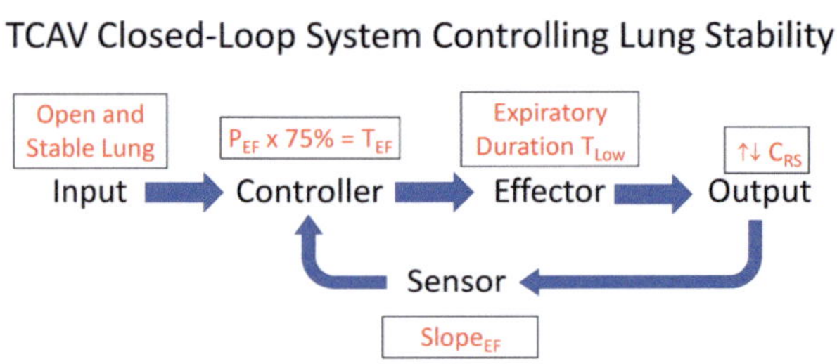

Fig. 8.10 The Time-controlled Adaptive Ventilation (TCAV) method uses a closed-loop system to maintain lung stability. The desired **Input** in our closed-loop system is an *Open and Stable Lung*. The **Controller** for our system is the equation used to set the expiratory duration (T_{Low}): *Peak Expiratory Flow* (P_{EF}) × *75%* = *Termination of Expiratory Flow* (T_{EF}). The **Effector** that will maintain an open and stable lung is the *Expiratory Duration* T_{Low} guided by the *Respiratory System Compliance* (C_{RS}), which is the **Output**. The C_{RS} is measured by the **Sensor**, which is the *Slope of the Expiratory Flow curve* ($Slope_{EF}$) that, in turn, adjusts the **Controller** (i.e., T_{EF}), which determines the expiratory duration, which is the **Effector**

The $Slope_{EF}$ acts as the sensor, adjusting the controller to maintain our chosen input, an Open & Stable Lung (Fig. 8.10).

This closed-loop system ensures dynamic adaptability, responding to real-time changes in respiratory mechanics and optimizing ventilator settings for individualized patient care (Fig. 8.10). A case progression from severe ARDS on conventional ventilation to early conversion to TCAV and eventual extubation demonstrates the effectiveness of the method in improving lung function and reducing ΔP (Fig. 8.9). The TCAV method provides a personalized and adaptive expiratory time, contributing to a closed-loop feedback system that aims to maintain an open and stable lung.

TCAV Mechanisms of Action—Extended Inspiratory Time

Lung tissue is viscoelastic in nature (Fig. 3.6, Video 3.5), and thus the longer the inspiratory time (Fig. 8.3, CPAP Phase), the more lung tissue will be reopened with each breath (Figs. 3.6 Viscoelastic Behavior Inspiration, 3.7, and 5.3, Videos 3.6, 5.1, and 8.1). If applying TCAV on a patient with severe ARDS who has a significant loss of EELV, the duration of the CPAP Phase will have to be significantly reduced. This is necessary to increase respiratory rate, and MVe to maintain an adequate level of minute ventilation (MVe) and acceptable $PaCO_2$. Since the V_T is determined by the expiratory duration (T_{Low}), which is critical to maintaining alveolar stability, the only safe way to reduce $PaCO_2$ is by increasing the respiratory rate. As the lung gradually reopens, the alveolar surface area for gas diffusion increases, and the CPAP Phase can be extended without increasing $PaCO_2$. Once the lung is fully reopened, the Inspiratory:Expiratory ratio (I:E) may be as high as 12:1 (Fig. 8.3, TCAV Method).

TCAV Mechanisms of Action—Inflate and Brake "Ratchet"

Inflating a small volume of tissue and preventing re-collapse (ratchet) are critical components of lung protection using the TCAV method (Fig. 8.8). Current lung recruitment methods attempt to forcibly open most of the lung in a brief time (seconds or minutes) and have not produced durable recruitment nor reduced ARDS-related mortality (Chap. 6). Opening a large volume of the collapsed lung with altered surfactant function and pulmonary edema is problematic. Even if the recruitment method transiently opens a large amount of collapsed tissue, which is difficult, [53] it would require extreme PEEP levels to maintain durable recruitment and lung stability. In addition, the best method to identify the correct amount of PEEP is still unclear [54], and it has been acknowledged that the "best PEEP" is impossible to identify [55].

Maybe we can take a lesson from nature's "playbook" and analyze how full-term newborns open their amnionic fluid-filled lungs. Tingay et al. analyzed the full-term newborn's first breaths at birth using electrical impedance tomography (EIT) and found that lung opening was a two-step process [56]. Lung tissue is aerated during the rapid, deep inspiration to begin a "cry." Now, the problem shifts to keeping the newly aerated tissue from reflooding. The newborn innately "brakes" expiratory flow by ceasing active contraction for the expiratory muscles and partially closing their glottis. These maneuvers defend the Functional Residual Capacity (FRC) and effectively "ratchet" open a small volume of lung tissue with each cry.

We postulate that the TCAV method, like the newborn, gradually ratchets open lung tissue using the same *inflate and brake* mechanism (Fig. 8.8). In addition, this braking results in lung water being displaced into the interstitium, similar to that in the newborn, where lung lymphatic vessels can clear lung edema [57]. The lung is rapidly reinflated at $T_{EF,}$ which will recruit more alveoli (Figs. 5.4 Inspiration APRV 75%, 5.8 Inspiration APRV 75%, Video 8.1 Peak Inspiration Hold 5 s), and re-collapse is prevented by the very brief expiratory time increasing EELV gradually with each breath (Figs. 5.4 Expiration APRV 75%, 5.8 Expiration APRV 75%, Video 8.2 TCAV P_{EF} 75%). More recently, it has been shown that premature infants, without a fully functioning surfactant system, modify the technique to open their fluid-filled lungs to a brake/hold breathing pattern. The premature infant holds their breath during inspiration, similar to the extended CPAP Phase using TCAV, and the brake must occur very early during expiration, similar to the brief Release Phase using TCAV, to grain functional residual capacity (Fig. 8.3, TCAV Method) [58].

Dissipated Mechanical Energy

From an engineering perspective, the lung can be considered a container with a specific limit to the amount of strain (change in size from the starting size) following an applied force until stress failure occurs. Amato et al. published the first major clinical paper that used the engineering principle of driving pressure ($\Delta P = V_T/C_{RS}$) as a marker of VILI and showed a strong correlation between a high ΔP and increased mortality [59]. This study demonstrated that it was not just the size of the V_T but also the size and pathophysiology of the lung, assessed as the change in C_{RS}, that the V_T was being delivered that made any ventilation strategy lung injurious or protective (Fig. 7.2). Multiple studies have confirmed that ΔP is a far better indicator of an injurious ventilation strategy than V_T size alone [60–62].

More recently, mechanical power (MP) being delivered to the lung may be a better measure of a ventilation strategy that may cause VILI [63–65]. All of the parameters that make up the MB_P contribute to the energy load exposed to the lung. When energy is expressed in unit/time, it will identify the mechanical power delivered to the lung (see equation below). However, the importance of mechanical power as a VILI mechanism is not universally accepted. Coppola et al. showed in a retrospective analysis of ARDS from seven published studies that there was no causal relationship between mechanical power and mortality. What did correlate with mortality was mechanical power normalized to C_{RS} and EELV, once again demonstrating the importance of lung pathophysiology to VILI development [66]. Danti et al. showed MP did not add better information on the risk of death from VILI compared with the V_T size or ΔP in a meta-regression in adults with ARDS [67]. In a pooled database of ARDS patients in six randomized trials of lung-protective ventilation and a large observational cohort of ARDS patients, it was found that higher MP was associated with increased mortality but was not superior to respiratory rate or ΔP [68].

MP is often calculated by multiplying each component of the motion equation by the change in lung volume (V) and respiratory rate (RR) ($\Delta V = V_T$, EL = elastance, R = resistance, aw = airways, rs = respiratory system I:E = inspiratory/expiratory ratio) [68]:

$$MP_{rs} = RR \bullet \left\{ \Delta V^2 \bullet \left[1/2 \bullet EL_{rs} + RR \bullet (1 + I:E)/60 \bullet I:E \bullet R_{aw} \right] + \Delta V \bullet PEEP \right\}$$

As discussed above, numerous studies have demonstrated that high MP correlates with worse outcomes [64, 68–71]. However, it was also shown that ΔP and respiratory rate (RR) are equally good at predicting outcomes and are much simpler to measure at the bedside [68]. Others have challenged the validity of MP as the primary mechanism of VILI [72]. Even if a high MP is delivered to the lung, if no energy is dissipated into the tissues, there can be no tissue damage. Thus, it is not the amount of MP delivered to the lung that causes VILI but rather the *dissipated* energy measured as the difference between the amount delivered during inspiration and the amount exhaled during expiration.

Energy is dissipated into the tissue by airflow resistance, by the stretch of viscoelastic tissue, and by surfactant and is measured by the hysteresis of the airway pressure-volume curve. These three components of dissipated energy are normal and do not cause tissue damage. A recent study in pigs showed that slowing the expiratory flow and thus reducing airflow resistance energy dissipation did not improve outcomes, supporting that the dissipated due to airflow resistance is not injurious [73]. However, this study was conducted in normal pigs with functional surfactant and stable alveoli thus, there was little to no energy dissipation due to alveolar recruitment, which would damage tissue (Figs. 4.2, 4.4, and 8.11, Videos 4.1 and 4.2).

Also, this study did not subdivide the dissipated energy into the three possible areas where it could occur (tissue stretch and surfactant hysteresis, airflow, and recruitment). Instead, it looked at total energy dissipation within the whole system (circuit + respiratory system), most of which is normal and not harmful [73]. They showed that reduced dissipated energy within the respiratory system did not reduce VILI but speculated that it might reduce VILI in the acutely injured lung. However, if alveoli are not prevented from collapsing during exhalation by slowing expiratory flow, then the energy dissipated when they reopen would cause VILI even if dissipated energy in the respiratory system was decreased.

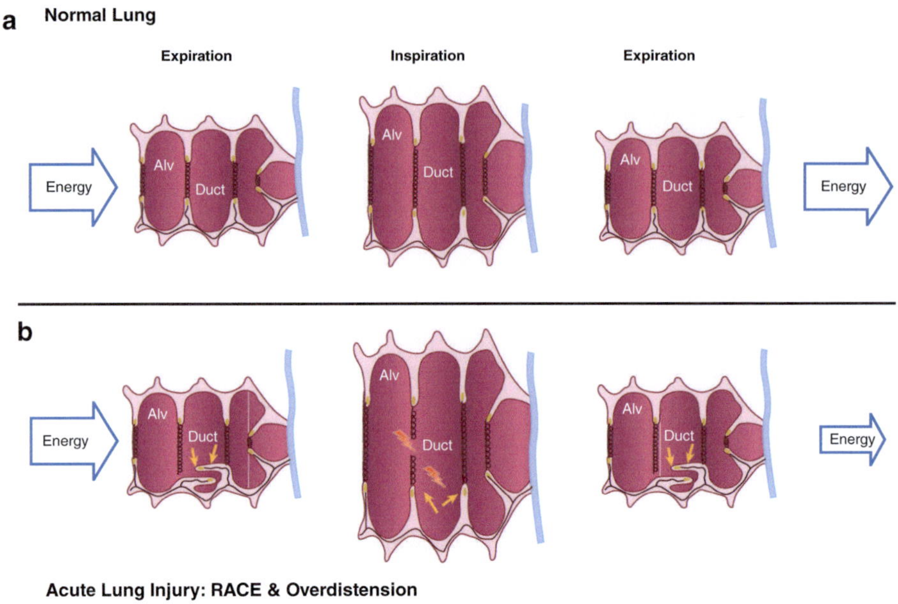

Fig. 8.11 Alveoli (Alv) and alveolar ducts (Duct) with elastic connective tissue (springs) during inflation and deflation in the normal and acutely injured lung. (**a**) In the *Normal Lung,* the energy dissipated during inspiration caused by tissue stretch, surfactant, and airflow hysteresis is evenly distributed and does not result in tissue injury. Alveolar walls do not collapse during expiration. The energy delieverd to the lung is nearly equal to the energy exhaled (same size arrow). (**b**) *Acute lung injury: RACE and Overdistension:* results in alveolar and alveolar duct flooding with edema and surfactant deactivation generating regional alveolar collapse and recruitment (Figs. 2.6, Videos 4.3 and 4.4) and overdistension (Fig. 5.8, Video 4.5). Alveolar walls collapse in apposition during expiration (gold arrows). During inspiration, a great deal of energy is dissipated as shear stress as the alveolar walls peel open (gold arrows, lightning bolt) (Figs. 4.6 and 8.11), and alveolar ducts are overdistended (broken spring, lightning bolt) in areas of alveolar instability and collapse due to stress multiplication (Figs. 2.7, 4.9, 4.10, and 4.11; Videos 2.1 and 4.5). The energy leaving the lung during exhalation is much small than that delivered (different sized arrows) during alveolar recruitment induced energy dissipation

Dissipated energy to the lung parenchyma was measured in a post hoc analysis of mechanically ventilated pediatric patients with and without pediatric acute respiratory distress syndrome (PARDS). [74] Mechanical power and derivatives (driving power, dynamic power, and mechanical energy) were calculated. The ΔP was better at distinguishing PARDS patients from non-PARDS patients than any of the MP calculations, and they suggest that the threshold of energy dissipated in the lungs that begins to cause VILI should be identified in future studies. It has also been shown that controlling airflow to be constant and continuous during inspiration and expiration can reduce dissipated energy, but as discussed above, dissipated energy by airflow does not cause lung tissue damage [75].

As collapsed alveoli with dysfunctional surfactant open, a shear or "peeling" stress is applied to the epithelial cells that dissipate heat as friction (Fig. 4.6) that can also occur as an air-bubble is forced into an edema-filled airway (Fig. 4.7).

Regional alveolar instability and collapse cause stress multipliers (Fig. 2.7, Video 2.1), resulting in overdistension of the adjacent open alveolar ducts causing energy dissipation during tissue rupture (Figs. 4.3, 4.9, 4.10, 4.11, and 5.8, Videos 4.4 and 4.5). In the normal lung, alveoli do not collapse at expiration, and alveolar ducts do not over-distend with homogenous alveolar inflation (Fig. 5.8c, Control). Acute lung injury causes the lung to become *time*- and *pressure*-dependent, causing regional alveolar collapse and instability (Chap. 5). Energy is dissipated as the alveolar walls in apposition are "peeled" apart (Fig. 4.6) as the alveolus recruits (Fig. 8.11, Acute Lung Injury Inspiration, red lightning bolts). In addition, alveolar ducts are overdistended, dissipating energy (red lightning bolt) due to overdistension-induced tissue tearing in ducts adjacent to regional alveolar collapse (Figs. 4.3, 4.9, 4.10, 4.11, and 8.11,Videos 4.3, 4.4, and 4.5).

In summary, the energy dissipated by viscoelastic tissue stretch, surfactant, and airflow is normal and does not cause tissue damage. The energy dissipated by focal and rapid recruitment of collapsed lung tissue and the overdistension of tissue adjacent to collapsed tissue are the mechanisms causing tissue damage (Fig. 8.11 Acute Lung Injury Inspiration, red lightning bolts). Thus, it is not the amount of power or energy *delivered* to the lung that causes VILI but rather the amount of a very specific *dissipated* energy secondary alveolar recruitment that does not return during exhalation, which causes tissue damage.

Evidence of TCAV Efficacy

There is a great deal of data demonstrating the efficacy of the TCAV method in animal physiologic and efficacy studies, computational modeling, clinical case studies, statistical analysis, and review papers. These are studies specifically using the TCAV method, not studies using the APRV mode that was set and adjusted using different techniques (Chap. 7). Multiple studies have analyzed the direct impact on dynamic subpleural alveolar mechanics in real time using in vivo microscopy (Fig. 5.4). In a rat surfactant deactivation ARDS model, the effect of two PEEP levels (5 and 16 cmH_2O) using LV_T conventional ventilation with APRV with the expiratory time (Fig. 8.3, Release Phase) set at $P_{EF} \times 75\% = T_{EF}$ (TCAV method) and at $P_{EF} \times 10\% = T_{EF}$, which would significantly increase the Release Phase time (see the *Expiratory time is personalized and adaptive* section) (Fig. 5.4). Fewer alveoli were recruited at inspiration in the conventional ventilation group at either PEEP. Many alveoli collapsed during expiration with PEEP 5, which was prevented by increasing PEEP to 16 (Fig. 5.4 PEEP5 PEEP 16). APRV with the extended inspiratory time (Fig. 8.3, CPAP Phase) recruited a large number of alveoli at inspiration (Fig. 5.4 Inspiration APRV 10%, APRV 75%) and with a very brief Release Phase ($P_{EF} \times 75\% = T_{EF}$) prevented alveolar re-collapse during exhalation (Fig. 5.4 Expiration APRV 75%). Extending the Release Phase ($P_{EF} \times 10\% = T_{EF}$) resulted in a significant alveolar collapse during exhalation (Fig. 5.4 Expiration APRV 10%) [29].

In a second study, dynamic alveolar heterogeneity was assessed using the same study groups. Higher PEEP resulted in alveolar recruitment and improved homogeneity, but alveolar size distribution differed significantly from control. A brief Release Phase ($P_{EF} \times 75\% = T_{EF}$) provided dynamic homogeneity and closely approximated alveoli's size and mechanics in the control uninjured group [52]. The impact on alveoli and alveolar ducts was assessed histologically using the same animal model and treatment groups. Alveolar ducts were greatly overdistended during inspiration using 5 and 16 cmH_2O of PEEP or with a long Release Phase ($P_{EF} \times 10\% = T_{EF}$). Conversely, both alveolar and alveolar duct size were close to the control uninjured group using a brief Release Phase ($P_{EF} \times 75\% = T_{EF}$) (Fig. 5.8 APRV 75%) [28].

Ventilating a normal rat with conventional ventilation with a V_T 10 cc/kg and PEEP 0.5 cmH_2O for 6 h caused a high permeability pulmonary edema, increase in lung IL-6, decrease in surfactant proteins SP-A and SP-B, and severe lung histopathology characteristic of ARDS. Ventilating with the TCAV method was highly lung protective, significantly reducing these lung pathologies [22]. In a trauma/hemorrhagic shock ARDS model, rats were ventilated with conventional ventilation using a V_T 10 cc/kg and a PEEP 0.5 for 6 h. There was a significant loss of lung function measured as the PaO_2/FiO_2 ratio (130 at 6 h), altered alveolar mechanics (RACE) assessed using in vivo microscopy, and severe histopathology. Once again, using the TCAV method, all of these pathologies were significantly reduced [35].

Using lung mechanics and *in vivo* microscopy in a rat ARDS model to train a computational lung mechanics model that contained tissue distension, the volume of open lung, and the presence of RACE. The computational model was fit to the MB_P of both conventional ventilation with LV_T and the APRV mode set using the TCAV method [40]. The model predicted that the TCAV method would be more effective at lung recruitment than LV_T without causing overdistension. Both LV_T with high PEEP (16 cmH_2O) and APRV with the Release Phase set using the equation $P_{EF} \times 75\% = T_{EF}$ stabilized alveolar showing minimal RACE (Fig. 5.4 Inspiration & Expiration APRV 75%, PEEP 16). Additionally, APRV 75% was very effective at lung recruitment with inflated alveoli over 50% of the microscopic field, whereas PEEP 16 had less than 30% of the field containing inflated alveoli. Other studies showed that TCAV was superior to PEEP at reducing RACE [22, 28, 29, 35, 52].

A second computational modeling study incorporated the temporal nature of both alveolar opening and collapse [20]. The study showed that LV_T with sufficiently high PEEP (>15 cmH_2O) and APRV with a sufficiently brief Release Phase (TCAV method) would prevent RACE. The tradeoff was that high PEEP could negatively impact hemodynamics, and a very brief Release Phase would reduce V_T and thus minute ventilation that may lead to hypercapnia. Using APRV, this problem can be easily corrected by shortening the CPAP Phase, effectively increasing the respiratory rate and MVe that will reduce $PaCO_2$. Lung recruitment and derecruitment depend on time and pressure, and thus, APRV does not prevent RACE solely by creating an intrinsic PEEP. Indeed, direct measurements of alveolar collapse show that a very brief expiratory time will more effectively stabilize alveoli than the same

PEEP held for a longer time (Figs. 5.6 and 5.7, Video 5.2), which has also been confirmed recently [41].

It was shown that APRV set using the TCAV method prevents VILI by two mechanisms: (1) maintaining a relatively normal EELV pulling the lung from the VILI vortex and (2) preventing RACE by not giving alveoli sufficient time to collapse during each Release Phase. These protective attributes are attained using a combination of airway time and pressure. In a computational model of lung fluid balance and edema formation, [21] it was suggested that the impact of the airway time and pressure profiles generated by TCAV on the interstitial pressure would reduce transvascular fluid flux and may be one of the mechanisms of reduced pulmonary edema accumulation seen in multiple studies [26, 34, 35].

In a porcine saline lavage-induced ARDS model comparing APRV with low V_T ventilation, it was shown that APRV set using the TCAV method preserved the alveolar-capillary barrier integrity, reduced pulmonary capillary permeability that translated to improved lung function and less histopathology [76]. In a translational clinically applicable porcine model of peritoneal sepsis (PS) and gut ischemia/reperfusion (I/R) injury-induced model of ARDS and multiple organ dysfunction syndrome (MODS), the TCAV method was compared with the ARMA LV_T and unprotective mechanical ventilation (V_T 10 cc/kg + PEEP 5 cmH_2O) method and control uninjured but ventilated group. In all three studies, the TCAV method completely protected the lung evidenced by lung function and mechanics, blood chemistry, inflammatory mediators, and histopathology [26, 34, 36]. At necropsy, lungs were inflated to 25 cmH_2O airway pressure and photographed. Gross photos of the lung 48 h following the initial PS + I/R injury in the TCAV group (Fig. 8.12a) and the LV_T group (Fig. 8.12b).

The TCAV lung is fully inflated without any visible atelectasis, whereas the LV_T lung has a severe heterogeneous injury with dense atelectasis (dark red) and normal (pink) tissue (Baby lung). The cut surface of the TCAV lung showed no evidence of interlobular or airway edema. In contrast, the LV_T lung showed edema-filled interlobular spaces and foamy airway edema, supported by a computational model of pulmonary edema formation [21]. The expiratory time (Fig. 8.3, Release Phase) set adjusted by changes in C_{RS} (Figs. 8.5, 8.6, and 8.7), prevents progressive lung collapse and maintains normal lung compliance (Fig. 8.12c). In the LV_T group, even though the V_T was 6 cc/kg, the ΔP was high at T48 (>25 cmH_2O) due to the low C_{RS} (Fig. 8.12d).

Using TCAV, the clinician does not set the V_T which changes with expiratory time (Video 8.3), is that controlled by the changes in C_{RS} measured as the $Slope_{EF}$ (Figs. 8.5, 8.6, and 8.7). The V_T is high (~12 cc/kg) at T48, but the ΔP is low (<10 cmH_2O) (Fig. 8.12d) because lung C_{RS} is normal (Fig. 8.12b) [17]. Video 8.4 illustrates how an extended expiratory time using conventional mechanical ventilation gives alveoli ample time to collapse during expiration, resulting in recruitment/derecruitment (R/D) with each breath. In contrast, the TCAV method averts R/D using a brief expiratory time. Using a very brief Release Phase followed by rapid reinflation back to the CPAP Phase (Fig. 8.3 CPAP Phase, Release Phase), R/D can be averted.

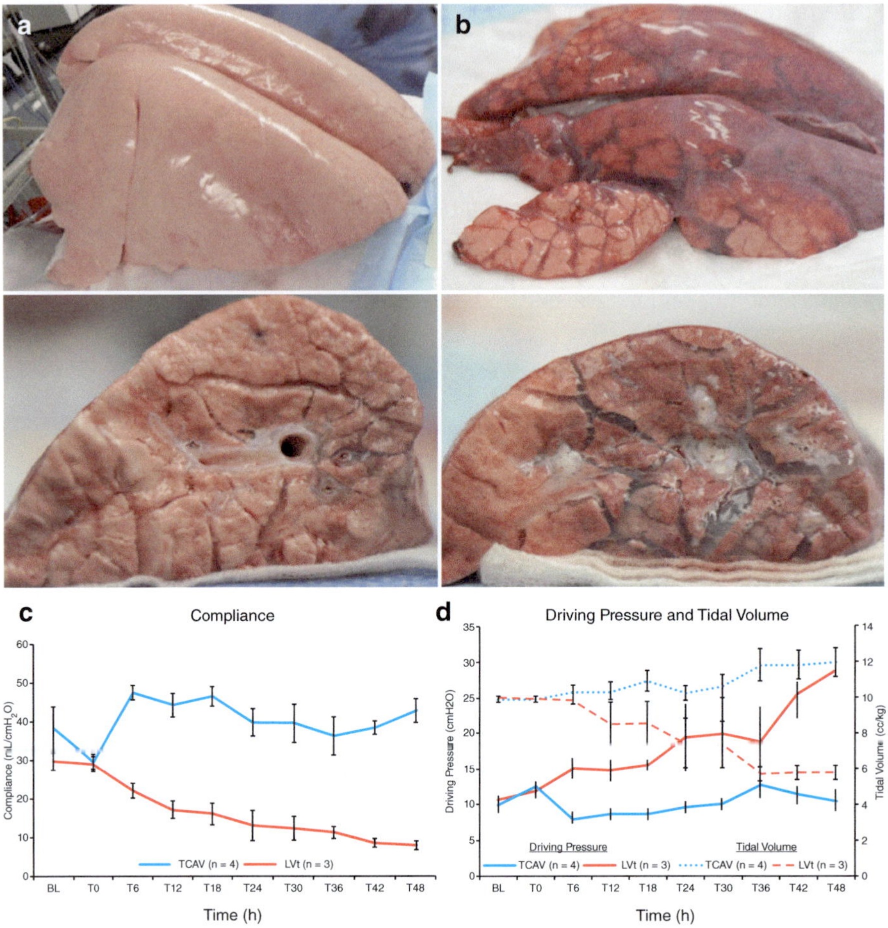

Fig. 8.12 Excised lungs, lung compliance, driving pressure (ΔP), and tidal volumes (V_T) in a clinically applicable 48-h porcine peritoneal sepsis and gut ischemia/reperfusion (PS + I/R) acute respiratory distress syndrome model. Whole lung (inflated to 25 cmH_2O) and cut lung surface of pigs ventilated with the TCAV method (**a**) and the ARDSnet low V_T method (LV_T) (**b**) 48 h follow PS + I/R injury. The lungs ventilated with TCAV are homogeneously inflated with no gross atelectasis, and the cut surface is edema-free. The ARDSnet lung has a severe heterogeneous injury with normal pink tissue (baby lung), inflamed red tissue, and dense atelectasis. The cut surface shows airway edema foam and interstitial edema as a jelly-like layer in the interstitium between lobules. (**c**) Lung compliance decreased progressively during the 48-h study period in the ARDSnet low V_T group, consistent with the pathologic findings of atelectasis and edema. Compliance in the TCAV group was higher than the baseline (BL) value at the end of the study (T48). (**d**) The V_T was progressively decreased in the ARDSnet LV_T group until ARDS criteria were met at T36, at which point V_T was fixed at 6 mL/kg. V_T using the TCAV method is not set but is a function of the CPAP Phase at high airway pressure (P_{High}) and the duration of the Release Phase (T_{Low}) (Figs. 8.4, 8.5, and 8.6). Since lung compliance increases, the slope of the expiratory flow curve ($Slope_{EF}$) becomes shallower, extending the expiratory duration and increasing V_T. Even with a V_T twice as high as the ARDSnet LV_T group, the ΔP was very low in the safe range, whereas the ARDSnet was very high and in the dangerous range. This is because $\Delta P = V_T/C_{RS}$, and the C_{RS} was much higher in the TCAV group (**c**) (Figs. 8.5, 8.6, and 8.9)

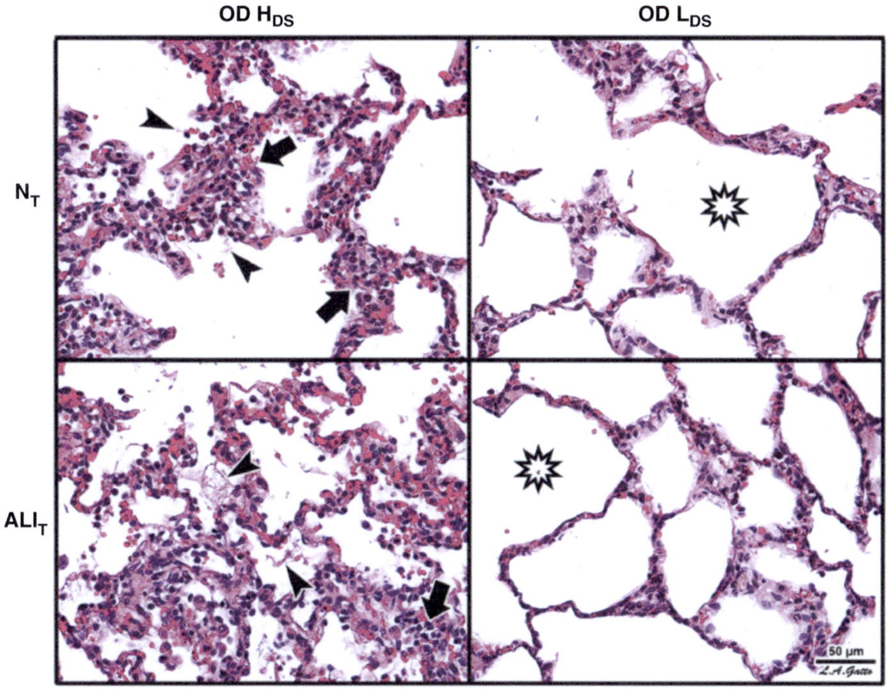

Fig. 8.13 Histopathology in a heterogeneous porcine acute lung injury model with normal "baby lung" tissue (N_T) or tissue with acute lung injury (ALI_T) cause by Tween instillation. Two groups were studied, both with a high airway pressure to cause overdistension (OD). Using the airway pressure release ventilation (APRV) mode, the expiratory duration (Fig. 8.3, Release Phase) was set according to the TCAV method using the equation: Peak expiratory flow (P_{EF}) L/min × 75% = Termination of expiratory flow (T_{EF}) L/min resulting in very brief Release Phase. A second group used the equation P_{EF} × 25% = T_{EF} that resulted in a significantly longer Release Phase. The short expiratory time would result in a low dynamic strain (L_{DS}), and the long expiratory time would result in a high dynamic strain (H_{DS}) caused by alveolar recruitment/derecruitment (R/D). High dynamic strain caused severe tissue damage in the N_T and ALI_T tissues, whereas with low dynamic strain, both tissue types were protected. In addition, this study showed that the baby lung (N_T) was not injured by OD as long as the dynamic strain was low (L_{DS}). *Arrows* show inflammatory cell infiltration, *Arrowheads* indicate the presence of fibrin deposits in airways, and *Stars* highlight open alveoli. The slide was analyzed by L.A. Gatto

Using a porcine heterogeneous surfactant deactivation lung injury model ventilated for 6 h, it was shown that overdistension (airway pressure 40 cmH_2O) in both normal and surfactant deactivated tissue was resistant to VILI as long that RACE was minimized with a brief expiratory time (P_{EF} × 75% = T_{EF}). However, if RACE was increased by increasing the expiratory time (P_{EF} × 25% = T_{EF}), serious VILI occurred in normal and surfactant-depleted tissues (Fig. 8.13) [23]. Video 8.5 shows a pig lung during the necropsy from the group with an extended Release Phase (P_{EF} × 25% = T_{EF}), resulting in lung collapse and reopening with each breath. This dynamic lung instability was eliminated in the brief Release Phase group (P_{EF} × 75% = T_{EF}) (Video 8.6) [23]. The difference in expiratory time was only 0.67 seconds demonstrating the precision necessary to prevent lung instability and collapse.

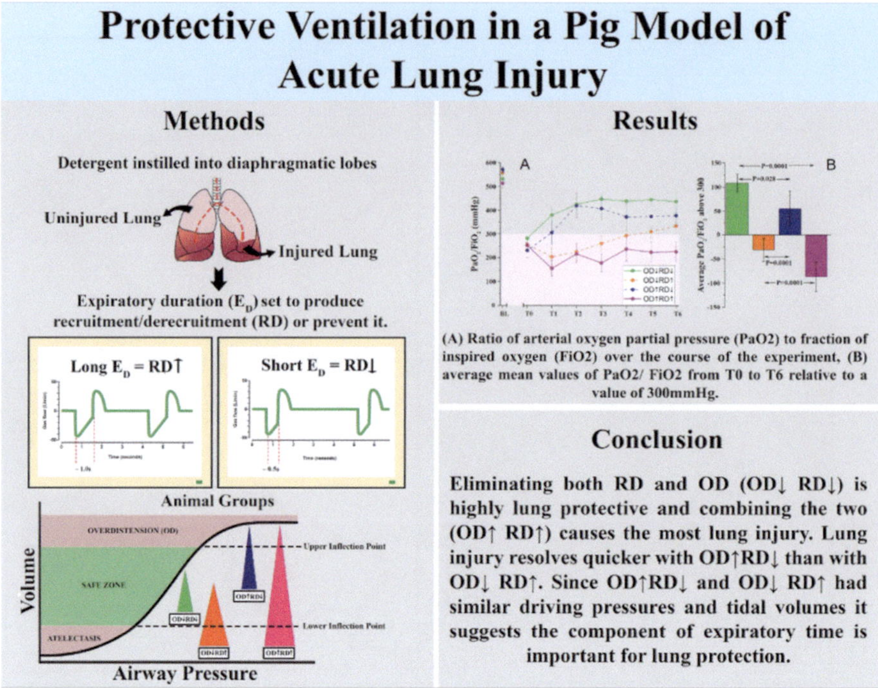

Fig. 8.14 The same porcine heterogeneous lung injury model was used in Fig. 8.13 to study four ventilation groups with all combinations of recruitment/derecruitment (RD) and overdistension (OD). Arrows indicate ventilator settings that increase (↑) or decrease (↓) RD and OD: OD↑RD↑; OD↑RD↓; OD↓RD↑; OD↓RD↓. Lung injury assessed by PaO_2/FiO_2 ratio showed that following injury eliminating OD and RD (OD↓RD↓) resulted in rapid lung improvement. In contrast, if ventilation was adjusted to cause OD and RD, the lung did not recover over 6 h, suggesting the two work synergistically to cause ventilator-induced lung injury (VILI). The OD only (OD↑RD↓) and the RD only (OD↓RD↑) had similar driving pressures and tidal volumes, suggesting that expiratory duration plays a role in lung protection or injury

A subsequent study using the same porcine heterogeneous ARDS model demonstrated that preventing both overdistension (airway pressure 28 cmH_2O) and RACE ($P_{EF} \times 75\%$) was highly lung protective, combining overdistension (airway pressure 40 cmH_2O) and RACE ($P_{EF} \times 25\%$) was synergistic in dissipating energy and damaging the lung (Fig. 8.14). Lung injury measured by PaO_2/FiO_2 ratio recovers more quickly in the OD-only group than in the RACE-only group. Since the ΔP and V_T were similar, the expiratory time must play a role in lung recovery (Fig. 8.14) [32].

Other studies using the TCAV method have shown significant lung protection in a neonatal porcine infant respiratory distress syndrome (IRDS) model compared to volume guarantee (VG) ventilation. TCAV improved oxygenation and lung C_{RS}, reduced inflammatory cell accumulation in the lung, and reduced mortality over a 24-h study period [27]. In a pneumonia rat model, TCAV was shown superior at lung protection as compared with volume-controlled ventilation (VCV) with a V_T of

8 cc/kg and PEEP set at the TC-PEEP level in the TCAV group or to an equivalent mean airway pressure level [37]. TCAV significantly reduced histopathology, blood bacteria counts, lung edema, and cytokine-induced neutrophil chemoattractant-1 gene expression compared to both VCV groups.

The TCAV method was compared with VCV (V_T 8 cc/kg, PEEP 2 cmH_2O) and non-ventilated animals (NV) in both pneumonia and secondary sepsis ARDS rat models. Histologic evidence of diffuse alveolar damage (DAD) was significantly reduced with TCAV over VCV and NV in both injury groups. In addition, VCV increased the expression of amphiregulin, vascular adhesion molecule-1, and metalloproteinase-9, whereas TCAV did not [37, 39]. TCAV was also shown to reduce VILI compared with pressure-controlled ventilation in a rat emphysema model when the Release Phase was lengthened ($P_{EF} \times 25\% = T_{EF}$). This allowed the slow emptying lung time to exhale sufficiently [39].

No clinical trials have been performed using the TCAV method [77, 78], and trials using the APRV mode have been lumped together for analysis regardless of the method used to set and adjust the mode [79]. As discussed in Chap. 7, it's not the mode that is lung-protective or injurious but rather how it is set and adjusted. Notwithstanding, recent APRV meta-analyses have shown the mode to be lung-protective [80–83] or no worse than the standard of care [84–86].

In a systematic review of observational data, the TCAV method compared outcomes to standard of care ventilation methods in 16 other surgical intensive care units (SICU). The main finding was that early application of the TCAV method significantly reduced ARDS incidence (14% vs. 1.3%) and in-hospital mortality (14.1% vs. 3.9%) (Fig. 8.15) [19]. A case report has been published using the TCAV method. More recently, the TCAV method was used on COVID-induced ARDS cases during the pandemic [33]. Janssen et al. used the TCAV method on a woman

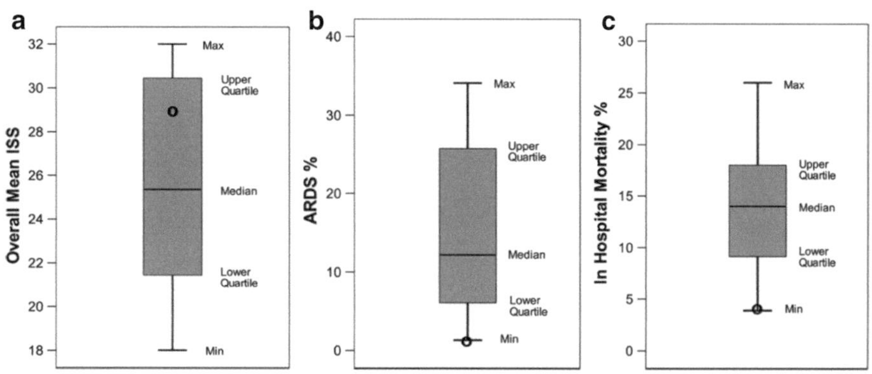

Fig. 8.15 Statistical comparison of patient outcomes in trauma centers using the TCAV method (**o**) versus 16 other SICUs using standard of care ventilation methods (bar and whiskers). The severity of injury (Injury Severity Score—ISS) was in the upper quartile for the TCAV patient; however, both the percent of patients that developed acute respiratory distress syndrome (ARDS %) and the in-hospital mortality were significantly lower using the TCAV method

with necrotizing pneumonia, and even in the presence of large bronchopleural fistulas, they were able to wean the patient from ECMO and mechanical ventilation. The patient was returned to the ICU with complications to close the fistula, was ventilated with TCAV, and once again weaned and extubated. The authors conclude that TCAV saved their patient from needing a lung transplant [24]. Besides the ability of the TCAV method to stabilize and gradually reopen the lung (Fig. 8.1), it may also reduce ventilator-associated pneumonia. A study on an excised pig lung showed that TCAV moved simulated mucus retrograde toward the ventilator, where it could be removed by suction. Thus, by improving pulmonary hygiene, the possibility exists that pneumonia will be reduced [25].

Lastly, there are many reviews on the physiologic method of TCAV efficacy and the scientific background behind the TCAV method to set and adjust in the APRV mode [12, 13, 15–17, 43]. Unfortunately, many myths and misconceptions have been written and published concerning the APRV mode that is not supported by solid science. In a recent review, ten common APRV myths are debunked using published literature, and some misconceptions about APRV clinical trials are also addressed by identifying the settings used to adjust the APRV mode were not physiologically sound [18].

TCAV Clinical Protocols

Settings for APRV using the TCAV method will be different when applied as a standard mode of ventilation rather than a rescue strategy. Although APRV is a form of CPAP that facilitates early spontaneous breathing, it can also be used in non-spontaneously breathing patients. Tables 8.1, 8.2, and 8.3 describe both the standard TCAV settings and rationale. Tables 8.4, 8.5, and 8.6 describe the Rescue TCAV settings and rationale when transferring a patient onto TCAV from a different mode. There are four parameters to set with APRV. Combined, the Pressure High (P_{High}) and the Time High (T_{High}) create the CPAP Phase, and the Low Pressure (P_{Low}) and Time (T_{Low}) create the Release Phase. NOTE: These guidelines in Tables 8.1, 8.2, and 8.3 are aimed toward patients with routine post-operative atelectasis or normal lungs, NOT as a rescue strategy (Tables 8.4, 8.5, and 8.6). As with any mode of mechanical ventilation, the settings for APRV using the TCAV method will be different when applied as a rescue strategy. Although APRV is a form of continuous positive airway pressure (CPAP) and can facilitate early spontaneous breathing, it can also be used in non-spontaneously breathing patients. This is a list of techniques to use to optimize TCAV:

- Decrease FiO_2 to 40% while maintaining a $SpO_2 \geq 95\%$
- The P_{High} is generally not decreased until FiO_2 is 60% with $SpO_2 \geq 95\%$ to maintain lung stability; however, if lung volume begins to exceed FRC but oxygenation remains an issue (i.e., V/Q matching), a pressure reduction may be necessary
- Optimize T_{High} by increasing 0.5–2 s to maintain normal PCO_2

A recent publication discusses the clinical application of the TCAV method [87].

Table 8.1 There are 4 parameters to set with APRV. Combined, the Pressure High (P_{High}) and the Time High (T_{High}) create the CPAP Phase and the Pressure Low (P_{Low}) and the Time Low (T_{Low}) create the Release Phase Standard protocol

Setting	Rationale
P_{High}	The P_{High} is set to maintain lung inflation along the steep portion of the pressure-volume curve [between end-expiratory lung volume (EELV) and total lung capacity (TLC)]. Before transitioning to TCAV, it is ideal to assess the patient's intravascular status to determine preload dependency. Data demonstrate patients with a positive preload dependency would respond favorably to a fluid bolus without generating pulmonary edema. **NOTE:** Lungs may recruit quickly. Therefore, monitor "lung volume" by assessing the curvature of the diaphragm (i.e., maximal curvature should be mid-clavicular) on chest radiograph. If diaphragms begin to flatten (i.e., maximal curvature deviates medially to lateral from mid-clavicle), consider reducing P_{High} 2–3 cmH_2O
P_{Low}	Unlike conventional ventilation modes with a PEEP set at 0 cmH_2O, a P_{Low} of 0 cmH_2O in TCAV will not result in alveolar instability and collapse when the T_{Low} is set to terminate (T_{EF}) at 75% of the expiratory flow peak (P_{EF}) ($P_{EF} \times 75\% = T_{EF}$). In conjunction with the release phase (T_{Low}), only a fraction of P_{High} is dissipated, thereby maintaining a static lung volume at a positive expiratory pressure. Time control rather than a set pressure (i.e., PEEP) is used for alveolar stability and captures the fastest closing time constant of the alveolus. Adding a P_{Low} >0 cmH_2O has been shown to increase PCO_2 and has a negative effect on secretion removal
T_{High}	The T_{High} controls bulk rate (convective) and alveolar (diffusive) ventilation. T_{High} also controls end- inspiratory lung volume and promotes alveolar stability to increase and maintain lung recruitment. The time dependent nature of recruitment dictates sufficient time at an optimal pressure in order to recruit alveoli and enhances CO2 clearance through diffusive ventilation. Alveolar recruitment increases alveolar Surface area and optimizes gas diffusion, which minimizes stress concentrators over a more homogenous lung. Using a T_{High} of 4–6 s is typical for patients with routine post-operative atelectasis or normal lungs ***but is generally inadequate when used as a rescue strategy***. **When using APRV-TCAV as a rescue strategy, it may be necessary to control the patient's ventilation until mechanical and gas exchange parameters improve to avoid excessive air hunger and breathing effort. Sedation should be continued and consideration of neuromuscular blocking agents to control respiratory drive if necessary.** In addition, the time-dependent nature of the increase in surface area for diffusive CO_2 clearance may not occur for 12–24 h. Therefore, when used as a rescue strategy, a briefer T_{High} is required to provide more bulk ventilation until the lung has recruited and stabilized. It is Important to make the distinction between alveolar recruitment and stability. Alveolar stability is time-dependent and make take more than 24 h to occur. **NOTE:** If the VT drops below 3 mL/kg after transitioning, it may be necessary to decrease T_{High} and increase P_{High} in order to maintain or exceed pre-transition minute ventilation (MVe)

(continued)

Table 8.1 (continued)

Setting	Rationale
T_{Low}	The T_{Low} is the duration of the release phase and controls the amount of airway pressure (P_{High}) and lung volume to be released. In addition, the termination of T_{Low} controls the amount of retained end-expiratory lung volume and pressure (release phase). The T_{Low} facilitates the transfer of potential to kinetic energy generated (recoil force) in the thoraco-abdominal cavity during the CPAP (P_{High}/P_{Low}) phase. Ideally, the T_{Low} is controlled in 1/100 s increments for precise adjustments.

During the release phase, expiratory gas flow through the artificial airway creates a slope angle of deceleration (*see* T_{Low} **Set and adjusted based on slope angle**). The resultant slope angle is analyzed as this reflects mechanical properties of the respiratory system. Although the release phase is ***protocolized*** to $P_{EF} \times 75\% = T_{EF}$, the time to achieve 75% is ***personalized*** to the patient and the time course of their respiratory mechanics. The $P_{EF} \times 75\% = T_{EF}$ has been clinically and experimentally validated to optimize alveolar stability (3).

Understanding the slope angle during the release phase

The TCAV method relies on the analysis of the slope angle of the expiratory flow-time curve as changes in the slope reflect changes in respiratory system elastance (compliance).

Slope analysis yields the following information:

1. Time to termination of the release phase
   (a) Dictates expiratory flow termination/expiratory peak flow ($P_{EF} \times 75\% = T_{EF}$)
2. Reflects elastance of the respiratory system
   (a) Provides real-time assessment of lung mechanics (6)
   (b) Matches Vt to changes in elastance (i.e., worsening or improving respiratory system mechanics)
   (c) Parallels residual lung aeration ("baby lung" size), which correlates with compliance rather than IBW (7)
   (d) Provides a bedside visual feedback loop as the physiologic condition of the respiratory system changes as determined by the slope angle

T_{Low} Set and adjusted based on slope angle

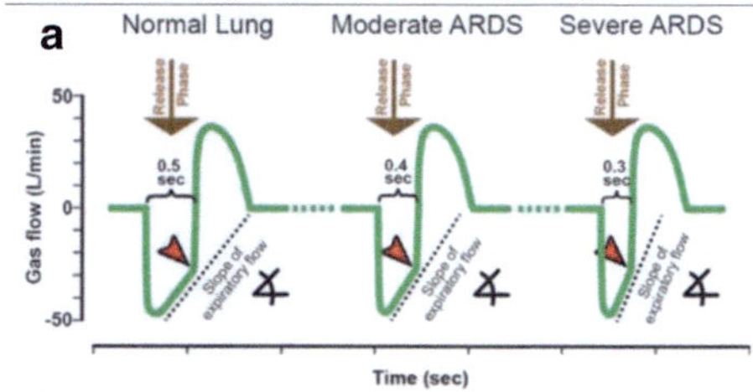

Example A:

Normal lung—T_{Low} is 0.5 s
Moderate ARDS—0.4 s
Severe ARDS—0.3 s

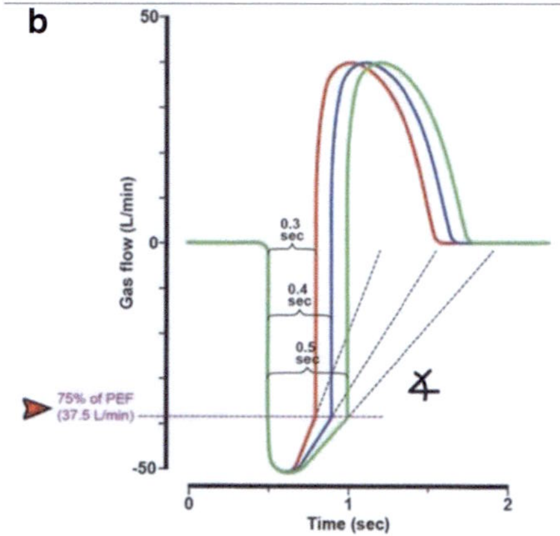

The release phase is protocolized to maintain $P_{EF} \times 75\% = T_{EF}$. However, the time to achieve 75% is ***personalized*** to each patient and the time course of their respiratory mechanics. **Example A** (left)**:** When the slope angle becomes more acute (<45°) as recoil forces intensify and elastance increases, a time reduction of T_{Low} is necessary if $P_{EF} \times 75\% = T_{EF}$. Conversely, as The lung recruits, the slope angle becomes less acute (>45°) a time increase in T_{Low} is necessary to maintain $P_{EF} \times 75\% = T_{EF}$.

Example B (left)**:** The release phase (T_{Low}) is calculated by expiratory flow terminating (T_{EF}) at 75% of the expiratory flow peak (P_{EF}) (red arrowhead).

In Example B, the $P_{EF} = -50$ L/min, so flow will be terminated (T_{EF}) at −37.5 L/min (−50 L/min × 75% = −37.5 L/min). Although the T_{EF} is always at −37.5 L/min in our example, the T_{Low} varies (0.3, 0.4, 0.5 s) due to changes in the slope angle. As elastance increases, the slope angle dictates a reduction in T_{Low} resulting in a lower VT; conversely, VT increases with decreasing elastance.

Note: TCAV used as a rescue on patients with increased elastance typically results in VT less than 6 mL/kg [frequently 3–5 mL/kg] resulting in lower minute ventilation (MVe). If this occurs, increase MVe by decreasing the T_{High}, i.e., (increasing rate) to achieve or exceed previous MVe. If VT is <3 mL/kg, consider increasing P_{High} or a combination of increased P_{High} and decreased T_{High}. As the lung recruits (compliance improves), MVe requirements decrease allowing the T_{High} to be increased. **DO NOT** increase MVe by increasing T_{Low} unless $P_{EF} \times 75\% = T_{EF}$ as this will decrease alveolar stability.

Table 8.2 Settings when transferred from other modes

Initial settings—Adjustment to settings is based on analysis of MVe, slope angle, and blood gases	From volume control mode	From pressure control mode	From dual targeted mode	From HFOV
P_{High} *(cmH₂O)**	Equal to plateau pressure	Equal to peak pressure	Equal to peak pressure	Mean airway pressure plus 2–4 cmH_2O
P_{Low} *(cmH₂O)*	0	0	0	0
T_{High} *(s)***	Set to match rate on mode transitioning from using the formula: (60/current rate) – T_{Low} (i.e., rate 26; (60/26) = 2.3 If T_{Low} is 0.5, then T_{High} would be set to 1.8 s			
T_{Low} *(s)**** set to P_{EF} × 75% = T_{EF}. **NOTE:** These ranges are a **starting point** and may require adjustment to achieve P_{EF} × 75% = T_{EF}.	0.4–0.6	0.4–0.6	0.4–0.6	0.4–0.6

* A High greater than 29 cmH_2O may be required depending on body habitus and increased chest wall elastane

** When transitioning to Rescue TCAV, V_T typically decreases to <6 ml/kg resultin in a lower minute ventilation (MVe). In this case increased the MVe bt decreasing T_{High} to increase the respiratory rate. Do Not increase MVe by increasing T_{Low} since this will increase alveolar instability. If VT is <3 ml/kg consider increasing P_{High} or a combination of increased P_{High} and decreased High

*** These are ranges for the intial T_{Low} settings

Table 8.3 Setting based on ARDS severity

Initial settings—Adjustment to settings is based on analysis of MVe, slope angle, and blood gases	Mild	Moderate	Severe
P_{High} *(cmH₂O)* based on Berlin criteria	20–24	25–29	26–30*
P_{Low} *(cmH₂O)*	0	0	0
T_{High} *(s)* Consider rate required based on respiratory/metabolic acidosis. NOTE: Use these ranges as a starting point and adjust based on blood gas.	2–4	2–3	1–3
T_{Low} *(s)*** set to P_{EF} × 75% = T_{EF}. **NOTE:** These ranges are a *starting point* and may require adjustment to achieve P_{EF} × 75% = T_{EF}.	0.4–0.6	0.3–0.5	0.2–0.4

Optimizing TCAV

- Decrease FiO_2 to 40% while maintaining a SpO_2 ≥95%
- The P_{High} is generally not decreased until FiO_2 is 40% with SpO_2 ≥95% in order to maintain lung stability; however, if lung volume begins to exceed functional residual capacity (FRC) but oxygenation remains an issue (i.e., V/Q matching) a pressure reduction may be necessary
- Optimize T_{High} by increasing 0.5–2 s to maintain normal PCO_2

* A High greater than 29 cmH_2O may be required depending on body habitus and increased chest wall elastane

** These are ranges for the intial T_{Low} settings

Table 8.4 Rescue protocol

Setting	Rationale
P_{High}	The P_{High} is set to maintain lung inflation along the steep portion of the pressure-volume curve (between end expiratory lung volume (EELV) and total lung capacity (TLC)). Before transitioning to TCAV, it is ideal to assess the patient's intravascular status to determine preload dependency. Data demonstrate patients with a positive preload dependency would respond favorably to a fluid bolus without generating pulmonary edema. **NOTE:** Lungs may recruit quickly. Therefore, monitor "lung volume" by assessing the curvature of the diaphragm (i.e., maximal curvature should be mid-clavicular) on chest radiograph. If diaphragms begin to flatten (i.e., maximal curvature deviates medial to lateral from mid-clavicle), consider reducing P_{High} 2–3 cmH_2O.
P_{Low}	Unlike conventional ventilation modes with a PEEP set at 0 cmH_2O, a P_{Low} of 0 cmH_2O in TCAV will not result in alveolar instability and collapse when the T_{Low} is set to terminate (T_{EF}) at 75% of the expiratory flow peak (P_{EF}) ($P_{EF} \times 75\% = T_{EF}$). In conjunction with the release phase (T_{Low}), only a fraction of P_{High} is dissipated, thereby maintaining a static lung volume at a positive expiratory pressure. Time control rather than a set pressure (i.e., PEEP) is used for alveolar stability and captures the fastest closing time constant of the alveolus. Adding a P_{Low} >0 cmH_2O has been shown to increase PCO2 and has a negative effect on secretion removal.
T_{High}	The T_{High} controls bulk rate (convective) and alveolar (diffusive) ventilation. T_{High} also controls end-inspiratory lung volume and promotes alveolar stability to increase and maintain lung recruitment. The time dependent nature of recruitment dictates sufficient time at an optimal pressure in order to recruit alveoli and enhances CO2 clearance through diffusive ventilation. Alveolar recruitment increases alveolar Surface area and optimizes gas diffusion, which minimizes stress-concentrators over a more homogenous lung. Using a T_{High} of 4–6 s is typical for patients with routine post-operative atelectasis or normal lungs ***but is generally inadequate when using as a rescue strategy***. **When using APRV-TCAV as a rescue strategy, it may be necessary to control the patient's ventilation until mechanical and gas exchange parameters improve to avoid excessive air hunger and breathing effort. Sedation should be continued and consideration of neuromuscular blocking agents to control respiratory drive if necessary.** In addition, the time-dependent nature of increase in surface area for diffusive CO_2 clearance may not occur for 12–24 h. Therefore, when using as a rescue strategy, a briefer T_{High} is required to provide more bulk ventilation until the lung has recruited and stabilized. It is Important to make the distinction between alveolar recruitment and stability. Alveolar stability is time-dependent and make take more than 24 h to occur. **NOTE:** If the Vt drops below 3 mL/kg after transitioning, it may be necessary to decrease T_{High} and increase P_{High} in order to maintain or exceed pre-transition minute ventilation (MVe).
T_{Low}	The T_{Low} is the duration of the release phase and controls the amount of airway pressure (P_{High}) and lung volume to be released. In addition, the termination of T_{Low} controls the amount of retained end-expiratory lung volume and pressure (release phase). The T_{Low} facilitates the transfer of potential to kinetic energy generated (recoil force) in the thoraco-abdominal cavity during the CPAP (P_{High}/P_{Low}) phase. Ideally, the T_{Low} is controlled in 1/100-s increments for precise adjustments.

(continued)

Table 8.4 (continued)

Setting	Rationale
	During the release phase, expiratory gas flow through the artificial airway creates a slope angle of deceleration (*see* T_{Low} **Set and adjusted based on slope angle**). The resultant slope angle is analyzed as this reflects mechanical properties of the respiratory system. Although the release phase is ***protocolized*** to $P_{EF} \times 75\% = T_{EF}$ the time to achieve 75% is ***personalized*** to the patient and the time course of their respiratory mechanics. The $P_{EF} \times 75\% = T_{EF}$ has been clinically and experimentally validated to optimize alveolar stability. *Understanding the slope angle during the release phase* The TCAV method relies on the analysis of the slope angle of the expiratory flow-time curve as changes in the slope reflect changes in respiratory system elastance (compliance). Slope analysis yields the following information: 1. Time to termination of the release phase (a) Dictates expiratory flow termination/expiratory peak flow $P_{EF} \times 75\% = T_{EF}$ 2. Reflects elastance of the respiratory system (a) Provides real-time assessment of lung mechanics (b) Matches Vt to changes in elastance (i.e., worsening or improving respiratory system mechanics) (c) Parallels residual lung aeration ("baby lung" size), which correlates with compliance rather than IBW (d) Provides a bedside visual feedback loop as the physiologic condition of the respiratory system changes as determined by the slope angle

Table 8.5 Settings when transferred from other modes

Initial settings—Adjustment to settings is based on analysis of MVe, slope angle, and blood gases	From volume control mode	From pressure control mode	From dual targeted mode	From HFOV
*P_{High} (cmH_2O)**	Equal to plateau pressure	Equal to peak pressure	Equal to peak pressure	Mean airway pressure plus 2–4 cmH_2O
P_{Low} (cmH_2O)	0	0	0	0
*T_{High} (s)***	Set to match rate on mode transitioning from using the formula: (60/current rate) – T_{Low} (i.e., rate 26; (60/26) = 2.3 If T_{Low} is 0.5, then T_{High} would be set to 1.8 s			
T_{Low} (s)*** set to $P_{EF} \times 75\% = T_{EF}$. **NOTE:** These ranges are a *starting point* and may require adjustment to achieve $P_{EF} \times 75\% = T_{EF}$.	0.4–0.6	0.4–0.6	0.4–0.6	0.4–0.6

* A High greater than 29 cmH_2O may be required depending on body habitus and increased chest wall elastane

** When transitioning to Rescue TCAV, V_T typically decreases to <6 ml/kg resultin in a lower minute ventilation (MVe). In this case increased the MVe bt decreasing T_{High} to increase the respiratory rate. Do Not increase MVe by increasing T_{Low} since this will increase alveolar instability. If VT is <3 ml/kg consider increasing P_{High} or a combination of increased P_{High} and decreased High

*** These are ranges for the intial T_{Low} settings

Table 8.6 Setting based on ARDS severity

Initial settings—Adjustment to settings is based on analysis of MVe, slope angle, and blood gases	Mild	Moderate	Severe
P_{High} (cmH_2O) based on Berlin criteria	20–24	25–29	26–30*
P_{Low} (cmH_2O)	0	0	0
T_{High} (s) Consider rate required based on respiratory/metabolic acidosis. NOTE: Use these ranges as a starting point and adjust based on blood gas.	2–4	2–3	1–3
T_{Low} (s)** set to $P_{EF} \times 75\% = T_{EF}$. **NOTE:** These Ranges are a ***starting point*** and may require adjustment to achieve $P_{EF} \times 75\% = T_{EF}$	0.4–0.6	0.3–0.5	0.2–0.4

* A High greater than 30 cmH_2O may be required depending on body habitus and icnreased chest wall elastane.

** These are ranges for the intial T_{Low} settings

Summary

In Chap. 1, we discuss how ARDS inflammatory pathology makes the lung susceptible to a secondary mechanical pathology caused by mechanical ventilation (Fig. 1.3). Subsequently, we explored the mechanisms of VILI in the ARDS lung, particularly the mechanical damage associated with VILI pathology (Fig. 1.3, VILI pathology). Chapters 1–7 comprehensively reviewed ARDS and VILI pathogenesis and the mechanical ventilation strategies used to minimize VILI to reduce ARDS-related mortality. The culmination of this understanding allowed us to answer the questions on the mechanisms of ARDS and VILI pathologies that we posed in Fig. 1.3, which is the basic science necessary to design a more effective protective mechanical breath (Fig. 8.16).

This dynamic understanding of VILI and alveolar physiology paved the way for designing a novel protective ventilation method known as TCAV. The TCAV method utilizes the MB_P component of inspiratory and expiratory *time* to stabilize and gradually reopen viscoelastic alveoli. The TCAV method is the most extensively studied method for setting and adjusting the APRV mode (Table 9.1). It is highly lung protection, substantially improving outcomes in studies that include clinically applicable animal models, case studies, small clinical trials, and statistical reviews. A comprehensive literature review has debunked the myths and misconceptions surrounding APRV [18].

The remaining step to establish TCAV as a primary ventilation strategy is a large RCT comparing TCAV to the current standard of care ventilation method. Based on the compelling evidence presented, there is a strong belief that the TCAV method can significantly reduce morbidity and mortality associated with ARDS.

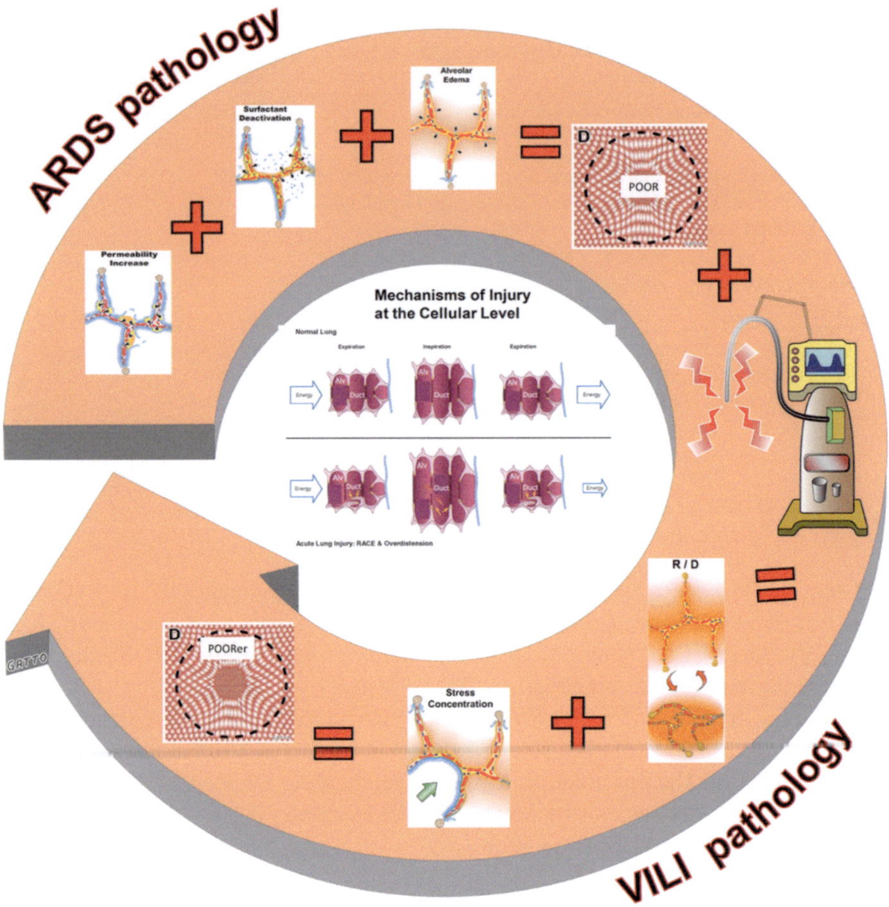

Fig. 8.16 Acute Respiratory Distress Syndrome (ARDS) pathology causes inflammatory injury that alters alveolar permeability, resulting in *Endothelial Leakage* of fluids into the alveolus, causing *Surfactant Deactivation* and *Alveolar Edema* (Fig. 1.1). This progressive pathology generates regional areas of collapsed and edema-filled tissue known as the Permeability-Originated Obstructive Response (*POOR*) response (Fig. 4.11). These lesions will spread and eventually cause sufficient hypoxemia to require mechanical ventilation. If the ventilator is set improperly, it can cause repetitive alveolar collapse and expansion (*RACE*—Atelectrauma) and stress multipliers (volutrauma), the engines driving VILI at the alveolar level. The underlying mechanisms of atelectrauma and volutrauma are energy dissipation during mechanical ventilation (Fig. 8.11). Using our knowledge of altered dynamic inflation and deflation with ARDS, our applied physiologic approach to breaking this cycle of lung tissue damage is to stabilize and then gradually reopen the POOR areas (Fig. 8.1) using the MB_P components of inspiratory and expiratory time

References

1. The Acute Respiratory Distress Syndrome Network. ARDSnet: ventilation with lower tidal volumes as compared with traditional tidal volumes for acute lung injury and the acute respiratory distress syndrome. N Engl J Med. 2000;342:1301–8.
2. Cui Y, Cao R, Wang Y, Li G. Lung recruitment maneuvers for ARDS patients: a systematic review and meta-analysis. Respiration. 2020;99:264–76.
3. Araos J, Alegria L, Garcia P, Cruces P, Soto D, Erranz B, Amthauer M, Salomon T, Medina T, Rodriguez F, et al. Near-apneic ventilation decreases lung injury and fibroproliferation in an acute respiratory distress syndrome model with extracorporeal membrane oxygenation. Am J Respir Crit Care Med. 2019;199:603–12.
4. Quintel M, Busana M, Gattinoni L. Breathing and ventilation during extracorporeal membrane oxygenation: how to find the balance between rest and load. Am J Respir Crit Care Med. 2019;200:954–6.
5. Schmidt M, Pham T, Arcadipane A, Agerstrand C, Ohshimo S, Pellegrino V, Vuylsteke A, Guervilly C, McGuinness S, Pierard S, et al. Mechanical ventilation management during extracorporeal membrane oxygenation for acute respiratory distress syndrome. An international multicenter prospective cohort. Am J Respir Crit Care Med. 2019;200:1002–12.
6. Marini JJ, Gattinoni L. Time course of evolving ventilator-induced lung injury: the "shrinking baby lung". Crit Care Med. 2020;48:1203–9.
7. Jamadar DA, Kazerooni EA, Cascade PN, Fazzalari FL, Vydareny KH, Bartlett RH. Extracorporeal membrane oxygenation in adults: radiographic findings and correlation of lung opacity with patient mortality. Radiology. 1996;198:693–8.
8. Bartlett RH. Physiology of extracorporeal gas exchange. Compr Physiol. 2020;10:879–91.
9. Spinelli E, Colussi G, Dal Santo G, Scotti E, Marongiu I, Garbelli E, Mazzucco A, Dondossola D, Maia R, Battistin M, et al. Atelectasis, shunt, and worsening oxygenation following reduction of respiratory rate in healthy pigs undergoing ECMO: an experimental lung imaging study. Front Physiol. 2021;12:663313.
10. Mc IRB, Timpa JG, Kurundkar AR, Holt DW, Kelly DR, Hartman YE, Neel ML, Karnatak RK, Schelonka RL, Anantharamaiah GM, et al. Plasma concentrations of inflammatory cytokines rise rapidly during ECMO-related SIRS due to the release of preformed stores in the intestine. Lab Investig. 2010;90:128–39.
11. Writing Group for the Alveolar Recruitment for Acute Respiratory Distress Syndrome Trial I, Cavalcanti AB, Suzumura EA, Laranjeira LN, Paisani DM, Damiani LP, Guimaraes HP, Romano ER, Regenga MM, Taniguchi LNT, et al. Effect of lung recruitment and titrated positive end-expiratory pressure (PEEP) vs low PEEP on mortality in patients with acute respiratory distress syndrome: a randomized clinical trial. JAMA. 2017;318:1335–45.
12. Nieman GF, Andrews P, Satalin J, Wilcox K, Kollisch-Singule M, Madden M, Aiash H, Blair SJ, Gatto LA, Habashi NM. Acute lung injury: how to stabilize a broken lung. Crit Care. 2018;22:136.
13. Habashi NM. Other approaches to open-lung ventilation: airway pressure release ventilation. Crit Care Med. 2005;33:S228–40.
14. Nieman GF, Satalin J, Andrews P, Aiash H, Habashi NM, Gatto LA. Personalizing mechanical ventilation according to physiologic parameters to stabilize alveoli and minimize ventilator induced lung injury (VILI). Intensive Care Med Exp. 2017;5:8.
15. Nieman GF, Al-Khalisy H, Kollisch-Singule M, Satalin J, Blair S, Trikha G, Andrews P, Madden M, Gatto LA, Habashi NM. A physiologically informed strategy to effectively open, stabilize, and protect the acutely injured lung. Front Physiol. 2020;11:227.

16. Nieman G, Kollisch-Singule M, Ramcharran H, Satalin J, Blair S, Gatto LA, Andrews P, Ghosh A, Kaczka DW, Gaver D, et al. Unshrinking the baby lung to calm the VILI vortex. Crit Care. 2022;26:242.
17. Nieman GF, Gatto LA, Andrews P, Satalin J, Camporota L, Daxon B, Blair SJ, Al-Khalisy H, Madden M, Kollisch-Singule M, et al. Prevention and treatment of acute lung injury with time-controlled adaptive ventilation: physiologically informed modification of airway pressure release ventilation. Ann Intensive Care. 2020;10:3.
18. Andrews P, Shiber J, Madden M, Nieman GF, Camporota L, Habashi NM. Myths and misconceptions of airway pressure release ventilation: getting past the noise and on to the signal. Front Physiol. 2022;13:928562.
19. Andrews PL, Shiber JR, Jaruga-Killeen E, Roy S, Sadowitz B, O'Toole RV, Gatto LA, Nieman GF, Scalea T, Habashi NM. Early application of airway pressure release ventilation may reduce mortality in high-risk trauma patients: a systematic review of observational trauma ARDS literature. J Trauma Acute Care Surg. 2013;75:635–41.
20. Bates JHT, Gaver DP, Habashi NM, Nieman GF. Atelectrauma vrsus volutrauma: a tale of two time-constants. Crit Care Explor. 2020;2:e0299.
21. Beretta E, Romano F, Sancini G, Grotberg JB, Nieman GF, Miserocchi G. Pulmonary interstitial matrix and lung fluid balance from Normal to the acutely injured lung. Front Physiol. 2021;12:781874.
22. Emr B, Gatto LA, Roy S, Satalin J, Ghosh A, Snyder K, Andrews P, Habashi N, Marx W, Ge L, et al. Airway pressure release ventilation prevents ventilator-induced lung injury in normal lungs. JAMA Surg. 2013;148:1005–12.
23. Jain SV, Kollisch-Singule M, Satalin J, Searles Q, Dombert L, Abdel-Razek O, Yepuri N, Leonard A, Gruessner A, Andrews P, et al. The role of high airway pressure and dynamic strain on ventilator-induced lung injury in a heterogeneous acute lung injury model. Intensive Care Med Exp. 2017;5:25.
24. Janssen M, Meeder JHJ, Seghers L, den Uil CA. Time controlled adaptive ventilation as conservative treatment of destroyed lung: an alternative to lung transplantation. BMC Pulm Med. 2021;21:176.
25. Mahajan M, DiStefano D, Satalin J, Andrews P, Al-Khalisy H, Baker S, Gatto LA, Nieman GF, Habashi NM. Time-controlled adaptive ventilation (TCAV) accelerates simulated mucus clearance via increased expiratory flow rate. Intensive Care Med Exp. 2019;7:27.
26. Kollisch-Singule M, Emr B, Jain SV, Andrews P, Satalin J, Liu J, Porcellio E, Kenyon V, Wang G, Marx W, et al. The effects of airway pressure release ventilation on respiratory mechanics in extrapulmonary lung injury. Intensive Care Med Exp. 2015;3:35.
27. Kollisch-Singule M, Jain SV, Satalin J, Andrews P, Searles Q, Liu Z, Zhou Y, Wang G, Meier AH, Gatto LA, et al. Limiting ventilator-associated lung injury in a preterm porcine neonatal model. J Pediatr Surg. 2017;52:50–5.
28. Kollisch-Singule M, Emr B, Smith B, Ruiz C, Roy S, Meng Q, Jain S, Satalin J, Snyder K, Ghosh A, et al. Airway pressure release ventilation reduces conducting airway micro-strain in lung injury. J Am Coll Surg. 2014;219:968–76.
29. Kollisch-Singule M, Emr B, Smith B, Roy S, Jain S, Satalin J, Snyder K, Andrews P, Habashi N, Bates J, et al. Mechanical breath profile of airway pressure release ventilation: the effect on alveolar recruitment and microstrain in acute lung injury. JAMA Surg. 2014;149:1138–45.
30. Nieman GF, Gatto LA, Habashi NM. Impact of mechanical ventilation on the pathophysiology of progressive acute lung injury. J Appl Physiol (1985). 2015;119:1245–61.
31. Nieman GF, Satalin J, Kollisch-Singule M, Andrews P, Aiash H, Habashi NM, Gatto LA. Physiology in medicine: understanding dynamic alveolar physiology to minimize ventilator-induced lung injury. J Appl Physiol (1985). 2017;122:1516–22.
32. Ramcharran H, Bates JHT, Satalin J, Blair S, Andrews PL, Gaver DP, Gatto LA, Wang G, Ghosh AJ, Robedee B, et al. Protective ventilation in a pig model of acute lung injury: timing is as important as pressure. J Appl Physiol (1985). 2022;133:1093–105.
33. Rola P, Daxon B. Airway pressure release ventilation with time-controlled adaptive ventilation (TCAV) in COVID-19: a community hospital's experience. Front Physiol. 2022;13:787231.

34. Roy S, Habashi N, Sadowitz B, Andrews P, Ge L, Wang G, Roy P, Ghosh A, Kuhn M, Satalin J, et al. Early airway pressure release ventilation prevents ARDS-a novel preventive approach to lung injury. Shock. 2013;39:28–38.
35. Roy SK, Emr B, Sadowitz B, Gatto LA, Ghosh A, Satalin JM, Snyder KP, Ge L, Wang G, Marx W, et al. Preemptive application of airway pressure release ventilation prevents development of acute respiratory distress syndrome in a rat traumatic hemorrhagic shock model. Shock. 2013;40:210–6.
36. Roy S, Sadowitz B, Andrews P, Gatto LA, Marx W, Ge L, Wang G, Lin X, Dean DA, Kuhn M, et al. Early stabilizing alveolar ventilation prevents acute respiratory distress syndrome: a novel timing-based ventilatory intervention to avert lung injury. J Trauma Acute Care Surg. 2012;73:391–400.
37. de Magalhaes RF, Cruz DG, Antunes MA, Fernandes MVS, Oliveira MV, Braga CL, Satalin J, Andrews P, Habashi N, Nieman G, et al. Time-controlled adaptive ventilation versus volume-controlled ventilation in experimental pneumonia. Crit Care Med. 2021;49:140–50.
38. Oliveira MV, Magalhaes RF, Rocha NN, Fernandes MV, Antunes MA, Morales MM, Capelozzi VL, Satalin J, Andrews P, Habashi NM, et al. Effects of time-controlled adaptive ventilation on cardiorespiratory parameters and inflammatory response in experimental emphysema. J Appl Physiol (1985). 2022;132:564–74.
39. Silva PL, Cruz FF, Samary CDS, Moraes L, de Magalhaes RF, Fernandes MVS, Bose R, Pelegati VB, Carvalho HF, Capelozzi VL, et al. Biological response to time-controlled adaptive ventilation depends on acute respiratory distress syndrome etiology. Crit Care Med. 2018;46:e609–17.
40. Smith BJ, Lundblad LK, Kollisch-Singule M, Satalin J, Nieman G, Habashi N, Bates JH. Predicting the response of the injured lung to the mechanical breath profile. J Appl Physiol (1985). 2015;118:932–40.
41. Ramcharran H, Wetmore G, Cooper S, Herrmann J, Cruz AF, Kaczka DW, Satalin J, Blair S, Andrews PL, Habashi NM, et al. Effects of lung injury and abdominal insufflation on respiratory mechanics and lung volume during time-controlled adaptive ventilation. Respir Care. 2024:respcare.11745.
42. Lutz MR, Charlamb J, Kenna JR, Smith A, Glatt SJ, Araos JD, Andrews PL, Habashi NM, Nieman GF, Ghosh AJ. Inconsistent methods used to set airway pressure release ventilation in acute respiratory distress syndrome: a systematic review and meta-regression analysis. J Clin Med. 2024;13:13.
43. Nieman G, Satalin J, Andrews P, Wilcox K, Aiash H, Baker S, Kollisch-Singule M, Madden M, Gatto L, Habashi N. Preemptive mechanical ventilation based on dynamic physiology in the alveolar microenvironment: novel considerations of time-dependent properties of the respiratory system. J Trauma Acute Care Surg. 2018;85:1081–91.
44. Nieman GF, Kaczka DW, Andrews PL, Ghosh A, Al-Khalisy H, Camporota L, Satalin J, Herrmann J, Habashi NM. First stabilize and then gradually recruit: a paradigm shift in protective mechanical ventilation for acute lung injury. J Clin Med. 2023;12:12.
45. Al-Khalisy H, Nieman GF, Kollisch-Singule M, Andrews P, Camporota L, Shiber J, Manougian T, Satalin J, Blair S, Ghosh A, et al. Time-controlled adaptive ventilation (TCAV): a personalized strategy for lung protection. Respir Res. 2024;25:37.
46. Nieman GF, Herrmann J, Satalin J, Kollisch-Singule M, Andrews PL, Habashi NM, Tingay DG, Gaver DP 3rd, Bates JHT, Kaczka DW. Ratchet recruitment in the acute respiratory distress syndrome: lessons from the newborn cry. Front Physiol. 2023;14:1287416.
47. Bersten AD, Davidson K, Nicholas TE, Doyle IR. Respiratory mechanics and surfactant in the acute respiratory distress syndrome. Clin Exp Pharmacol Physiol. 1998;25:955–63.
48. Hess DR. Respiratory mechanics in mechanically ventilated patients. Respir Care. 2014;59:1773–94.
49. Pellegrini M, Hedenstierna G, Roneus A, Segelsjo M, Larsson A, Perchiazzi G. The diaphragm acts as a brake during expiration to prevent lung collapse. Am J Respir Crit Care Med. 2017;195:1608–16.

50. Baumgardner JE. (Airway) closure, at last! Crit Care Med. 2019;47:1281–2.
51. Syring RS, Otto CM, Spivack RE, Markstaller K, Baumgardner JE. Maintenance of end-expiratory recruitment with increased respiratory rate after saline-lavage lung injury. J Appl Physiol (1985). 2007;102:331–9.
52. Kollisch-Singule M, Jain S, Andrews P, Smith BJ, Hamlington-Smith KL, Roy S, DiStefano D, Nuss E, Satalin J, Meng Q, et al. Effect of airway pressure release ventilation on dynamic alveolar heterogeneity. JAMA Surg. 2016;151:64–72.
53. Gattinoni L, Caironi P, Cressoni M, Chiumello D, Ranieri VM, Quintel M, Russo S, Patroniti N, Cornejo R, Bugedo G. Lung recruitment in patients with the acute respiratory distress syndrome. N Engl J Med. 2006;354:1775–86.
54. Hess DR. Recruitment maneuvers and PEEP titration. Respir Care. 2015;60:1688–704.
55. Millington SJ, Cardinal P, Brochard L. Setting and titrating positive end-expiratory pressure. Chest. 2022;161:1566–75.
56. Tingay DG, Farrell O, Thomson J, Perkins EJ, Pereira-Fantini PM, Waldmann AD, Ruegger C, Adler A, Davis PG, Frerichs I. Imaging the respiratory transition at birth: unraveling the complexities of the first breaths of life. Am J Respir Crit Care Med. 2021;204:82–91.
57. Hooper SB, Te Pas AB, Kitchen MJ. Respiratory transition in the newborn: a three-phase process. Arch Dis Child Fetal Neonatal Ed. 2016;101:F266–71.
58. Gaertner VD, Buchler VL, Waldmann A, Bassler D, Ruegger CM. Deciphering mechanisms of respiratory fetal-to-neonatal transition in very preterm infants. Am J Respir Crit Care Med. 2024;209:738–47.
59. Amato MB, Meade MO, Slutsky AS, Brochard L, Costa EL, Schoenfeld DA, Stewart TE, Briel M, Talmor D, Mercat A, et al. Driving pressure and survival in the acute respiratory distress syndrome. N Engl J Med. 2015;372:747–55.
60. Chiumello D, Carlesso E, Brioni M, Cressoni M. Airway driving pressure and lung stress in ARDS patients. Crit Care. 2016;20:276.
61. Guerin C, Papazian L, Reignier J, Ayzac L, Loundou A, Forel JM. Investigators of the A, Proseva t: effect of driving pressure on mortality in ARDS patients during lung protective mechanical ventilation in two randomized controlled trials. Crit Care. 2016;20:384.
62. Goligher EC, Costa ELV, Yarnell CJ, Brochard LJ, Stewart TE, Tomlinson G, Brower RG, Slutsky AS, Amato MPB. Effect of lowering Vt on mortality in acute respiratory distress syndrome varies with respiratory system elastance. Am J Respir Crit Care Med. 2021;203:1378–85.
63. Gattinoni L, Tonetti T, Cressoni M, Cadringher P, Herrmann P, Moerer O, Protti A, Gotti M, Chiurazzi C, Carlesso E, et al. Ventilator-related causes of lung injury: the mechanical power. Intensive Care Med. 2016;42:1567–75.
64. Marini JJ, Rocco PRM, Gattinoni L. Static and dynamic contributors to ventilator-induced lung injury in clinical practice. Pressure, energy, and power. Am J Respir Crit Care Med. 2020;201:767–74.
65. Marini JJ, Thornton LT, Rocco PRM, Gattinoni L, Crooke PS. Practical assessment of risk of VILI from ventilating power: a conceptual model. Crit Care. 2023;27:157.
66. Coppola S, Caccioppola A, Froio S, Formenti P, De Giorgis V, Galanti V, Consonni D, Chiumello D. Effect of mechanical power on intensive care mortality in ARDS patients. Crit Care. 2020;24:246.
67. Dianti J, Matelski J, Tisminetzky M, Walkey AJ, Munshi L, Del Sorbo L, Fan E, Costa EL, Hodgson CL, Brochard L, Goligher EC. Comparing the effects of tidal volume, driving pressure, and mechanical power on mortality in trials of lung-protective mechanical ventilation. Respir Care. 2021;66:221–7.
68. Costa ELV, Slutsky AS, Brochard LJ, Brower R, Serpa-Neto A, Cavalcanti AB, Mercat A, Meade M, Morais CCA, Goligher E, et al. Ventilatory variables and mechanical power in patients with acute respiratory distress syndrome. Am J Respir Crit Care Med. 2021;204:303–11.
69. Cressoni M, Gotti M, Chiurazzi C, Massari D, Algieri I, Amini M, Cammaroto A, Brioni M, Montaruli C, Nikolla K, et al. Mechanical power and development of ventilator-induced lung injury. Anesthesiology. 2016;124:1100–8.

70. Romitti F, Busana M, Palumbo MM, Bonifazi M, Giosa L, Vassalli F, Gatta A, Collino F, Steinberg I, Gattarello S, et al. Mechanical power thresholds during mechanical ventilation: an experimental study. Physiol Rep. 2022;10:e15225.
71. Tonetti T, Vasques F, Rapetti F, Maiolo G, Collino F, Romitti F, Camporota L, Cressoni M, Cadringher P, Quintel M, Gattinoni L. Driving pressure and mechanical power: new targets for VILI prevention. Ann Transl Med. 2017;5:286.
72. Huhle R, Serpa Neto A, Schultz MJ, Gama de Abreu M. Is mechanical power the final word on ventilator-induced lung injury?-no. Ann Transl Med. 2018;6:394.
73. Busana M, Zinnato C, Romitti F, Palumbo M, Gattarello S, Sonzogni A, Gersmann AK, Richter A, Herrmann P, Hahn G, et al. Energy dissipation during expiration and ventilator-induced lung injury: an experimental animal study. J Appl Physiol (1985). 2022;133:1212–9.
74. Diaz F, Gonzalez-Dambrauskas S, Cristiani F, Casanova DR, Cruces P. Driving pressure and normalized energy transmission calculations in mechanically ventilated children without lung disease and pediatric acute respiratory distress syndrome. Pediatr Crit Care Med. 2021;22:870–8.
75. Barnes T, van Asseldonk D, Enk D. Minimisation of dissipated energy in the airways during mechanical ventilation by using constant inspiratory and expiratory flows—flow-controlled ventilation (FCV). Med Hypotheses. 2018;121:167–76.
76. Cheng J, Yang J, Ma A, Dong M, Yang J, Wang P, Xue Y, Zhou Y, Kang Y. The effects of airway pressure release ventilation on pulmonary permeability in severe acute respiratory distress syndrome pig models. Front Physiol. 2022;13:927507.
77. Katzenschlager S, Simon CM, Rehn P, Grilli M, Fiedler MO, Muller M, Weigand MA, Neetz B. Time-controlled adaptive ventilation in patients with ARDS-lack of protocol adherence: a systematic review. Crit Care. 2023;27:57.
78. Miller AG, Gentile MA, Davies JD, MacIntyre NR. Clinical management strategies for airway pressure release ventilation: a survey of clinical practice. Respir Care. 2017;62:1264–8.
79. Jain SV, Kollisch-Singule M, Sadowitz B, Dombert L, Satalin J, Andrews P, Gatto LA, Nieman GF, Habashi NM. The 30-year evolution of airway pressure release ventilation (APRV). Intensive Care Med Exp. 2016;4:11.
80. Carsetti A, Damiani E, Domizi R, Scorcella C, Pantanetti S, Falcetta S, Donati A, Adrario E. Airway pressure release ventilation during acute hypoxemic respiratory failure: a systematic review and meta-analysis of randomized controlled trials. Ann Intensive Care. 2019;9:44.
81. Chen C, Zhen J, Gong S, Yan J, Li L. Efficacy of airway pressure release ventilation for acute respiratory distress syndrome: a systematic review with meta-analysis. Ann Palliat Med. 2021;10:10349–59.
82. Lim J, Litton E. Airway pressure release ventilation in adult patients with acute hypoxemic respiratory failure: a systematic review and meta-analysis. Crit Care Med. 2019;47:1794–9.
83. Zhong X, Wu Q, Yang H, Dong W, Wang B, Zhang Z, Liang G. Airway pressure release ventilation versus low tidal volume ventilation for patients with acute respiratory distress syndrome/acute lung injury: a meta-analysis of randomized clinical trials. Ann Transl Med. 2020;8:1641.
84. Othman F, Alsagami N, Alharbi R, Almuammer Y, Alshahrani S, Ismaeil T. The efficacy of airway pressure release ventilation in acute respiratory distress syndrome adult patients: a meta-analysis of clinical trials. Ann Thorac Med. 2021;16:245–52.
85. Roshdy A, Elsayed AS, Saleh AS. Airway pressure release ventilation for acute respiratory failure due to coronavirus disease 2019: a systematic review and meta-analysis. J Intensive Care Med. 2023;38:160–8.
86. Sun X, Liu Y, Li N, You D, Zhao Y. The safety and efficacy of airway pressure release ventilation in acute respiratory distress syndrome patients: a PRISMA-compliant systematic review and meta-analysis. Medicine (Baltimore). 2020;99:e18586.
87. Camporota L, Rose L, Andrews PL, Nieman GF, Habashi NM. Airway pressure release ventilation for lung protection in acute respiratory distress syndrome: an alternative way to recruit the lungs. Curr Opin Crit Care. 2024;30:76–84.

Chapter 9
Adaptive Dynamic Sub-tidal Ventilation (ADSV *Technology*): Lung Protection by Millisecond Adjustments in Gas Flow, Volume, and Pressure at the Alveolar Level

Introduction

The Conundrum of Ventilating the Acutely Injured Lung

Ventilating the acutely injured lung poses a conundrum due to the complex pathophysiology associated with acute respiratory distress syndrome (ARDS) (Fig. 1.1). ARDS causes a heterogeneous injury throughout the lung (Fig. 2.5) known as "hidden micro-atelectasis" (Fig. 2.8). These structural changes result in repetitive alveolar collapse and expansion (RACE) (Fig. 2.6) and stress multipliers (Fig. 2.7, Video 2.1), causing both volutrauma (Fig. 4.3, Video 4.4) and atelectrauma (Fig. 4.9, Video 4.5). As a result of these structural changes, the lung becomes *time*- and *pressure*-dependent, meaning that it will take more time for the lung to open (Fig. 5.3, Video 4.1) and less time for it to collapse (Fig. 5.6, Video 5.3) at any given airway pressure. Consequently, the conundrum is finding a suitable ventilation strategy to adequately oxygenate and ventilate a lung with regional normal, unstable, and collapsed tissues without causing volutrauma or atelectrauma.

Since lung tissue opens and collapses as a viscoelastic system, both inspiratory and expiratory *time* play a crucial role in facilitating alveolar recruitment (Fig. 5.3, Video 5.1) and preventing collapse (Fig. 5.6, Video 5.3). To address this conundrum, the time-controlled adaptive ventilation (TCAV) method is employed, which utilizes the airway pressure release ventilation (APRV) mode with exact expiratory time settings directed by lung pathophysiology (i.e., respiratory system compliance—C_{RS}) (Chap. 8). Briefly, an extended time at inspiration recruits viscoelastic tissue, followed by a very brief expiratory time to prevent re-collapse. These

Supplementary Information The online version contains supplementary material available at https://doi.org/10.1007/978-3-031-66352-9_9.

© The Author(s), under exclusive license to Springer Nature Switzerland AG 2024

G. F. Nieman, N. M. Habashi, *Applied Physiology to Reduce Ventilator Induced Lung Injury*, https://doi.org/10.1007/978-3-031-66352-9_9

combined ventilation times and appropriate airway pressures stabilize and gradually reopen the ARDS lung (Fig. 8.3 TCAV Method).

Using the TCAV method, the brief expiratory time acts as a "brake," preventing alveoli with fast collapse time constants from de-recruiting. Simultaneously, the prolonged inspiratory time, combined with an inflate and brake "ratchet" effect, facilitates the gradual reopening of collapsed alveoli, one breath at a time (Fig. 8.3 TCAV Method, 8.8). Since the expiratory time is set based on C_{RS}, the TCAV method is personalized and adaptive to the patient's lung pathophysiology.

Applied physiology strongly suggests the TCAV method would effectively safeguard the acutely injured lung (Chap. 8), further supported by basic and clinical science (Table 9.1). However, to be optimally effective, volume and pressure should be instantly (milliseconds) changed as the resistance and elastance change to effectively recruit collapsed tissue (higher pressure and lower volume) and prevent derecruitment without overdistension (lower pressure and higher volume).

Table 9.1 Publications supporting the Applied Physiology of Airway Pressure Release Ventilation (APRV) mode set and adjusted using the Time-Controlled Adaptive Ventilation (TCAV) method

Al-Khalisy H. *Resp Res* 2024;25:37	https://doi.org/10.1186/s12931-023-02615-y
Andrews P. *J Trauma ACS* 2013;75:635	https://doi.org/10.1097/TA.0b013e31829d3504
Andrews P. *Frontiers Physiol* 2022;13	https://doi.org/10.3389/fphys.2022.928562
Bates JHT. *Crit Care Explor* 2020;2	https://doi.org/10.1097/CCE.0000000000000299
Bates JHT. *Ann Biomed Eng* 2023	https://doi.org/10.1007/s10439-023-03186-1
Bates JHT *AJRCCM* 2024;209	https://doi.org/10.1164/rccm.202307-1292VP
Beretta E. *Front Physiol* 2021;12	https://doi.org/10.3389/fphys.2021.781874
Camporota L. *Curr Opin Crit Care* 2023;30	https://doi.org/10.1097/MCC.0000000000001123
Emr B. *JAMA Surg* 2013	https://doi.org/10.1001/jamasurg.2013.3746
Habashi N. *Crit Care Med* 2005;33	https://doi.org/10.1097/01.CCM.0000155920.11893.37
Habashi N. *JAP* 2021;130	https://doi.org/10.1152/japplphysiol.00742.2020
Habashi N. *Crit Care Med* 2022;50	https://doi.org/10.1097/CCM.0000000000005403
Habashi N. *Crit Care Med* 2023	https://doi.org/10.1097/CCM.0000000000006018
Jain S. *Inten Care Med Exp* 2016;4	https://doi.org/10.1186/s40635-016-0085-2
Jain. S. *Inten Care Med Exp* 2017;5	https://doi.org/10.1186/s40635-017-0138-1
Kingsley J. *Perfusion* 2024;0:1	https://doi.org/10.1177/02676591241227167
Janssen M. *BMC Pulm Med* 2021;21	https://doi.org/10.1186/s12890-021-01545-z
Kollisch M. *JACS* 2014;219	https://doi.org/10.1016/j.jamcollsurg.2014.09.011
Kollisch M. *JAMA Surg* 2014, 149	https://doi.org/10.1001/jamasurg.2014.1829
Kollisch M. *Care Med Exp* 2015;3	https://doi.org/10.1186/s40635-015-0071-0
Kollisch M. *J Ped Surg* 2016;52	https://doi.org/10.1016/j.jpedsurg.2016.10.020
Kollisch M. *JAMA Surg* 2015, 151	https://doi.org/10.1001/jamasurg.2015.2683
Magalhaes R. *Crit Care Med* 2021	https://doi.org/10.1097/CCM.0000000000004675
Mahajan M. *Inten Care Med Exp* 2019;7:27	https://doi.org/10.1186/s40635-019-0250-5

(continued)

Table 9.1 (continued)

Ma H. *Front Netw Physiol* 2023;3	https://doi.org/10.3389/fnetp.2023.1257710
Nieman G. *Crit Care Med* 2013;41	https://doi.org/10.1097/CCM.0b013e31828ce91b
Nieman G. *J Appl Physiol* 2015;119	https://doi.org/10.1152/japplphysiol.00659.2015
Nieman G. *Inten Care Med Exp* 2017;5	https://doi.org/10.1186/s40635-017-0121-x
Nieman G. *J Appl Physiol* 2017;122	https://doi.org/10.1152/japplphysiol.00123.2017
Nieman G. *Crit Care* 2018;22	https://doi.org/10.1186/s13054-018-2051-8
Nieman G. *J Trauma ACS* 2018;85	https://doi.org/10.1097/TA.0000000000002050
Nieman G. *Frontiers Physiol* 2020;11	https://doi.org/10.3389/fphys.2020.00227
Nieman G. *Ann Inten Care*. 2020;10	https://doi.org/10.1186/s13613-019-0619-3
Nieman G. *Crit Care* 2022;26	https://doi.org/10.1186/s13054-022-04105-x
Nieman G. *J Clin Med* 2023;12	https://doi.org/10.3390/jcm12144633
Nieman G. *Front Physiol* 2023;14	https://doi.org/10.3389/fphys.2023.1287416
Oliveira M. *J Appl Physiol* 2022;132	https://doi.org/10.1152/japplphysiol.00689.2021
Ramcharran H. *J Appl Physiol* 2022	https://doi.org/10.1152/japplphysiol.00312.2022
Rancharran H. *Resp Care* 2024	https://doi.org/10.4187/respcare.11745
Rola P. *Front Physiol* 2022;13	https://doi.org/10.3389/fphys.2022.787231
Roy S. *Shock* 2013;39	https://doi.org/10.1097/SHK.0b013e31827b47bb
Roy S. *Shock* 2013;40	https://doi.org/10.1097/SHK.0b013e31829efb06
Roy S. *J Trauma ACS* 2012;73	https://doi.org/10.1097/TA.0b013e31825c7a82
Satalin J. *Trends Anaesth Crit Care* 2018;22	https://doi.org/10.1016/j.tacc.2018.05.007
Silva P. *Crit Care Med* 2018; 46	https://doi.org/10.1097/CCM.0000000000003078
Silva P. *Crit Care Med* 2018	https://doi.org/10.1097/CCM.0000000000003078
Smith B. *J Appl Physiol* 2015;118	https://doi.org/10.1152/japplphysiol.00902.2014

What Must the Mechanical breath Do to Solve This Conundrum?

The dynamic elastic properties of pulmonary structures enable the uniform ventilation of numerous alveoli, even when airways vary in caliber, length, and patency (Chap. 3). Delivering a constant tidal volume (V_T) to patients with near homogeneous, uniformly compliant lungs will distribute gas evenly throughout most of the lung. However, in cases of acute lung injury, the lung develops regional heterogeneous injuries in multiple areas throughout the lung, presenting with very different pulmonary resistance and elastance (Fig. 2.5). In this condition, managing flow and pressure relationships and the mechanical energy necessary to inflate the lungs becomes problematic. In response to these pathologic alterations, the gas volume, pressure, and the rate of the inspiratory airflow into and out of the lungs must interface with this changing pattern of pulmonary inspiratory and expiratory resistances in milliseconds for optimal gas distribution in the microenvironment.

Applying a positive pressure of adequate magnitude is essential to deliver a V_T against the elastic and non-elastic resistances within the lungs. The mean inspiratory flow rate against these intrapulmonary resistances determines the necessary pressure rise to establish an inspiratory flow gradient from the proximal to distal pulmonary airways, overcoming the intrapulmonary resistance to inflow.

The ideal mechanical breath profile (MB_P), consisting of all airway pressures, volumes, flows, rates, and the time they are delivered during inspiration and expiration, necessary to ventilate a heterogeneously injured lung would preferentially deliver a higher pressure to recruit and a lower volume to minimize volutrauma to collapsed areas, while delivering a low pressure and higher volume to inflated areas. Then, to support the newly recruited tissue, the MB_P components of pressure and volume would reverse instantaneously, delivering a higher volume and lower pressure to prevent both re-collapse and OD of the newly opened tissue. To accomplish the above goals, the ventilator much be novel (Fig. 9.1) and the MB_P must:

- Operate at a high rate (millisecond) to deliver sub-tidal volume pulses of gas with the pressure and volume adjusted based on R_{RS} to gas flow and elastance (Flow × Resistance = Pressure). This ensures that the volume and pressure will differ at each sub-tidal breath depending on lung tissue elastance and resistance (high pressure and low volume in high resistance/elastance tissue and reversed in low resistance/elastance tissue). The high rate of inspiratory gas pulses creates a "river" of gas flowing into the lung in the central portion of the airway and back out along the airway walls. Thus, gas continuously flows into and out of the lung, similar to a high-velocity stream of water flowing from a faucet into a glass and splashing back along the walls (Fig. 9.2).
- This novel MB_P must differ from classical ventilators in that it must be capable of cycling at high rates without generating auto-PEEP.

Addressing the Conundrum of Ventilating the Acutely Injured Lung: Adaptive Dynamic Sub-tidal Ventilation (ADSV) Technology

ADSV is a modification of the High-Frequency Percussive Ventilation (HFPV) method. [2] Few publications demonstrate the HFPV method's effectiveness for ARDS patients. However, the unique MB_P components and our understanding of VILI mechanisms at the alveolar level (Chaps. 4 and 5) warrant a thorough investigation [1–6]. Although much research will be necessary to identify the efficacy of ADSV technology for acute and chronic lung injury, applied physiology, and the physics of gas flow suggest a high potential for success. Thus, this chapter will focus on the unique physics of this ventilation method and speculate on its potential efficacy in managing patients with acute lung injury based on our understanding of dynamic alveolar mechanics and gas flow physics (Chap. 4).

Anatomy of ADSV Technology

A cross-sectional view of the Sliding Venturi (I) and the physics of gas flow (II) used in ADSV technology (Fig. 9.3II). ADSV Technology uses the Bernoulli (Fig. 9.4) and Venturi (Fig. 9.5) effects to modify gas volume, flow, and pressure in response to changes in downstream R_{RS}. Gas pulses are represented by the red line, and entrainment gas by the black dotted line. Using ADSV technology (Fig. 9.3I, II) the higher the rate at which the lines strike the wall of the Sliding Venturi, the higher the airway pressure and vice versa. Short lines represent high velocity, while longer lines represent slower velocity. The physician sets the high-frequency pressure pulses of gas to enter the venturi through the narrow tube (**A**, red line). These pulses then go into the entrainment chamber (**B**). The fall in airway pressure (Bernoulli effect, see Fig. 9.4) caused by the narrow tube (**A**) through which the gas pulse enters the entrainment chamber (**B**) causes gas to be entrained (Venturi effect, see Fig. 9.5) into the Sliding Venturi. The volume of gas entrained is a function of the R_{RS}. The higher the R_{RS}, the lower the entrainment and vice versa. The sub-tidal volume (S-V_T) is a combination of the pulse (red line) and entrainment (black dotted line) volume. This S-V_T then enters the thin portion of the Sliding Venturi (**C**), increasing the gas flow velocity and decreasing airway pressure to improve gas mixing. Finally, the S-V_T enters the tapered distal end of the venturi tube (**D**), which will reduce flow velocity and increase airway pressure. ADSV technology uses the Bernoulli and Venturi effects to automatically adjust delivered volume and pressure based on the physics of gas flow directed by changes in downstream resistance and elastance of the lung being ventilated (Bernoulli and Venturi effects, see Figs. 9.4 and 9.5).

The Bernoulli and Venturi Effects

According to the first law of thermodynamics, energy cannot be created or destroyed; it is conserved and transformed from one form to another. When considering gas moving through a tube, the total energy includes kinetic energy (forward movement) and static energy (the force exerted against the walls of the tube). This can be expressed as:

$$E_{\mathrm{T}} = E_{\mathrm{K}} + E_{\mathrm{S}} = \mathrm{Cte}$$

$$E_{\mathrm{K}} = \tfrac{1}{2}mv^2$$

where E_T is the total energy, E_K = kinetic energy (m = the mass, and v = gas velocity), E_S = the static energy expressed as the pressure on airway walls, and Cte = E_T remains constant. When a tapering or restriction occurs within the tube, the energy related to forward movement increases, and then, to conserve total energy, the static pressure must decrease. This phenomenon is known as the Bernoulli effect (Fig. 9.4A–C). If the driving pressure is kept constant, a larger tube diameter (**A**) has a relativity lower gas flow velocity (V) and a higher pressure (P) than a small diameter tube (**B**, **C**). Three different tube constrictions are shown (Fig. 9.4A–C). The size of the tube leading up to the constriction is the same, so the pressures (P1,

48 cmH_2O) and velocity (V1) are all the same (Fig. 9.4A–C). As the size of the tube is narrowed (A > B > C), the pressure falls (A = 35 cmH_2O, B = 28 cmH_2O, C = 12 cmH_2O) as the gas velocity increases. Thus V4 > V3 > V2 > V1 and P1 > P2 > P3 > P4 (Fig. 9.4A–C).

The Venturi effect is shown in Fig. 9.5. A large tube (**A**) is constricted (**B**) and then returned to the same diameter as before the constriction (**C**). A small entrainment port is connected to the constricted portion of the tube. The sizes of the tubes leading up to the constriction (**A**) and after the constriction (**C**) are the same, so the pressures (P1 & P3, 48 cmH_2O) and velocity (V1, V3) will be the same after the constriction (Fig. 9.2A–C). If the driving pressure is kept constant, reducing the tube size (**B**) will increase the gas flow velocity (V2) and decrease the pressure (P2) (**B**). Additional gas enters the entrainment port in the Venturi throat due to the lower pressure (P2) (**B** arrows).

The Sliding Venturi (Figs. 9.1 and 9.3) uses the following two Venturi effects to personalize gas delivery to the pathophysiology of the patient's lung: *Venturi Effect*

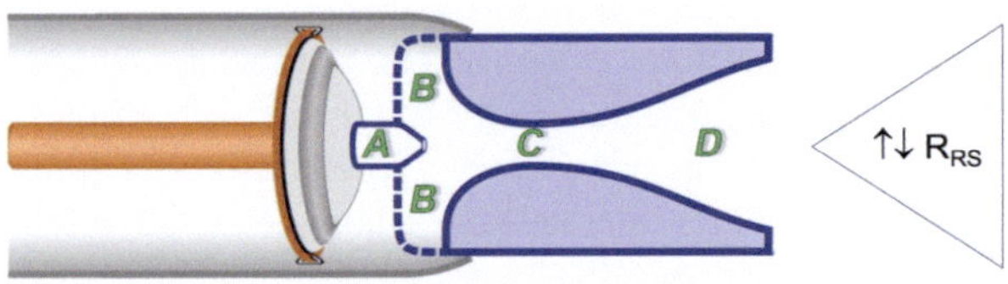

Fig. 9.1 The cross sectional view of the ADSV's Sliding Venturi tube. The Sliding Venturi is designed based on the principles of Bernoulli (Fig. 9.4) and Venturi (Fig. 9.5). A gas pulse is injected into the Sliding Venturi (**A**) through a narrow orifice. The gas pulse enters a much broader chamber in which additional gas can be entrained (**B**), then moves into the narrow portion of the Venturi tube where the gas pulse and entrainment gas are mixed (**C**) and finally into the wide portion of the Venturi tube where gas flow velocity decreases and airway pressure increases (**D**). The amount of entrained gas is regulated by lung physiology. The respiratory system resistance (R_{RS}) in the normal lung would be low (↓$\mathbf{R_{RS}}$), and thus, back pressure in the entrainment chamber (**B**) would be low, establishing a significant pressure drop, and a relatively large volume of gas would be entrained. In the acutely injured lung, RRS would be high (↑$\mathbf{R_{RS}}$); thus, back pressure in the entrainment chamber (**B**) would also be high, the pressure drops low, and a relatively small volume of gas would be entrained
There are two main Venturi effects used by ADSV technology: **(1)** *Venturi Effect 1*—Reducing the diameter of the tube where the pressured pulses of gas enter the Sliding Venturi (**A**) accelerates gas flow and drops airway pressure, causing entrainment of gas into the Sliding Venturi **(B).** *Venturi Effect 2*—A decrease or increase in downstream backpressure (Triangle ↓↑$\mathbf{R_{RS}}$) will increase or decrease the sub-tidal volume (S-VT) size, respectively. Elevated back pressure could be caused by increased $\mathbf{R_{RS}}$ or elastance or both secondary to acute lung injury with surfactant deactivation, edema, and lung collapse. The increased backpressure will increase airway pressure in the entrainment chamber, reducing the volume of entrained gas and the size of **the S-$\mathbf{V_T}$**
A significant feature of ADSV technology is that it is personalized and adaptive to changes in lung pathophysiology on a millisecond basis. When backpressure is applied downstream to the outflow tract of the Sliding Venturi (triangle), the pressure will increase inside the tube to the level of the entrainment port **(B).** Consequently, gas entrainment and the delivered sub-tidal volumes will decrease in milliseconds due to the *Venturi Effect 2***.** When translated into clinical application, the following will occur. In diseased lungs (high R_{RS} and elastance), gas entrainment will instantaneously drop, reducing the size of the S-V_T and preventing lung overinflation. When the lungs improve (decrease in R_{RS} and elastance), gas entrainment will instantaneously increase and augment the size of S-V_T, stabilizing the newly recruited lung tissue

1: Airway pressure decreases, and gas velocity increases as the gas moves into the narrow portion of the Venturi causing gas entrainment. *Venturi Effect 2:* The airway pressure necessary to ventilate the lung will be reflected from the lungs back into the Sliding Venturi. The higher the $R_{RS,}$ the less gas entrainment and vice versa. Combined, these two Venturi effects personalize the size of the S-V_T to lung pathophysiology—Normal lung with low airway resistance and elastance, more extensive gas entrainment resulting in a higher S-V_T; ARDS lung with high airway resistance and elastance, smaller gas entrainment, reducing the S-V_T.

ADSV Technology and Gas Flow Physics

The main principles used by ADSV technology are the Venturi effect to convert flow to pressure and pressure to flow in milliseconds as intrapulmonary resistance to inspiratory flow constantly changes. The Sliding Venturi has two flow gradients: (1) the positive flow gradient produced by gas flowing from the jet orifice and (2) the sub-atmospheric entrainment gradient produced by flow velocity through the Venturi throat (Fig. 9.3A). The Venturi body is sized to slide within the breathing circuit interface within a specific range (1 to 2 mm) (Video 9.1). The diaphragm carries a hollow stem connected to the jet cage, forming a sealed interface (Fig. 9.1).

ADSV technology regulates inspiratory flow rates during a time-cycled programmed high-frequency S-V_T exchange and delivers a millisecond-based inspiration/expiration cycle. As previously discussed, the Sliding Venturi uses the Bernoulli and Venturi effects (Figs. 9.4 and 9.5). Gas would expand in the Venturi tube's distal end, slowing its forward movement and increasing proximal pressures, creating a pressure gradient to deliver gas into the airways (Fig. 9.3II, D). When intrapulmonary resistance and elastance (R_{RS}) oppose flow downstream of the Venturi tube, it causes back pressure into the entrainment chamber (Fig. 9.3II, B), reducing the pressure gradient or driving pressure (ΔP) from the Venturi into the lungs. The variations in ΔP, secondary to lung recruitment (higher) or collapse (lower), result in millisecond changes in entrainment volume (Fig. 9.3B, black dotted lines). Thus, with equal inspiratory pressures, the ΔP will be lower in an injured lung with high R_{RS} because of the back pressure.

A "River" of Gas into and out of the Lung: ADSV technology delivers a high-frequency percussive breath (0.5–20 Hz) usually set to generate a sinusoidal convective breath waved form (0–70 breaths/min). This innovative concept uses a pneumatic, high-energy percussive breath (Fig. 9.6). Inspiration (Big I) is a progressive accumulation of sub-tidal volume breaths that gradually increase both airway pressure and volume, leading to an oscillatory plateau followed by passive exhalation (Big E) (Fig. 9.6). Thus, using S-V_T gas pulses, convective lung volume changes in a sinusoidal waveform form. The pulses are stopped or reduced to lower airway pressure and flow (Big E) to facilitate $PaCO_2$ removal. However, this would not be necessary for an acutely injured lung once it was reinflated and the CO_2 diffusion area increased.

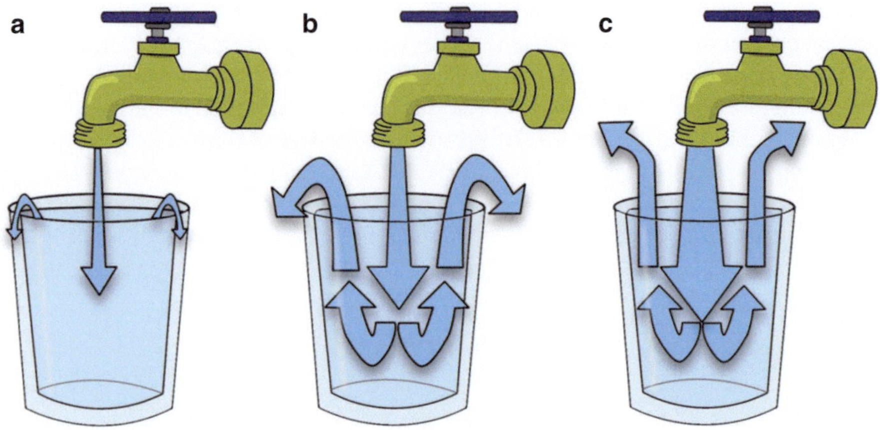

Fig. 9.2 Conceptual simulation of the postulated gas flow into and out of the lung using ADSV technology based on Newton's Third Law of Motion. Water is injected into the center of the glass with increasing energy (**A**–**C**). (**A**) If a low-energy stream of water is directed into the glass, it fills and then slowly overflows. (**B**) When the energy is sufficient, there will be a bidirectional flow of water into the center of the glass and water flowing out of the glass along the glass walls. (**C**) A very high-energy stream of water will cause the water to return from the glass to the height of the source. We postulate that ADSV technology generates a similar gas flow *into* and *out of* the lung, forming a bidirectional "river" of gas flow

Each pulse has an inspiratory phase (Little i) and an expiratory phase (Little e) (Fig. 9.6). The high-energy gas pulses form a continuous "river" of gas flowing simultaneously into and out of the lung. An analogy would be turning a water facet in full force and directing the stream into an empty glass (Fig. 9.2). In this conceptual diagram, a water stream with increasing hydraulic energy is directed into the center of the glass. As the velocity and energy of the stream progressively increase, a point is reached where the force becomes sufficient to facilitate counterflow, ultimately leading to outflux from the glass. Thus, water is flowing into and out of the glass simultaneously. We postulate that this same bidirectional gas flow occurs during ADSV technology in the lung's airways. The gas flowing into the lung would deliver oxygen, while the gas flowing back out would remove CO_2. This "river" of gas would oxygenate and ventilate without significantly changing lung volume between inspiration and expiration.

Volume, Flow, and Pressure Delivered by the Sliding Venturi

By having separate opening and closing speed controls, the electro-valves will allow a wide selection of pulse sizes (i:e) and inspiratory/expiratory (I:E) ratios, as well as an accurate titration of the time and flow delivered to the breathing circuit interface (Fig. 9.6). The repeated opening and closing of their internal orifice in response to signals from the digital controller create a pulsatile flow over an extensive range of frequencies and pressures (Fig. 9.6, Video 9.1). By controlling the delivered pulses at a high rate, the scheduled expiratory time is insufficient to allow the previously delivered S-V_T to be exhaled before the next tidal injection occurs (Fig. 9.7a, b, Volume/Time Curve, IN and OUT, Video 9.1). Thus, the slight initial increase in dynamic end-expiratory lung volume (EELV) is constantly maintained.

The volume, flow, and pressure delivered during the Big I differ depending on lung compliance measures as the R_{RS} (Fig. 9.3II, ↑↓R_{RS}). The ARDS lung has a large volume of collapse and low-compliant tissue with a small amount of remaining normal lung ("Baby Lung") (Figs. 9.8 and 9.9). At the beginning of inspiration, the S-V_T delivered volume (IN) is larger than the volume exhaled (OUT) as the normal "Baby Lung" fills. However, the small volume of normal tissue fills so that the IN and OUT volumes rapidly equilibrate. As the R_{RS} increases after the "Baby Lung" fills, entrainment is reduced, lowering the size of the S-V_T (Fig. 9.7). The normal

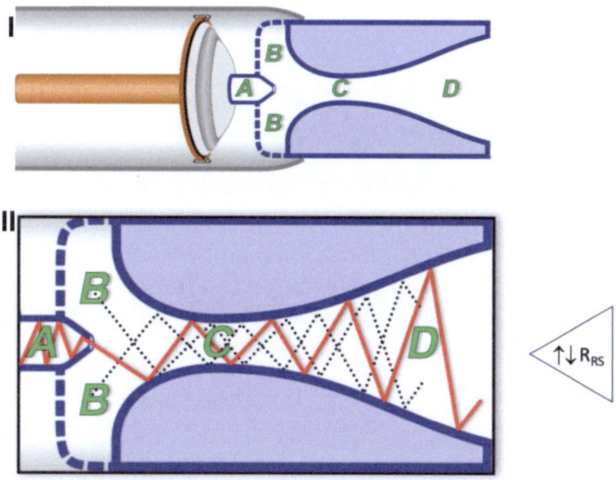

Fig. 9.3 Cross section of the Sliding Venturi (**I**) and a diagram of how a change in tube diameter impacts gas volume and pressure within the tube (**II**). (**A**) Intermittent pulses of high-energy gas are delivered to the orifice of the Sliding Venturi (red line), and the reduced diameter of the circuit generates the Bernoulli effect, accelerating primary gas flow (longer red line) and reducing the airway pressure (number of times the red line hits the tube wall). (**B**) This high-velocity, low-pressure gas enters the Venturi's entrainment port. The airway pressure at this point is lower than that outside the port, and thus, additional gas is entrained into the gas stream. This secondary gas combines with the primary gas and becomes the sub-tidal volume (black dotted line). (**C**) The narrow portion of the Venturi's throat section is the merging zone of the primary and secondary gas, where flow acceleration is maintained to amplify gas mixing. (**D**) The increased diameter in the distal section or cone of the Venturi will decelerate the flow and increase airway pressure in conformance with the equation of conservation of energy. Pressure on the airway walls is represented by the number of times the injected primary flow gas (red solid line) and the entrained secondary gas (black dotted line) strike the wall of the airways. Thus, the Venturi tube allows gas entrainment to increase gas flow and volume and to restore delivered lateral pressure to the airway walls

lung continues to fill throughout inspiration, and the S-V_T IN is always higher than that returning OUT. Like the volume, the flow and pressure equilibrate more quickly in the ARDS lung than in the normal lung (Fig. 9.7).

ADSV Technology and the Lung

The venturi slider functions as a flow-to-pressure and pressure-to-flow converter, and the interrupter electro-valves, together, allow the control of the inspiratory flow gradient and indirectly the delivered sub-tidal volume (Fig. 9.8). Pressurized respiratory gases are delivered into the patient's airway through a breathing circuit (Fig. 9.8, A red line). As the patient's lungs are inflated to the programmed peak inspiratory pressure, R_{RS} will increase with lung inflation and be transmitted back through the breathing circuit into the venturi as a back pressure (Fig. 9.8, R_{RS}), thus regulating the volume of gas entrainment (Fig. 9.8, B arrows). In the normal lung (Fig. 9.8I), the R_{RS} is low (small triangle), the back pressure in the entrainment chamber is low, and the volume of entrained gas is high (Fig. 9.8I, B large black arrows and thick black dotted lines). The result is a high gas volume delivery at low airway pressure.

In the ARDS lung, the R_{RS} is high (large triangle), the back pressure in the entrainment chamber is high, and the entrainment volume is small (Fig. 9.8II, B small black arrows and thin black dotted lines). The result is a low gas volume delivery at high airway pressure. Thus, the normal and ARDS lung received the correct gas volume and pressure for their physiologic condition. The normal lung is large with a low R_{RS}, so it needs a high gas volume delivered at a low airway pressure. The ARDS lung is small with a high R_{RS}, so it needs a low gas volume (so as not to overdistend) delivered at a high airway pressure (necessary to recruit collapsed tissue).

Location of the Sliding Venturi

Placing the Sliding Venturi at the patient's proximal airway eliminates gas compression in ventilator tubing and reduces dead space, significantly reducing the reaction time; therefore, the Venturi response to changing inflow or outflow R_{RS} and elastance is almost immediate. The Sliding Venturi is contained within a breathing circuit housing and allows for near-instantaneous venting of exhaled gas at the proximal airway because of the atmospheric pressures at the exhalation port. Inspiration will not dampen the expiratory flow (Video 9.1). Therefore, the forward S-V_T injection is synchronized with the expired gas pulse by a near-immediate retraction of the Sliding Venturi, venting an expired gas pulse after the venturi depressurizes. There is no positive end-expiratory pressure (PEEP) at the exhalation port, so atmospheric pressure is employed as an expiratory flow gradient constant through the breathing circuit interface. During the millisecond expiratory pauses between repeated cyclic injections allow the progressive recruitment of lung volume one sub-tidal breath at a time, with a portion but not all of each sub-tidal volume being exhaled after each pulse (Fig. 9.7 Volume/Time curves, In & Out).

The stepwise increase in airway pressure with ADSV allows a progressive increase in lung volume (Fig. 9.7 Volume/Time curves). This gradual application of sub-tidal volume inspiration and expiration can avoid overdistension of lung tissues, which can occur with a single large V_T. The Sliding Venturi proximal to the patient's airways, with inspiratory gas injection and expiratory atmospheric release combined in a single stroke, more precisely controls the inflow and outflow gradients within the pulmonary airways during the ventilatory process while protecting the pulmonary structures.

The Sliding Venturi is designed to provide a pressure-flow and flow-pressure conversion, where the first pulses of gas generate maximal entrainment, and the delivered sub-tidal volumes of gas to the patient's airway are relativity large (~70 mL) (Fig. 9.7 Volume/Time curves, In & Out). Subsequently, the progressive increase in R_{RS} and elastance as the lung fills will generate a back pressure reflected into the Sliding Venturi (Fig. 9.8II, R_{RS}). This will increase the pressure inside the Sliding Venturi, decreasing gas entrainment. Thus, the delivered sub-tidal volumes of gas become smaller (~30 mL) (Fig. 9.8II, B small black arrow), and the gas in and out stabilizes during the equilibrium (Fig. 9.7a Volume/Time curves Equal IN & OUT).

ADSV Technology in the Lung Microenvironment

Despite the absence of direct scientific evidence, our comprehension of the principles governing gas flow, specifically the Bernoulli and Venturi effects (Figs. 9.4 and 9.5), enables us to propose a logical science-based hypothesis of ADSV technology gas flow dynamics in the lung microenvironment (i.e., small airways, alveolar ducts, and alveoli). ADSV technology gas flows into and out of the lung and can be conceptualized as a high-velocity stream of water into the center of glass (Fig. 9.2). Initially, at low velocity, water fills the glass gradually until it overflows (Fig. 9.2A). With increased water velocity, a counter-current flow pattern emerges, where a stream of water enters the center of the glass and exits simultaneously along the glass walls, based on Newton's Third Law of Motion (Fig. 9.2B, C). The higher the entry velocity, the faster and further the water will move out of the glass.

We postulate that this phenomenon occurs in the lung when high-velocity pulses and entrained gas volume are injected (Fig. 9.9B). Acute lung injury causes regional heterogeneous tissue damage throughout the lung, resulting in thousands of different lung R_{RS} and compliances. The blue arrows moving into the lung down the center of the airways represent the high-velocity pluses and entrained flow (analogous to the water coming out of the faucet—Fig. 9.2). As the high-velocity gas pulse reaches the terminal alveoli, it reverses and flows back toward the trachea along the airway walls (indicated by small tan arrows), similar to the water flowing out of the

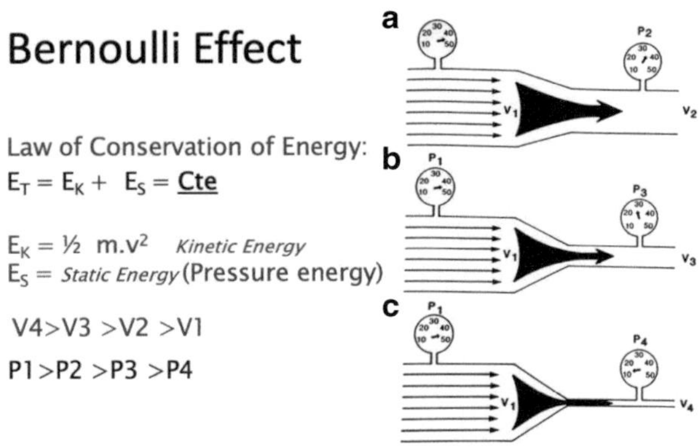

Fig. 9.4 An example of the Bernoulli effect. As the forward velocity of a gas moving through a tube increases, the lateral wall pressure of the tube decreases. Thus, in a large tube, pressure is high (P1–45 cmH_2O), and the velocity is low (V1–10 L/min). (**A**) A slight constriction in the cylinder results in a decrease in pressure (P_2–38 cmH_2O) and an increase in velocity (V_2—50 L/min). Further constrictions in the cylinder (**B**, **C**) amplify the decrease in pressure (P_3_28 cmH_2O, P_4_12 cmH_2O) and the increase in velocity (V_3—80 L/min, V_4—100 L/min) such that $V_4 > V_3 > V_2 > V_1$ and $P_1 > P_2 > P_3 > P_4$. This Bernoulli effect is based on the Law of Conservation of Energy
E_T is the total energy, E_K = kinetic energy, E_S = the static energy (pressure energy) expressed as the lateral pressure, m = the mass, v = the velocity, and Cte = E_T remains constant

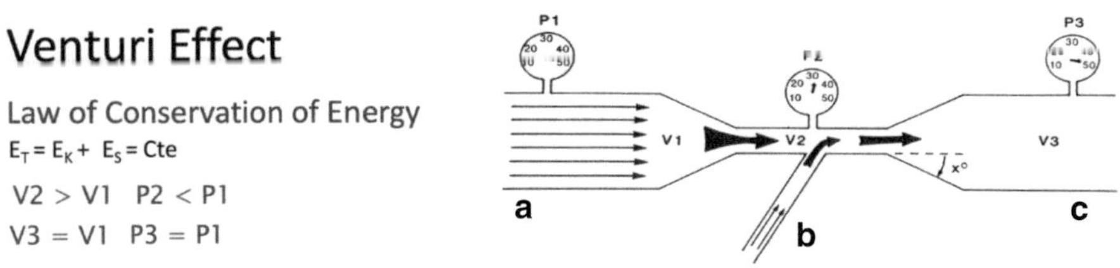

Fig. 9.5 An example of the Venturi effect is an extension of the Bernoulli effect. It states that the initial pressure drop, as the gas flows through the tube constriction, can be restored to the pre-constriction pressure if a tube with a gradual increase in diameter, not higher than 15% (X°), is added distal to the constriction. *Venturi Effect 1:* A tube (**A**) is constricted (**B**) [the Bernoulli tube] and then returned to the original size (**C**). Gas pressure (P_1, P_3–48 cmH_2O) and velocity (V_1, V_3–10 L/min) are equal because the tube size is identical (**A**, **C**). In the constricted portion of the tube (**B**), the pressure (P_2_32 cmH_2O) is lower, and the velocity (V_2—50 L/min) is higher than in the larger tube (**A**, **C**). When a side port is created at the constriction (**B**) level, the pressure drop P2 (32 cmH_2O) will entrain gas from outside the cylinder that will mix with the main flow of gas. Thus, the Venturi tube causes an increase in the flow and the volume (entrainment) of gas while restoring "lateral"pressure. *Venturi Effect 2:* If the outflow gas meets high respiratory system resistance (R_{RS}) or elastance, backpressure will be transmitted back into the Venturi entrainment chamber, increasing the airway pressure and reducing the volume of entrained gas (Fig. 9.3). The Venturi effect is based on the Law of Conservation of Energy
E_T is the total energy, E_K = kinetic energy, E_S = the static energy (pressure energy) expressed as the lateral pressure, m = the mass, v = the velocity, and Cte = E_T remains constant

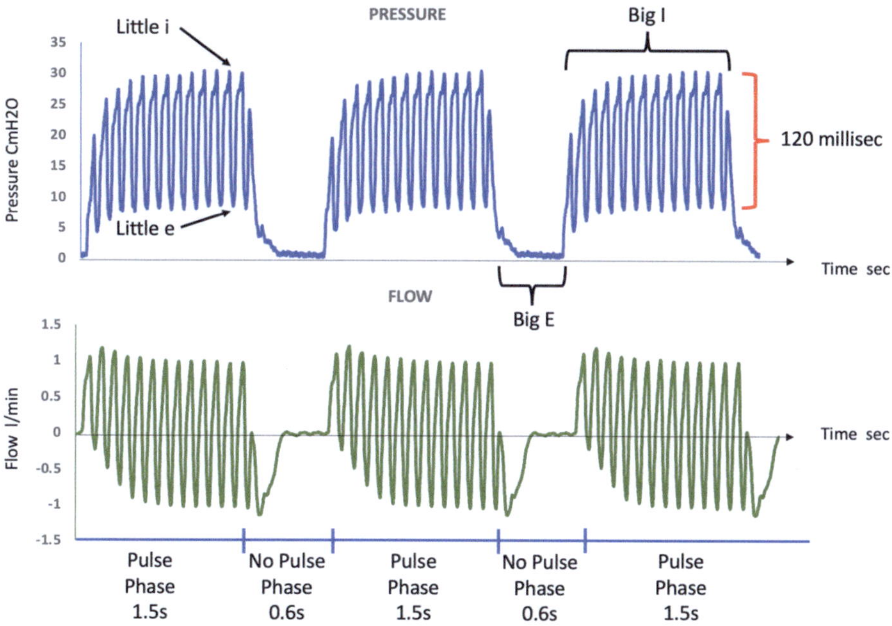

Fig. 9.6 A typical ADSV technology pressure/time and flow/time curve shows the pressure and flow pulses that generate the sinusoidal convectional waveform. The physician can control and modify the inspiratory *Pulse Phase* (Big I) during which the pulses are applied and the length of the expiratory *No Pulse Phase* (Big E). The physician also controls the pulse cycles/minute. In this example, the *Pulse Phase* is for 1.5 s, and the *No Pulse Phase* is for 0.6 s. The frequency and amplitude of the individual pulses are adjusted using an electro-valved interrupter to generate a pulse inspiration (Little i) and a pulse expiration (Little e) phase. In this example, the pulse rate was set at 500 cycles/min, so each cycle is approximately 120 ms. The inspiratory time of each pulse was 30–50 ms, and the expiratory time was 50–80 ms

glass (Fig. 9.2). The flow-no-flow with each gas pulse (Video 9.1) creates a pressure-no-pressure zone along the airways and has a peristaltic-like effect, enhancing airway recruitment during gas flow in (Fig. 9.9, Blue gas pulses) and removing secretion along the airway wall with the gas flowing out (Fig. 9.9, tan gas pulses).

The size, R_{RS}, and elastance of the airways and tissue differ significantly in the heterogeneously injured ARDS lung (Fig. 9.9, Gross lung photo). In the normal tissue, flow (f) and resistance (r) will be high because the resistance is low (f1r1). With progressive lung injury, the resistance will increase, and the flow decreases (f2r2, f3r3). However, flow × resistance will be equal in all tissues due to the Law of Conservation of Energy. This relationship will result in a high gas volume at lower pressure delivered to the normal lung tissue (f1r1) and a lower volume at a higher pressure (f2r2, f3r3) delivered to the acutely injured lung since Flow × Resistance = Pressure. The inspired gas pulses (blue arrow) are returned to the Sliding Venturi (tan arrows) along the airway walls, and a pulse of gas will be exhaled following each pulse of inhaled gas (Video 9.1).

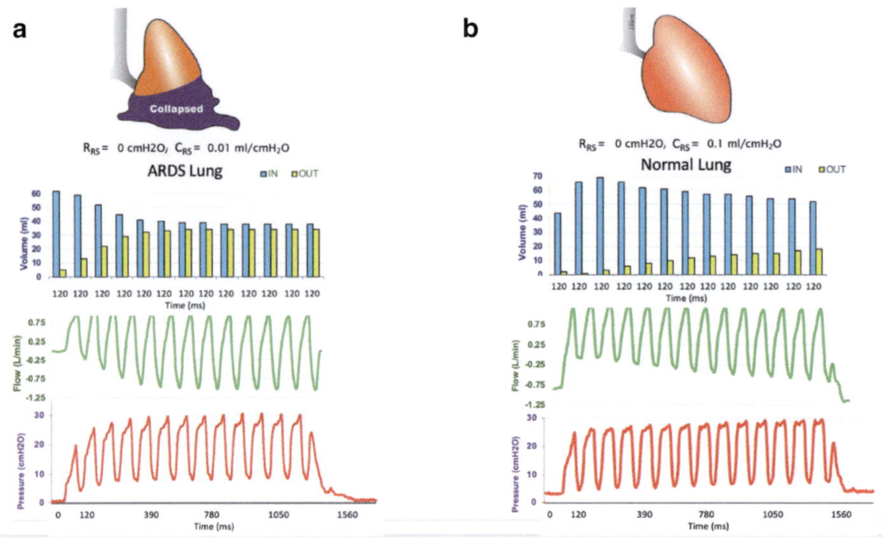

Fig. 9.7 The impact of decreased respiratory system compliance (C_{RS}) with the same lung respiratory system resistance (R_{RS}) on the Volume/, Flow/, and Pressure/Time curves. (**a**) In the ARDS lung with low C_{RS} (0.01 mL/cmH_2O), the sub-tidal volume (S-V_T) "IN" (blue bar) and "OUT" (yellow bar) equalize rapidly after the small amount of normal tissue fully inflates. The Flow/Time and Pressure/Time also rapidly stabilize during the inspiration. (**b**) In a normal lung with high C_{RS} (0.1 mL/cmH_2O), the S-V_T "IN" is higher than in the ARDS lung and remains higher during the entire inspiratory cycle Pulse Phase cycle (Fig. 9.6). The sub-tidal volume "OUT" never equilibrates with the volume "IN" such that the large normal lung inflates during the entire inspiratory cycle. Pressure also continues to increase throughout inspiration

ADSV technology operates on the fundamental principle of preventing the administration of an S-V_T pulse greater than the anatomical dead space. The millisecond cyclic energy released into the Sliding Venturi required for a sub-tidal volume intrapulmonary delivery of a gas pulse generates a shock wave. When a high-pressure gas is rapidly released, it can suddenly disturb the surrounding area, forming mini-shock waves. A rapid increase in pressure and velocity in these localized areas characterizes these mini-shock waves that will assist in lung recruitment, airway clearance, and mucus removal [7, 8].

As R_{RS} causes the sub-atmospheric pressures within the venturi throat to become ambient, the entrainment gradient is reduced to zero (Fig. 9.3II B small black arrow). The lung volume gradually increases in conformance with the set peak pressure. There is no flow through the venturi throat, and a total reverse flow from the venturi through the venturi entrainment port commences. Therefore, the primary advantage of delivering inspiratory gases into the lung through an adequately designed venturi relates to the instantaneous change in flow gradient and, thus, gas entrainment governed by the difference in the back pressure.

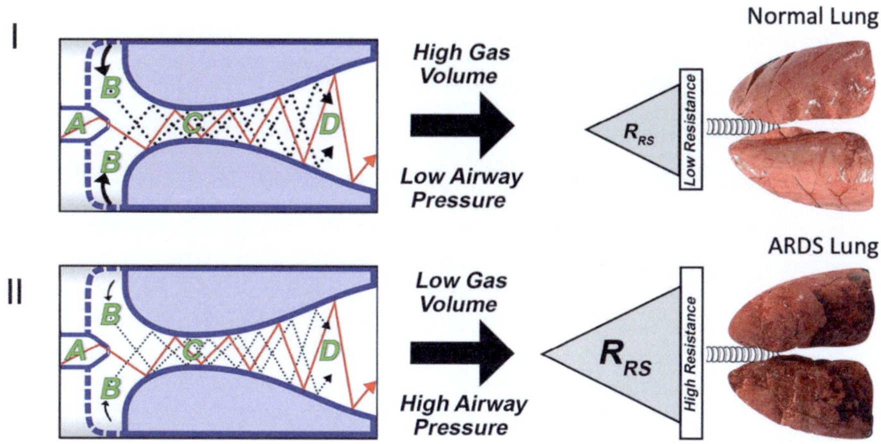

Fig. 9.8 The impact of lung pathophysiology on delivered gas volume and pressure based on the Venturi effects. *Venturi Effect 1:* If a tube through which gas flows is constricted, the velocity of the gas increases, and the airway pressure decreases. If an entrainment port is placed in the narrow portion of the tubing, the reduced airway pressure will result in gas entrainment (Fig. 9.3II, B black dotted line). *Venturi Effect 2:* A change in lung backpressure will increase (low backpressure) or decrease (high backpressure) gas entrainment (Fig. 9.3II Triangle ↑↓R_{RS}), changing the size of the sub-tidal volume (S-V_T). (**I**) In the normal lung, R_{RS} and elastance are low (small triangle), generating low back pressure. This will allow for a relatively large gas entrainment (B, large black arrows, and thick dotted lines) and increase the size of the S-V_T. (**II**) The R_{RS} and elastance are high (large triangle) in the ARDS lung, generating high backpressure. This causes a relatively small gas entrainment (B, small black arrows, and a thin dotted line) and reduces the size of the S-V_T. Thus, the normal lung will receive high gas volumes and low airway pressure, whereas the ARDS lung will receive lower gas volumes and higher airway pressure (Flow × Resistance = Pressure)

Conclusions

ADSV technology is an entirely different mode of mechanical ventilation. Applied physiology suggests that, like the TCAV method, it can eliminate both RACE and stress multipliers, the mechanical mechanisms causing VILI, using the component of inspiratory and expiratory time. The physician controls the rate and pressure of the high-velocity pulses of gas, but the gas entrainment is controlled by lung pathophysiology. An acutely injured lung with high airway R_{RS} and elastance will receive a lower volume and higher pressure breath to avoid volutrauma while assisting in lung recruitment. As the lung heals and reopens, the gas volume will increase, and the airway pressure will lower. Thus, ADSV technology is personalized and adaptive to the patient's lung pathology (Fig. 9.10). Much study is necessary before ADSV technology becomes a primary mode of ventilating the ARDS patient. However, the novel use of dynamic gas flow physics makes it a promising new tool for preventing VILI.

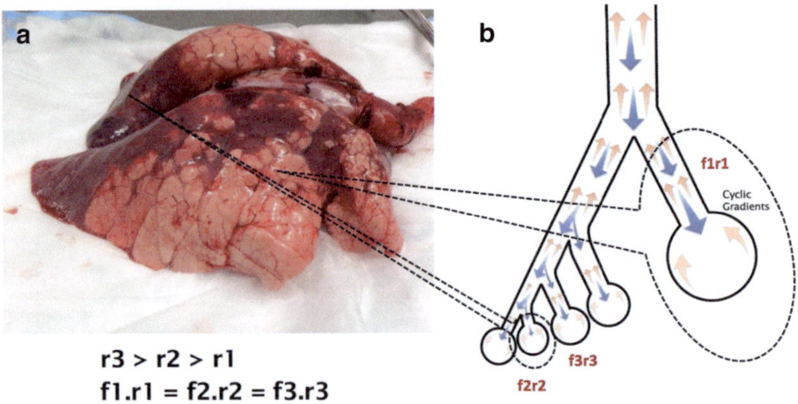

Fig. 9.9 The impact of heterogeneous changes in lung tissue pathophysiology on gas flow, volume, and pressure in the microenvironment with acutely injured lung. High-velocity inspiratory pluses are represented by blue arrows moving into the lung down the center of the airways. As the high-velocity gas pulse reaches the terminal alveoli, it reverses direction and flows back toward the trachea along the airway walls (small tan arrows), similar to the water flowing out of the glass (Fig. 9.4). The millisecond cyclic energy released into the Sliding Venturi generates a shock wave along the airway walls. When the resistance (r) is low (f1), the flow (f) will be high (f1). With increasing resistance, the flow will be reduced (f2.r2 and f3.r3). Areas with the highest airway resistance (r3) will be the areas that generate the highest Back Pressure (Flow ×Resistance = Pressure) that will be reflected in milliseconds back to the Venturi entrainment chamber (Fig. 9.3II, B). This will reduce gas entrainment and the delivered sub-tidal volume, protecting the lung from over-distending

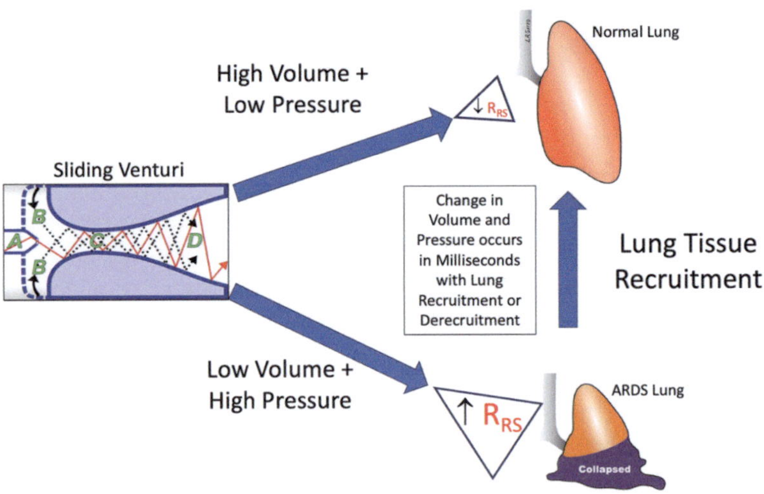

Fig. 9.10 The key to ADSV technology efficacy is personalizing delivered gas volume and pressure based on lung pathophysiology. Normal lung low resistance and elastance will generate a low pressure (↓R_{RSP}) that will increase the volume and reduce the airway pressure delivered to the lung (High Volume + Low Pressure). The ARDS lung with high resistance and elastance will generate high back pressure (↑R_{RSP}), reducing the volume and increasing the airway pressure delivered to the lung (Low Volume + High Pressure). The Low Volume will prevent overdistension and the High Pressure will result in Lung Tissue Recruitment

References

1. Kunugiyama SK, Schulman CS. High-frequency percussive ventilation using the VDR-4 ventilator: an effective strategy for patients with refractory hypoxemia. AACN Adv Crit Care. 2012;23:370–80.
2. Bougatef A, Casteels A, Cools F, De Wolf D. High frequency percussive ventilation: principle and 15 years of experience in preterm infants with respiratory distress syndrome. Cuidados Respiratorios y Tecnologias Aplicadas J Respir Care Appl Technol. 2007;2:39–50.
3. Allardet-Servent J, Bregeon F, Delpierre S, Steinberg JG, Payan MJ, Ravailhe S, Papazian L. High-frequency percussive ventilation attenuates lung injury in a rabbit model of gastric juice aspiration. Intensive Care Med. 2008;34:91–100.
4. Velmahos GC, Chan LS, Tatevossian R, Cornwell EE 3rd, Dougherty WR, Escudero J, Demetriades D. High-frequency percussive ventilation improves oxygenation in patients with ARDS. Chest. 1999;116:440–6.
5. Wang D, Zwischenberger JB, Savage C, Miller L, Deyo DJ, Alpard S, Cardenas VJ Jr. High-frequency percussive ventilation with systemic heparin improves short-term survival in a LD100 sheep model of acute respiratory distress syndrome. J Burn Care Res. 2006;27:463–71.
6. Michaels AJ, Hill JG, Sperley BP, Young BP, Ogston TL, Wiles CL, Rycus P, Shanks TR, Long WB, Morgan LJ, Bartlett RH. Use of HFPV for adults with ARDS: the protocolized use of high-frequency percussive ventilation for adults with acute respiratory failure treated with extracorporeal membrane oxygenation. ASAIO J. 2015;61:345–9.
7. Dmello D, Nayak RP, Matuschak GM. High-frequency percussive ventilation for airway clearance in cystic fibrosis: a brief report. Lung. 2010;188:511–3.
8. Fernandez-Restrepo L, Shaffer L, Amalakuhan B, Restrepo MI, Peters J, Restrepo R. Effects of intrapulmonary percussive ventilation on airway mucus clearance: a bench model. World J Crit Care Med. 2017;6:164–71.

Epilogue

Applied Physiology to Reduce Ventilator-Induced Lung Injury: Epilogue

We began the book asking the following questions: (1) Why does ARDS make the lung susceptible to ventilator-induced lung injury (VILI) and (2) What are the mechanisms of VILI in the ARDS lung (Fig 1.3)? As we conclude our book, we reflect on the high mortality associated with acute respiratory distress syndrome (ARDS) and many attempts to lower this mortality using multiple protective mechanical ventilation strategies. Our dedication to this field stems from our understanding that it is possible to significantly improve patient outcomes today by simply properly adjusting mechanical ventilator settings. Such progress owes its gratitude to the trailblazing giants of Science and Medicine whose contributions paved the way for the insights presented in this work.

Throughout our book, we have harnessed the power of applied physiology to formulate a unifying hypothesis, shedding light on the mechanisms of ARDS-induced pathophysiology and how the changes in alveolar micromechanics drive VILI. We use this knowledge to analyze the reasons that low tidal volume Protect the Lung Approach and the Open Lung Approach have not been successful at further reducing ARDS-related mortality.

The book details normal alveolar and alveolar duct (acinar) mechanics and how acute lung injury-induced pulmonary edema and surfactant deactivation result in regional alveolar instability and collapse, generating stress multipliers that cause both volutrauma and atelectrauma. Lung tissue changes volume as a viscoelastic system with a time lag after the airway pressure is delivered (inspiration) or removed (expiration) before there is a change in tissue volume. Using this understanding, we have proposed a novel approach to protective mechanical ventilation.

© The Editor(s) (if applicable) and The Author(s), under exclusive license to Springer Nature Switzerland AG 2024

G. F. Nieman, N. M. Habashi, *Applied Physiology to Reduce Ventilator Induced Lung Injury*, https://doi.org/10.1007/978-3-031-66352-9

In addition, acute lung injury renders the lung time- and pressure-dependent, meaning that it will take more time for the viscoelastic lung to open and less time for it to collapse at any given airway pressure. Thus, it is critical in the design of protective mechanical ventilation strategies to greatly extend the inspiratory time and use a very brief expiratory time to counteract these pathologic changes in opening and collapse time constants necessary to stabilize and then gradually reopen the lung. We conclude the book by filling in the ARDS pathophysiology, which are the mechanisms of VILI (Fig 8.16) that allow the design of logical lung-protective ventilation strategy based on this applied physiology.

Applying this physiology suggests that the airway pressure release ventilation (APRV) mode would be ideal to increase inspiratory and reduce expiratory times necessary to recruit and stabilize pathologic lung tissue that has become time- and pressure-dependent. However, it is also critical to understand that it is not just the mode but the way you set and adjust the mode that is vital for lung protection.

The time-controlled adaptive ventilation (TCAV) method is the most studied method to set the APRV mode and is personalized and adaptive as the lung gets better or worse (Table 9.1). A large volume of published literature using clinically applicable animal ARDS models supports the efficacy of TCAV as a highly lung-protective strategy. Moreover, case studies, small clinical trials, clinical expertise, and statistical analyses support the effectiveness of TCAV on ARDS patients. Importantly, a large randomized controlled trial testing TCAV versus the standard-of-care low tidal volume method has been funded in the United Kingdom and will be completed in approximately 4 years (Dr. Luigi Camporota, Principal Investigator).

A highly novel ventilation method, adaptive dynamic sub-tidal volume technology (ADSV technology), offers new horizons in protective ventilation, offering millisecond adjustments in gas flow, volume, and pressure at the alveolar level. This technology holds great potential in addressing the conundrum of ventilation in the acutely injured lung, leveraging the Bernoulli and Venturi effects to optimize gas flow physics and lung function.

Our primary goal throughout this book has been to enhance patient care and reduce the morbidity and mortality associated with ARDS and VILI. It is our hope that the insights provided within these chapters serve as a foundation for further research, collaboration, and innovation in the field of applied pulmonary physiology.

In closing, we extend our gratitude to all those who have contributed to this work, including researchers, clinicians, and medical professionals who continue to dedicate themselves to advancing the understanding and practice of lung-protective mechanical ventilation. Together, we can strive toward better outcomes for our patients and improve the quality of critical care medicine.

It is our hope that this book will inspire the next generation of critical care scientists and clinicians as we work together to finally reduce the unacceptably high mortality associated with ARDS.

Sincerely,

Gary F. Nieman and Nader M. Habashi

Index

© The Editor(s) (if applicable) and The Author(s), under exclusive license to Springer Nature Switzerland AG 2024
G. F. Nieman, N. M. Habashi, *Applied Physiology to Reduce Ventilator Induced Lung Injury*, https://doi.org/10.1007/978-3-031-66352-9

MIX
Papier aus verantwortungsvollen Quellen
Paper from responsible sources
FSC® C105338

If you have any concerns about our products,
you can contact us on
ProductSafety@springernature.com

In case Publisher is established outside the EU,
the EU authorized representative is:
Springer Nature Customer Service Center GmbH
Europaplatz 3, 69115 Heidelberg, Germany

Printed by Libri Plureos GmbH
in Hamburg, Germany